THE PROCESS
OF
HAZARD CONTROL

THE PROCESS
OF
HAZARD CONTROL

Robert J. Firenze

Hazard Control Consultant
R J F Associates, Inc.
Occupational & Environmental Affairs
Consultants, Bloomington, Indiana

KENDALL/HUNT PUBLISHING COMPANY
2460 Kerper Boulevard,
Dubuque, Iowa 52001

C 408002 01

To Pat, Bob, and Doug

For Sacrificing the Many
Weekends We Could Have Been
Together

Contents

Preface

Now, more than any time in the history of American society, an increasing awareness exists of the need for organizational hazard and loss reduction. Along with this awareness has come the concommitant need for additional knowledge to facilitate the understanding of how workers are injured, diseased and killed, and how other precious organizational resources are lost.

When I conceived this book, I saw the opportunity to organize and record ideas, philosophies and techniques acquired and developed during my own professional experiences, in addition to those of my most respected colleagues. It seemed plausible that if these ideas could be assembled whereby the reader could acquire a clear picture of how others think about and approach various aspects of hazard control, such information might serve as the catalyst to solidify the reader's own thinking about the course of action to be taken in organizing and administering his own hazard control program.

This book's primary purpose is to assist those in hazard control positions in understanding the dimensions of hazard control programming and how such programming fits into and becomes part of an organization's total management system. Additionally, the book is well-suited for the classroom setting where the new student can obtain a perspective of how others perceive the overall business of hazard control. The book presents the entire spectrum of the hazard control process in clear terms. It explores human and situational error as well as environmental factors associated with death, injury, and occupational illness. It offers an understanding of the role of hazard control as an integral part of the overall management process. It lists the essential elements of programs designed to reduce hazards. And finally, it demonstrates the application of diagnostic techniques for locating and assessing problems in management and operational systems which are contributing to hazards and losses. Related subjects such as techniques of accident investigation, monitoring the workplace for hazards, product safety, and the role of labor and management relations in hazard control are not neglected. Of additional value is the comprehensive bibliography at the end of each chapter.

In my opinion, the terms "safety" and "accident prevention" are not functional titles for programs dealing with the conservation of an organization's human, physical, and economic resources. However, since these terms are popularly used, I will incorporate them within the text. The person designated to administer such programs will be referred to hereinafter as the hazard control specialist. To provide consistency in the use of terms, a special glossary has been provided.

No book is the work of a single author. To my colleagues, friends, and critics I owe a special debt of gratitude. Special appreciation is given to the McGraw-Hill Book company, Charles C. Thomas Book Company, John Wiley and Sons Book Company, Richard D. Irwin Book Company, Mine Safety Appliances Company, Marsh-McLennan Inc., the Royal Globe Insurance Company, Western Electric Company, Boeing Company, Dr. Joseph Zuzick, and the Questor Corporation for granting me permission to reproduce information from their publications. Special appreciation is given to Frank E. McElroy of the National Safety Council for his cooperation in procuring many of the illustrations that appear in this book; Dr. Richard G. Pearson and Dr. Mahmound Ayoub of North Carolina State University and the American Institute of Industrial Engineering for permission to use their material on ergonomics; Dr. Robert Nertney, E. G. & G., Idaho, Inc. for his contributions to Chapter 6; Dr. William E. Tarrants of the National Highway Traffic Safety administration who permitted the use of his ideas in Chapter 4; L. W. Rook and the Sandia Corporation; Dennis Skinner of the U.S. Department of Energy for his information on Accident Investigation; Dr. Jack Mickle of Iowa State University for his efforts in applying the Construction Hazard Analysis techniques; Wayne Christensen of Rust Engineering Company for reviewing the manuscript; Joe Adam of the United Association, Hunter Wharton, and Ben Hill of the IUOE for their assistance in reviewing and offering suggestions for Chapter 11; Walter Lambert and Michael Smith of the International Association of Fire Fighters who provided me with the opportunity to conduct research into accident and injury reporting systems; Dr. Thomas Tuttle, PSYCON, Inc., for his contributions on organizational diagnosis in Chapter 5; the Dravo Corporation for its assistance in obtaining information on policy statements; President Robert A. Georgine and Jim E. Lapping of the Building and Construction Trades Department, AFL-CIO, who provided me with information and assistance during the writing of this book; to my friend and mentor Mr. William Dalton at New York University who offered sound direction and advice during the early design of this book; and to my colleague and good friend, Dr. Ronald D. Baker who I owe a special debt of gratitude for sharpening the manuscript and encouraging me to publish this book.

Scope

My intent is to provide the new hazard control specialist and the student with a comprehensive overview of the reasons for, benefits of, and activities related to hazard control programming. I have strived to provide ideas and demonstrate techniques within this book that can be used in the organizational and classroom setting.

The book is divided into twelve chapters.

Chapter 1 looks at the evolution of hazard control in the United States. For the future, it addresses recommendations for reform and specific objectives to be accomplished.

Chapter 2 acquaints the reader with some traditional theories and models of accident causation. This assists him in solidifying his ideas on the problems associated with human and situationally caused errors.

Chapter 3 demonstrates how hazard control fits into the overall management process. It examines various management people's participation toward the goal of conserving their organization's human, physical and economic resources.

Chapter 4 examines the elements of a comprehensive hazard control program, from the standpoint of how hazard data are acquired and classified, how decisions are made, control alternatives selected, improvements monitored, and effectiveness of overall program effort evaluated.

Chapter 5 discusses the diagnostic process in an attempt to locate hazard potential situations in both management procedures and operational systems. Emphasis is placed on organizational characteristics, the physical work environment, tools, machinery and equipment, and individual/job compatibility. This chapter includes criteria for an organizational hazard diagnosis.

Chapter 6 acquaints the reader with popular hazard analytical techniques while demonstrating the capabilities and limitations of each in the actual problem-solving process.

Chapter 7 considers the role of ergonomics in the total hazard control process. Explored are the roles of equipment design, worker/machine relationships, environmental task stress, and other relevent human factors areas.

Chapter 8 devotes an in-depth look at the accident investigation process from the standpoint of which accidents should be investigated, the specific techniques employed, the use of hazard analysis as an accident investigative tool, and how to get the most out of accident investigation forms and reports.

Chapter 9 illustrates the process of setting-up and conducting a program for hazard inspections. This chapter includes information sheets and audit forms for practical application.

Chapter 10 provides the reader with an overview of the product safety/product liability issue. It gives the recommended steps taken at the organizational level to assure against product hazards and their resultant losses.

Chapter 11 shows the importance of labor and management cooperation in effecting high levels of hazard control. It examines cooperation in enforcing the law, in inspections, in bargaining table discussions and in standards adoption, deletion, and modification.

Chapter 12 includes technical topics I consider important. Areas such as occupational health, hazardous materials, fire protection and machine guarding are discussed.

Terms Commonly Used Throughout This Text

Accident: Any event which interrupts the normal work process caused by human, situational, and environmental factors or any combination of these factors which may or may not result in personal injury, death, property damage, and other undesired events, but which has the potential to do so.

Effect: An event or condition which results from a problem situation.

Failure: The inability of a system or portion of a system to perform as specified under the specific conditions, for the specific time, when installed, operated, maintained and supported as specified.

Goal: A general statement of intent.

Hazard: An existing or potential condition in the workplace which by itself, or in combination with other factors, has the capacity to result in the undesired events of deaths, injuries, diseases, damage, and mission loss.

Hazard control specialist: A staff member of an organization whose expertise lies in the total spectrum of hazard reduction activities including hazard identification and evaluation, problem solving and decision making, recommending controls, monitoring the workplace for hazards, and measuring hazard control program effectiveness.

Injury: The bodily hurt sustained as the result of an accident—such as lacerations, sprains, broken bones, amputations, etc.

Liability: An obligation to rectify or recompense any injury or damage for which the employer is held responsible.

Negligence: Failure to exercise a reasonable amount of care or failure to carry out a legal duty so that injury or property damage occurs to another.

Objective: Objectives operationalize goals. They are statements of actions and performances which must take place in order to reach the wishes and intentions expressed in goals.

Occupational disease: Any abnormal condition or disorder, other than one resulting from an occupational injury, caused by exposure to environmental factors associated with employment. It includes acute and chronic illnesses or diseases which may be caused by inhalation, absorption, ingestion, or from stresses affecting the entire body such as heat and vibration.

Problem: A situation which has the potential for modification via one or more alternative courses of action.

Risk: The product of the amount to be lost times the probability of losing it.

Safe workplace: One in which the likelihood of all identifiable undesired events are maintained at an acceptable level.

Unsafe act: The human act of commission or omission which departed from hazard controlled procedures or practices, or which caused unnecessary exposure to a hazard.

Unsafe condition (General Definition): Those physical and environmental conditions in the workplace resulting from defects, errors in design, faulty planning, and/or omission of essential minimum hazard controls that have the capacity to cause injuries, deaths, damage, and reduced operational performance.

Setting the Theme 1

In recent years, as the result of pressure created from federal health and safety laws, people throughout industry have discovered the emergence of a startling new idea: hazard control. Actually, a closer examination of the whole concept behind locating and controlling or eliminating hazards in the workplace dates well back beyond recent times.

If we trace the history of programs which dealt directly or indirectly with preventing hazards in industry, we find that Fredrick W. Taylor (1910), the Father of Scientific Management, was employing hazard control practices in the operation of his production lines to locate problems with the potential to cause losses in time, material, and personnel, because he saw such problems as deterrents to efficiency and profits. While Taylor may not have realized the complexity and full benefits to be derived from hazard control programming as we do today, he did see that a need existed within the control segment of his management system to locate and remove—wherever possible— obstacles that could reduce his estimated number of production items per hour and the income these items would bring. The whole notion behind decreasing loss-producing situations while increasing productivity, whether instituted by Taylor or by anybody else, is sound business. The philosophy of increasing operational effectiveness through hazard control will form the basis upon which this book is written.

A close examination of almost every program designed to eliminate or reduce hazards in the workplace, reveals one significant flaw. These programs have focused their attention on correcting hazards *after* they resulted in the unwanted events of accidents, deaths, injuries and damage. These traditional safety programs have been, for the most part, post-facto-oriented. Essentially,

Past Approaches to Accident Control

they have been oriented toward counting accidents, attempting to determine cause, and providing solutions after accidents occur, rather than evaluating the hazard potential of work activities before the accidents' occurrence. Study of many safety programs further reveals that, in many instances, these programs have centered around mechanical improvements and technical problem-solving, with little or no attempt to establish workable relationships between those performing the "safety" work and those members of the management system who have control over the industrial processes. Finally, as embarrassing as it is to admit, many safety programs have relied on superficial approaches to achieve their ends. These flashing-light and magic mirror methods have done little more than create a facsimile of a safety program and, in most cases have done more harm than good. The employees working under such programs are apt to lose respect for the entire concept of hazard recognition and control on the job, and sometimes are turned off by the entire issue of safety itself.

The Need for Reform Was Apparent

In attempt to reduce the vast numbers of deaths, injuries and occupational diseases which are affecting the nation's workforce, interested people in the private, industrial, and governmental sectors have begun to offer their recommendations. These recommendations are grouped into two categories.

In Category I, we find recommendations oriented toward the philosophy that methods are needed to identify and assess the nature and effects of hazards in the workplace before accidents occur and workers are killed, injured, or diseased. Instead of stalking off in a haphazard manner correcting problems as they found them, the proponents of this philosophy are willing to take the time to assess carefully the hazard potential associated with various types of work activities, in order to establish priorities for solutions.

In Category II, we find recommendations which call for legislating hazards out of the workplace. The proponents of this philosophy feel that the only way the vast number of work-related deaths, injuries and occupational diseases could be minimized is to establish federal legislation which mandates that such reductions happen. Of course, these people know that such legislation requires four important ingredients if their idea is ever to work, namely: (1) it has to be adequately funded; (2) it needs a strong enforcement system behind it; (3) it requires competent, well-trained people to administer it; and (4) it requires reliable data to guide standards development. Today, seven years after the passage of the federal OSHA law, there is great doubt as to how successful the federal government has been in blending these four ingredients into a viable program. If the numbers of injuries and deaths reduced were the yardstick by which success is measured, then the program could not boast of being very effective. On the other hand, if the amount of interest generated among industry was the criterion by which the OSHA program were judged, then perhaps the law has had some favorable impact.

The most important question to answer, however, is how much has the "interest" on behalf of the nation's employers actually accomplished in making a significant improvement to the death, injury and illness problem throughout the nation?

Those who are most pessimistic about the success of federal regulations in safety and health voice the opinion that these regulations did not represent the awaited cure all and have limited attention to the monitoring or compliance aspects of the issue instead of providing assistance to employers so that they could more capably recognize, assess, and control hazards which have significant impact on their workplaces. Many of those less enthused over the results of the law feel that the Pareto principle is at work in full force[1]—that the OSHA law is concentrating more energy on catering to the trivial many problems in the nation's workplaces than in concentrating on the vital few problems which have the most undesirable impact ramifications.

In Chapters 4 and 6 the issue of risk and hazard evaluation is addressed with specific emphasis on how the hazard control specialist and other members of his or her management team can sort, and prioritize hazards by virtue of their consequential effects and the impact of these effects on the overall hazard control mission.

The impetus behind worker safety and health reform is based on several other factors. The first factor involves the rising costs of accidents in the workplace. These costs comprise the direct expenses stemming from Workers' Compensation premium increases and medical expenses, along with the indirect expenses associated with down-time, material waste, supervision, and so forth. Today's accelerated production and construction schedules makes down-time more costly than ever before.

The second factor is the complexity of today's industrial processes. Along with highly complex industrial processes have come hazards which may not be obvious. New processes, materials, and methods require a planned, purposeful approach to the location of hazards which may have adverse affects on workers as well as overall operational performance. No longer can an inspector go out into the workplace and by the "seat of his pants" locate problem areas or intuitively predict the presence of job hazards which have high destructive capacity.

The third factor concerns society's response to accidents. We can see this response coming from many fronts including the public as well as the governmental sectors. Essentially, people do not want to see other people killed, injured or diseased, while they are producing products or providing services for the benefit of society at large. Of course, such societal influences are more intense at times of prosperity, when a nation can stretch out and work on issues not pertaining to its immediate survival. On the other hand, when the belt gets tightened, and the umbrella of austerity is drawn over an economy, the desire to spend money on social issues diminishes in intensity. People learn that change costs money and, like it or not, money has to be spent on a priorities basis. Today, before any significant change intended to assure "safety" and better health for workers is made, its cost to, and whether society evaluates the role of perceived risk in the same frame of reference and with the same priorities as do those who seek the change must be considered. The commonly-used word to describe this relationship is "economic impact"—a phrase which, by its very nature, suggests careful evaluation of the cost/benefit aspects of any improvement for society at large.

The fourth factor entails the enormous amount of pressure from consumer groups requiring that products and services be hazard-free or at least adequately controlled. Investigations by members of these groups have indicated that some of the same problems responsible for deaths, injuries, and illnesses to the workers who make the products are likewise responsible for a large number of injuries and deaths to the consumers who use the products. Gone are the days when a manufacturer could design, produce and turn his products loose on society without taking realistic precautions to identify hazards, safeguard the product, and protect the consumer from unreasonable risk. In Chapter 10, an examination of the issue of product safety and product liability will be made with focus on the role of the hazard control specialist in the overall product safety effort.

Arguments of Interest

An interesting observation made by one faction of people involved in hazard control is that this field is in the same state the medical profession was in 100 years ago. What these people mean is that 100 years ago, the medical doctor, like the hazard control specialist of today, had to perform his work with a lot less knowledge and technical advances working in his favor than do physicians performing their work today. Although this statement is, to a certain extent, reasonable, it holds one critical flaw. The medical community has always had one element working in its favor—it has an empirical base of knowledge on which to base its approaches. While the medical profession may have been in its infancy a century ago, there nevertheless existed some fundamental elements and laws in the sciences of chemistry, biology, etc. upon which the physician could base his decisions and take action. Hazard control, unlike medicine, is not now nor ever has been considered a science in its own right. Instead, it can be visualized as a specialty area which utilizes many sciences to carry out its mission. Thus, without fundamental principles and laws to provide consistent interpretation and application of hazard control information and methods, it would be very misleading to purport hazard control as a scientific activity. At best, it might qualify as an art. The business of hazard control takes on many interpretations—not consistent across organizations—it is carried out in many ways with varied objectives and with different techniques and methods. Lacking universal standards of operation, methods of accomplishing hazard control objectives, and instituting and evaluating program effectiveness, each person responsible for hazard reduction programs has, nevertheless, the latitude to choose his own methods and techniques and to operate fairly much on his own perception of what has to be done and how to do it. Wide variation among ideas and approaches to reduce hazards and increase operational performance, has provided a wide variation in program results— some good and some inferior.

One of the most perplexing issues that faces the field of hazard control is those working in the field have traditionally made errors in identifying and assessing significant hazards produced by the human, physical, and environmental components of the workplace. An analysis of these errors reveals that instead of attacking the problems of importance, the practitioner oriented his efforts and resources toward the attack of the visible "effects" of the real problem issue. Such intervention is both costly and sometimes counterproductive. Most importantly, though, is the fact that the problem which spawned the "effect" is allowed to survive—with the potential for producing other undesirable "effects" in the future. To a certain extent, the hazard control specialist is very much like the man who was looking busily under a lamppost. When asked by a passerby what he is doing, he says he is looking for his keys. The man begins to help him and after awhile, the following exchange ensues:

Passerby: "Well, where did you actually drop them?"

Man: "Over there in that dark alleyway."

Passerby: "Why are you looking here?"

Man: "This is where the light is."[2]

The hazard control specialist often finds that it is easier for him to address issues on the basis of what he knows, and what is practical and easy to do. It does not, of course, always solve the true problem.

Most traditional organizational thinking has been "control"-oriented, focussing on the prevention of bad changes. It was mentioned earlier in this chapter that Fredrick Taylor did whatever he could to prevent any change from occurring which was not part of the norm he had set for operation of his production lines. While there is a place for such thinking, it can and will, unless something is done to prevent it, keep organizational people so tied up preventing the things they know about from going wrong that they are not able to discover new problems and devise remedies to have both immediate and long-range favorable impact on organizational operations. Such measures are known as *"breakthrough"* techniques. While there is a definite need for applying control to prevent bad changes in a system, there is the simultaneous need for an

Where We Are Going—What We Will Need to Get There

organization to be able to look out beyond day-to-day control-oriented activities to the creation of new and necessary changes—changes which will allow an organization to grow, remain viable, and stand a better chance of surviving and competing in the marketplace. The relationship between *control* and *breakthrough* oriented activities introduced by Juran[3] will be discussed further in Chapter 3.

In hazard control there is a pressing need for well-organized and competent control procedures as well as for new and valid information and methodologies to assure the overall success of organizational operations.

When we consider what it will require to mobilize our efforts for breakthrough in the hazard control area, it becomes clear that such reforms will be made by reaching out beyond the narrow disciplines traditionally associated with hazard control—to other disciplines which can provide significant contributions. It becomes obvious that many solutions will emerge, and benefits produced from the efforts of task forces representing diverse professional skills. In summary, there is a need to concentrate greater efforts on the discovery of new knowledge, applying this new knowledge to the solution of old and new problems affecting workers and worker-performances as they arise, and effectively communicating this new knowledge to those who can use it. It should be obvious that we have our work cut out for us.

The Areas for Breakthrough

Among the considerations of what must be done to increase overall hazard reduction are:

1. A more thorough definition of the important safety and health requirements of the worker on the job. The time has come to determine how and to what extent hazards in the workplace affect workers, and rank these hazards according to a hierarchy of importance, before we can intelligently set out to solve problems in a meaningful way. In addition, emphasis will have to be placed on a more careful differentiating of human error from management-caused error. The issue is of critical importance, as it holds the key to the direction which the hazard control specialist will direct his concentration and emphasis.

2. The increased application and incorporation of systems engineering methods and analytical methodologies to define, extract, and evaluate hazards in work operations during the conceptual, design and operational phases of its life cycle. Greater emphasis needs to be placed on simplifying some of the existing hazard analytical procedures and getting these procedures into the hands of the people who can use them effectively in their respective industries. Chapter 6 will address this issue by presenting those analytical approaches which are both understandable as well as useful in extracting meaningful hazard information.

3. The need to bring together members of an organization's management system and organized labor to blend their knowledge and experiences for the solution of safety and health problems. This subject will be dealt with again in Chapter 3 and Chapter 11 when the role of management systems in the hazard control process and the role of labor/management relations will be discussed in greater detail.

4. The need to explore better ways of gaining worker acceptance of procedures designed to increase their effectiveness on the job while reducing their chances of being killed, injured or occupationally diseased.

5. The need for more precise data on the toxicity and hazards of industrial chemicals, materials, and substances found in the workplace. These data must be not only acquired, but simplified, then put into the hands of those who need it, and who are in the position to use it.

6. The study of a worker's relation to his work from the standpoint of ergonomics and the design and operation of effective and safe workplaces. Among the specific areas of concentration might be:

   a. *Job Matching* where consideration will be given to the assignment of individuals to jobs based on the favorable match between the psychological, physiological, and physical requirements of the job and the similar characteristics of the workers. In addition to reducing job-related injuries and deaths, spinoff benefits in the form of improved work quality, increased work output and increased worker satisfaction may be expected.

   b. *Preventing Worker Overload* where emphasis should be placed on factors of worker fatigue and the determination of whether the system demands are exceeding worker capabilities.

   c. *Anthropometric Designing* where aspects of the workplace including tools, equipment, machinery and protective devices are made compatible with the anatomical and functional dimensions of the worker population.

   d. *Suiting Safety Devices to the Work to be Done and the Hazard Present*—Here is an area which deserves a great deal of emphasis. Many of our existing "protective" systems, on close evaluation, are not protective at all. In fact, they may even be the direct cause of accidents on the job. We can see many examples of this problem in the area of machine guarding, and personal protective equipment.

7. Comparing Organization Progress to Employee Attitudes—Although an organization may be looking ahead to change, their workers may be "set" in their thinking and feeling against such changes. Emphasis will have to be placed on defining the precise attitudes, and introducing ideas and methods credible enough to make the worker want to shape his beliefs and actions toward the direction of favorable change. It cannot be over-emphasized here

that credible, meaningful behavioral approaches must be utilized if such change is ever to take place.

8. Acquiring and Utilizing Accurate Safety and Health Data—Breakthrough in the field of hazard reduction, as with breakthroughs in any other area of endeavor, necessitates accurate base line data from which good decisions can be made. Looking back on some of the issues which adversely affected progress in hazard control it is often found that half true, untrue, inaccurate, or conflicting information was at the base of poorly solved problems and their resultant solution alternatives. If advances in the field of hazard control are to be made, then it is imperative that we acquire and utilize more accurate hazard and risk information for decision-making purposes.

For those hazard control specialists, working at a company level, it will be mandatory for them to define precisely where and how hazards may enter their workplaces, including those junctures where problems occur. This includes both careful analysis and evaluation of the physical workplace and its components, as well as the social, psychological, and physiological dimensions of the problem. In addition, greater demands must be placed on the federal safety and health information systems, and those who are compiling data for these systems, to produce valuable information. The principle of collecting data for data's sake must terminate; it is too costly, time-consuming, and most important of all, insufficiently helpful in coping with and solving the issues which are paramount to us today, and will be important to us tomorrow.

9. Safety and Health Standards—Another area for breakthrough over the next decade will entail a very careful and intelligent appraisal of existing safety and health standards to determine whether such standards are actually contributing to a reduction in the injuries, deaths, and damage to which they were meant to address. Some standards—if followed to the letter, may be adding to the risk of accident situations which we are trying to avoid. This is the reason why reforms of standards are needed. The second problem is that of "consensus" or generally accepted standards. When we speak of consensus standards, we do so with a knowledge that such standards have emerged as the result of a collaborative effort; an effort which perhaps may have resulted in a compromise among those who developed the standard. Thus, the standard by its very construction may not be designed to yield the highest level of performance. Economics can often be blamed for most compromises in standards adaptation. An example would be: why should be adopt an 85 decible noise standard, a standard which will provide the degree of protection needed to significantly reduce hearing loss, when the nation's industry is not presently able to comply with the existing 90 decible noise limit specified in the present standard? Beyond the fact that there are limitations in the standards themselves, another major fault lies in the fact that compliance with a standard according to the letter by which it was written, under all circumstances,

may prove to be a counterproductive. An example of this would be the safety latch required by the OSHA standards for all hooks used on cranes and other similar materials handling equipment. If one were to analyze the reason behind this standard, it would become obvious that under most conditions where hooks are used, the safety latch serves a very valuable role. It prevents accidents by reducing the possibility of loads slipping off the hook due to vibration, impact, or some other reason. However, there are specific instance when complying with this particular standard could increase risk and actually contribute to causing the deaths and injuries we are seeking to eliminate. A case in point would be when a materials handling operator raises steel to the upper levels of a building structure. Using a safety hook, to prevent loads from falling on people or on expensive equipment or materials below, the ironworkers above are required to walk out on to the steel and unhook the hook from its choker repeatedly throughout the work day. Each time, they expose themselves to the possibility of slipping and falling to their death below. How the worker feels that day (as dictated by his physiological and psychological state), the physical condition of the steel, weather conditions, and a host of other circumstances enter the picture, possibly increasing the worker's chances of falling off the beam, each time he is forced to walk out and unhook. The hook with the safety latch, a very valuable risk-reducing aid for most operations most of the time, in this instance, actually contributes to the risk associated with the ironworker's job in this mode of operation. From the standpoint of injury and death reduction, we have a problem: The standard in this one configuration of construction isn't doing its job. Is there any alternative ways of solving the problem? Possibly the following situation holds part of the answer: Suppose the contractor, having appraised the true nature of the risk to the ironworker, decides that the raising of the steel could be accomplished with a hook without a safety latch. Now the steel could be raised, lowered, and detached by the operating engineer on the ground—reducing the risk to the ironworkers above. If such an alternative were opted for, the contractor would have to take other precautions to assure the safety of the workers. One alternative would be barricading the area beneath the portion of the building where the lifting process is taking place. This modification in the interpretation and use of standard serves a very valuable and useful purpose, in that the work situation now is less likely to precipitate the very injury situation we are trying to avoid.

The point of this discussion is that throughout industry, in various forms of manufacturing, and construction activities, other situations similar to this one exist requiring more effective solution alternatives.

In order to achieve this type of intelligent use of existing and new safety and health standards, we must bring together a mixture of people in injury and accident reduction, federal government, and most important, people who are thoroughly and intimately familiar with the systems and job tasks which the standards are addressing themselves to collaborate, and reach conclusions on methods of standards innovations to reach higher levels of safe work performance. Many of the standards which exist today were not created by people who really knew the operations to which the standards were meant to address themselves. Close examination reveals that so many of today's standards were designed by people who were party to the system involved, but not necessarily familiar with job, job tasks, and job demands. Consequently, when the standard was actually applied in operations, it proved less than effective. In some cases, the standard became so impossible to use that the people who were responsible for using it were forced to innovate on it or not use it at all, because the standard hindered the accomplishment of productive effort.

Standards must be evaluated as they relate to job situations and be provided with provisions for their intelligent use, to increase operational performance. Variations and modifications to any standards package are not intended to let people "off the hook" or to degrade the purpose—the protection of the worker—the standard is instead to provide workers with the highest degree of safety possible, within today's production, construction and service processes.

10. The Issue of Training and Educating Tomorrow's Workers—Perhaps one of the major areas for breakthrough, in achieving a reduction in injuries, deaths, and occupational diseases concerns those responsible for training and educating the nation's youth—the workers of tomorrow. Before and since the establishment of the OSHA law, industry has spent millions of dollars attempting to acquaint workers with the hazards associated with their trades. The effectiveness of such programs, on the basis of their favorable impact on reducing deaths and injuries is questionable. Although industry's implementation of control measures for physical and environmental hazards presents difficulties in iteslf, the most profound difficulties are realized when efforts are made to modify worker attitudes and work techniques to coincide with acceptable and hazard controlled procedures. To compound the problem of reshaping the work styles of their existing employees to make them more sensitive to recognizing and avoiding hazards associated with their work, industry has been faced with the dilemma of being forced to acquire, on a steady basis, new workers graduated from secondary and vocational schools. These new employees often hold set opinions, attitudes, and work styles running contrary to the safety and health requirements of their employers.

Since the passage of the OSHA Act one of the single most critical errors made has been that too much emphasis is placed on the control of physical and environmental components of the workplace, at the sacrifice of understanding worker-workplace relationships, particularly those relationships which are formed during a workers learning process,—during his formative years in school.

A student's perception of job safety and health, coupled with his work habits acquired via contact with and exposure to school curriculums, instructional methods, etc., are likely to prove very powerful influences on his future hazard recognition and avoidance capacity. Clearly, at the training level, a high future payoff may be realized if the student's behavior is shaped toward a sound philosophy of safe work practices and methods. Also, at this point in the student's developmental cycle, his knowledge of industry's requirements for safe work performance and of his role in a hazard controlled worker/machine system will prove to be highly beneficial. We can't divorce hazard recognition from skill attainment.

To alter our current approach to preparing a young person to be both perceptive and knowledgeable of safety and health problems as well as positive in his attitude toward the benefits of safe work practices, a collaborative effort among the federal government, industry, vocational schools, apprentice programs, and state offices of education must be established. The results of such an activity may well justify the effort.

Specifically, there is a need to: understand better the depth and quality of student and educator-thinking about the role of safety and health; include hazard recognition and avoidance inputs in the skill training process; integrate industry's safety and health worker recognition needs into student understanding and respect for health and safety countermeasures.

The Vocational Educator and Administrator, must address the problem by: gaining a broader perspective of industry's needs with respect to safety and health training and educational requirements; being able to identify significant industrial models which would create a more favorable student attitude toward safety and health; acquiring specific data to introduce into school shop laboratories, vocational curriculums, instructional methods, etc; gaining industry's support as a resource for inputs to vocational educational curriculums, as well as acquiring industry's professional expertise for the development and/or modification of curriculums and instructional methods; acquiring assistance from industry in integrating hazard recognition and avoidance into overall student learning objectives, as well as in selecting those methods and strategies which have the most favorable impact on school/industry relationships.

In concluding our discussion of areas of breakthrough, it is indeed appropriate to discuss what is perhaps one of the most important areas—that of increasing the hazard control specialist and his management's capacity to define and analyze hazard-producing problems for the purpose of deciding upon and implementing the most effective solution alternatives

Today, more than any time before, professionals in the field of hazard control require assistance in addressing problem situations and decisions arising in

Assistance in Problem-solving and Decision-making

normal and exceptional operations. During recent years the hazard control field has generated many useful techniques and methods to assist in solving hazard and loss problems. Along with the development of these techniques aimed at hazard identification and risk analysis, has come the concommitant over-reliance on these approaches to do what they never were designed to do—that is, to think for the person using them. Oftentimes, the hazard analyst selects and uses techniques for the purpose of defining problems when in fact, all that the techniques can yield is information about a problem's effects. As new techniques grow in their sophistication and useability, the need will become increasingly apparent for methods aimed at assisting the hazard control specialist in problem identification, as the effective use of these techniques will depend upon the thoroughness of problem specification.

Hazard and loss control is outcome-oriented. Hazard control specialists equipped with sophisticated analytical methods often fail to examine carefully the problem before them, or to review and evaluate the process which led them to choose a particular analytical technique. Because the hazard control specialist is frequently working under pressure to respond to a dangerous, perhaps costly, situation, he often finds himself seeking ready made answers. Under such stress, he may neglect critical elements of problem-solving needed to achieve sound decisions.

"Problem" and "problem-solving" are terms so casually used their definitions and the logic of their process are masked. In a presentation to hazard control professionals at the National Safety Management Society and Wichita State University Inaugural Conference, "State of the Art in Safety Management Concepts," Bethesda, Maryland, November 1977, Firenze, Robert J. and Baker, Ronald D. in a presentation entitled "Decision Strategies in the Hazard Control Process," illustrated the difficulties arising from inadequate analyses of problem situations, determination of effect and recognition of key decision points in the problem-solving process.

The hazard control specialist will require a strengthening of his ability to select and utilize more effectively, available hazard analytical techniques for hazard control purposes. A need exists to demonstrate to the problem-solver how the available qualitative and quantitative techniques may assist his thinking process, but should not be used as methods which do the thinking and deciding for him.

Each of the areas for breakthrough, talked about in this Chapter need ample time to given them the attention they deserve. So, this book cannot address them all. Instead, the author has chosen to let these major themes wherever appropriate, guide the discussion in the chapters to follow. As this book has been written primarily for the newcomer to the field of hazard control, the author would like the reader to consider the themes of this Chapter along with those discussed in the chapters to follow during the formulation of his own hazard control philosophies.

There are some hazard control professionals who voice the opinion that their job is to evaluate how management manages. Challengers of this philosophy contend that such thinking leads to the development of programs and work styles which have proven to be counterproductive. In light of the fact that the hazard control specialist is a mutually inclusive part of the total management system, it is diffitult to see why he would want to set himself up as the company auditor. Instead, the hazard control specialist's most important contribution is to collaborate with and assist each member of the management team in attaining the highest levels of performance, by locating and countering hazards capable of lowering operational performance. The hazard control specialist is not to be thought of as a watchdog, but instead as a viable contributor in enabling an organization to reach its goals and objectives. This theme has been carefully intertwined throughout each chapter of this book. It has been emphasized and reemphasized in many configurations because the author deeply believes that the goal of hazard reduction cannot be accomplished by a single person or a select group, but instead by the cooperative efforts of each member of an organization working in concert.

Another idea worthy of examination is that hazard control is a management process unto itself, and that the skills of those performing the hazard control function should be management oriented not technical/engineering oriented.

In response to the first part of this theme, it can be said with fair certainty, that anyone who convinces himself or his organization that hazard control is a separate management activity is kidding himself. It is this very line of reasoning that causes many stresses between hazard control and the line departments in organizations. In light of what has already been said, the one thing that we can no longer tolerate, is any situation—whether it be actual or perceived—which will prevent the favorable interaction and cooperation among organizational members toward the common hazard control goal.

In response to the second part of this theme, as the pages which follow will substantiate, the people performing the hazard control function must have a good grasp of both managerial skills and knowledge of the technical areas which constitute the major part of their contribution to their organization. This statement is supported by a recent NIOSH study[4] which demonstrated that a factor associated with hazard control programs in companies with low incidences of accidental injuries and deaths, was that such a company maintained a better balance between engineering and non-engineering approaches toward overall hazard reduction.

This book approaches hazard reduction as an activity which requires that the skills and knowledge both of management and engineering be blended in the proportions necessary to address and to offer viable solutions for the problems at hand.

Bibliography   Juran, J. M., "Managerial Breakthrough," McGraw-Hill Book Company, New York, 1964.

Omaya, A. K., "Critique of Neural Trauma Research: Status and Solutions," A Paper presented to NIOSH, May, 1950.

"Safety Program Practices in High Versus Low Accident Rate Companies," An Interim Report, U.S. Department HEW, National Institute for Occupational Safety and Health, June 1975.

Notes   1. J. M. Juran, "Managerial Breakthrough," McGraw-Hill Book Company, New York, 1964.

2. A. K. Omaya, "Critique of Neural Trauma Research: Status and Solutions," A paper presented to NIOSH, May 1950.

3. J. M. Juran, "Managerial Breakthrough," McGraw-Hill Book Company, New York, 1964.

4. "Safety Program Practices in High Versus Low Accident Rate Companies," An Interim Report, U.S. Department HEW, National Institute for Occupational Safety and Health, June 1975.

The Phenomenon of Accident Causation 2

This chapter is designed to introduce the reader to the accident problem from the standpoint of its underlying etiologies. Its purpose is to take the reader through the various accident causation theories in order that a clearer perspective can be obtained and erected into a framework in which principles, methods, and techniques of hazard control will fit.

Throughout this book we have continuously used the word "safety" to describe certain behavior conditions or management programs.

If ever a word were classified as nondefinitive, confusing, and in some cases actually misleading, "safety" would head the list. If one were to ask a representative number of people how they define safety, the results would be interesting and perhaps even disturbing. The author has tried similar experiments over the years and concluded that as many interpretations of the word safety exist as people who can pronounce it. Although most of the definitions differ for various reasons, a single factor consistently implied by most people, is that safety is associated with accidents. In some cases, the researcher may find that the mere mention of the word "safety" triggers a negative response on behalf of the person questioned. The term therefore has not been conceived in general, as being attractive or popular.

The perplexing thing about this little experiment is that if so many people have so many varied ideas about what safety is, or in fact whether such a phenomenon exists at all, then how does an organization get programs they have named with the word safety to accomplish what needs to be done? Some may argue that the definition of safety is really a matter of semantics, that people know what the organization is trying to do, and therefore do go along with the program.

On this point it may be said that the author's experience demonstrates the fact that in organizations where the workers and other organizational personnel do not understand the intent of management's programs aimed at hazard and loss reduction, the degree of effectiveness of these programs is minimized. In some cases, they can even be counterproductive.

One lesson of our experiment is that before any hazard control program can make headway in the conservation of human, physical, and environmental resources, time must be spent to ascertain that the intent of the program and the specific behavior management expects of its organizational personnel are being conveyed to and interpreted without distortion by the organizational personnel. One way of accomplishing this is to be sure the words and terms used are understood, and carry consistent meanings.

Among all the definitions of safety, the one stated by Eddie Rickenbacker[1] is one worth considering. Rickenbacker stated that *"he never liked to use the word 'safe' in connection with the entire transportation field, he preferred the word 'reliable.' For whenever motion is involved, there can be no condition of absolute safety. The only time man is safe is when he is completely static, in a box underground. With motion comes the inexorable possibility of accidents. It is the price we pay for motion."*

When it comes to the issue of providing work systems which are as free from costly error as possible—"reliable systems" if you will—then we must concentrate our efforts on locating and defining those causal factors which have the capacity to produce the undesired results, the basis for any hazard control program.

The Concept of Accident

"Accident," like "safety" is difficult to define by the rank and file. Webster's Third New International Dictionary defines it as: *"Event or condition occurring by chance or arising from unknown or remote causes,"* and also as *"sudden event or chance occurring without intent or volition through carelessness, unawareness, ignorance, or a combination of causes producing an unfortuante result."* These definitions contain some interesting words which may not suit the thinking of those in hazard control work. To begin with, it may be debated that accidents are not caused by chance but instead exists as the result of a chain of definable causal factors. Secondly, while some accidents are caused by remote causes, the great majority are caused by problems, on which information does exist. Thirdly, carelessness, unawareness, and ignorance are leveled at the human component. That is to say that the accident phenomena is more closely associated with human fallibility than with the fallibility of the system with which the human must contend.

Suchman[2] has analyzed the meaning of "accident" and conluded that the term requires an operational definition in terms of probabilities. He goes on to say that *"an accident may be defined as that class of events which involves a low level of expectedness, avoidability, and intention.''* The term "accident" is more likely to be used, the more the event manifests the following three characteristics (1) Degree of Unexpectedness—the less the event could have been anticipated, the more likely it is to be labeled an accident; (2) Degree of Avoidability—The less the event could be avoided, the more likely it is to be labeled an accident; (3) Degree of Intention—The less the event was the result of deliberate action, the more likely it is to be labeled an accident. Suchman's analysis of the definition enabled him to understand the reasons behind calling certain situations "accidents" and others not.

The psychologist, Arbous[3] defines an accident with a little different twist. He conceptualizes the term this way: *"In a chain of events each of which is planned or controlled, there occurs an unplanned event, which being the result of some nonadjustive act on the part of the individual (variously caused) may or may not result in injury."* In this definition Arbous, introduces the point that the unplanned, undesired or uncontrolled event doesn't have to result in any injury situation. Essentially, blood does not have to flow before an accident potential situation may be recognized. While the author of this book agrees with this point, agreement is not so readily reached on the idea that the accident situation is dependent solely on the human element. This point will be developed further, when an examination is made of the workplace as system, and of the various contributory elements in a workplace which either directly or indirectly influence the accident situation.

Schulzinger,[4] in his work on accident causation and the subject of accident proneness, defines "accident" in the following manner. He states that *"An accident with or without injury, is in the main a morbid phenomenon resulting from the integration of a dynamic variable constellation of forces and occurs as a sudden, unplanned, and uncontrolled event."* Schulzinger, in his definition of "accident" has introduced the fact that the undesirable consequences of the accident situation are the result of many factors and conditions with which the person must contend. We will return to Schulzinger's work again on page 31 when an examination of "accident syndrome" is made.

Tarrants[5] conceives the phenomena of "accident" as having a *"close relationship to notions of personal vulnerability and invulnerability, reminiscent of the supernatural and prescientific."* Tarrants, in his conceptualization of "accidents" points out the fact that "the term gives no indication of associated causal factors or results and thus, since it is not appropriate for describing the situation surrounding it, should be replaced by descriptions of the injuries and other undesirable outcome events along with the causal factors responsible for their occurrence."

While Tarrant's suggestion would help to reduce some of the confusion and ambiguity surrounding accident situations, it nevertheless is not a suggestion which is likely to happen tomorrow—and for good reasons. Perhaps the best reason of all is the fact that the term "accident" has become so ingrained in the minds of the populace that any attempt at getting people to change their perception of the term would require a long and tedious effort.

It would seem then that perhaps one way for the hazard control specialist to deal with "accident" as it relates to his own organization, is to define it in terms of the elements which are necessary for investigation, reporting, analysis and control purposes.

In so doing, within the bounds of a single organization "accident" will take on a meaning understood by those required to perform some function under the umbrella of the organization's total hazard control effort.

The author's definition of "accident" which will be adhered to throughout this text is *"any event which interrupts the normal work process caused by human, situational, and environmental factors, or any combination of these factors which may or may not result in personal injury, death, property damage and other undesired events—but which has the potential to do so."* This definition will be explored further on page 23.

Human Error and Accidents

In Chapter 4 we will explore the concept of human error from the standpoint of its contrast with a situation which will be defined as "workplace induced, or management error." In this Chapter, we will examine the human element as a controlling factor in the worker/machine system.

Over the years considerable research has been conducted on error-reduction programs. For the most part, the results of the research depicted two main subject areas worth addressing. One concerns modifying people, and the other concerns modifying situations. Rook[6] explains that one way of describing the two alternatives would be to group them into situational and motivational categories.

Situational Aspects[7]

The degree to which errors can be reduced and quality improved by changing environmental situations is virtually unlimited. By pin-pointing error-likely situations and designing around them, almost any error can be reduced to a tolerable level. The permanent gains "motivational" programs make are, to a large extent, the result of such situational pin-pointing. When concern for errors is high, more error-likely situations are noted, and more effort is devoted to changing them. Tarrants[8] points this out with the use of the "Critical Incident Technique"—a personal observation method, designed to identify failures resulting situationally—caused error which have the potential to cause accidents. The most significant point to be made about situational changes is that they are relatively permanent. Permanence is not typically attainable, however, with purely motivational efforts.

Motivation of People

There is a real limit to the extent that improvement can be effected by purely motivational efforts. Rook explains that this can be readily seen if it is realized that, in any normal production situation, we normally find all levels of motivation. That is, at any given time one would expect to find, among any large group of production workers, some that are well motivated and some that are poorly motivated, with the majority falling in-between. This being the case, it is obvious that as we attempt to increase motivation of the group as a whole, we will produce relatively little effect among the highly motivated because they are already enthused. Most of the gains come from a shifting upwards of the lower end of the distribution of motivation, the effect increasing as we move upward. Motivational campaigns work by squeezing the lower end upward toward the top, thus shifting the mean and decreasing the variance. But this obviously has limits.

It has been observed many times, that, in typical situations the best workers are almost never more than three times better than the worst workers.[9] In fact, a ratio of two to one is more typical. If the range of inter-person variability in performance is no greater than a ratio of three to one, and if we make the reasonable assumption that an all-out motivational program will increase the performance of the best worker about 10 percent and will bring the worst worker up to the previous level of the average worker, we will find that the mean has shifted about 25 to 45 percent upward (with an average shift of about 30 percent). This is the figure that is almost always the result of any new demonstration by management of great interest in workers. The first of the many investigations which have shown such results were the famous studies conducted at the Hawthorne Plant of Western Electric in the 1920's[10] As a result of these studies this phenomenon has become widely known as the ''Hawthorne Affect.''

This is not to belittle a gain of 45 percent. It is merely to point out that this is about all that can be obtained by motivation alone, no matter how it is done. Another consideration is that the results are usually transient. Even if the program is maintained at the level which initially produced the increase, it is almost inevitable that satiation will cause a gradual decline in performance back toward its original level. the only way to maintain continued high motivation is to continually change motivational methods.

Training as a Factor

The process of training may be thought of as both situational and motivational. In paying attention to a person, by instructing him, we motivate him. The Hawthorne studies demonstrated this. By giving him new methods of knowledge with which to work, we modify the situation. The later effects will persist, the former will be transient.

In summarizing these findings surrounding the modification of people or situations, it would be easy although perhaps ill-advised for the reader to conclude that permanent gains are typically produced only by situational changes. If such a conclusion were accurate, then it would be exceedingly concerning that over the past seven years during which federal safety and health agencies imposed standards and regulations to upgrade the situational aspects of the workplaces in industry, the national disabling injury and death rates have been barely affected.

Is Human Error a Factor of Concern?

A problem that has proven to be of serious concern in the evaluation of workplace operations is the role of human error. For example, Willis[11] estimates "that 40 percent of the problems uncovered in missile testing derive from the human element. In 63.6 percent of (shipboard) collisions, flooding and grounding could be blamed upon human error. Reports produced by the United States Air Force indicate that human error was responsible for 234 of 313 aircraft accidents during 1961." Shapero[12] et al (1960) estimated that between 20 percent to 50 percent of all equipment failures result from human mistakes.

The results indicated by these researchers leaves one important question to be answered. That is, were the data used to compute the results valid and reliable? The flaws in accident and injury data reporting mentioned in Chapter 4 raise some doubt over this question. The author's experiences reveals that in a great number of failure situations attributed to the human element, close examination discloses underlying situational factors which were the primary initiators. So before any error-reduction program is undertaken, those in command must be confident they are chasing the real problem.

The relative impact of human error on the overall reliability of a system is shown graphically by Meister and Rabideau[13] Figure 1 demonstrates the relationship between human reliability R_H and equipment R_E, and their contribution to overall system reliability R_S. Thus, an R_E of .85 coupled with an R_H of .90 produces an R_S of approximately .78. If we were to lower the human reliability to .30 with the same equipment reliability of .85, the system reliability would now be lowered to .25. "It is apparent, therefore, that anything which decreases R_H must be a primary concern of the human engineer. It is assumed that much of this error results from inadequacies in system design which incite accidents."

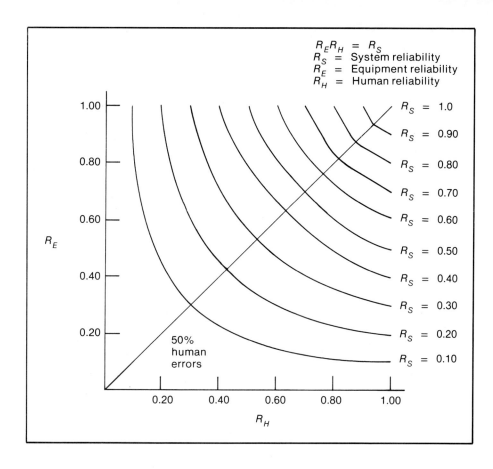

Figure 1. Effect of human and equipment reliability on system reliability, $R_E \times R_H = R_S$. (With permission of John Wiley & Sons, Inc., New York, New York. From "Human Evaluation in System Development" Meister & Rabideau, 1965.)

Overmotivation and Human Error

The results of typical motivational programs are indicated in Figure 2. These results are not in need of documentation since they may be found in any elementary textbook on industrial psychology.[14] The relationship between motivational efforts and performance gains are within the usual limits, represented by a rising, negatively accelerated curve. The less widely known fact is, however, if the motivational efforts are increased beyond those usually found in real life situations, the performance curve begins to decline and may sink below its original level, as anxiety and stress build up. This later effect is seldom observed outside the laboratory, since management seldom exerts enough effort toward motivating workers to cause such a decline. Further, even in those cases where extreme pressure is exerted, workers can be relied on to devise ways to prevent declines from being apparent.

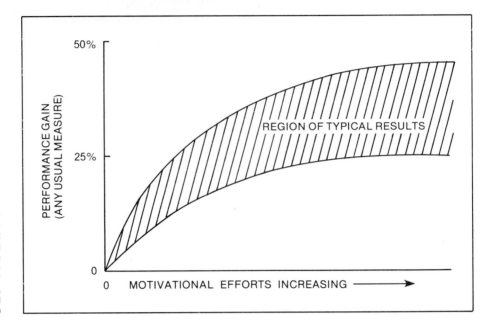

Figure 2. Typical relationship between performance gain and effort toward motivating workers. (With permission of "Principles of Industrial Psychology" Ryan, T. A., and Smith, P. C., New York, Ronald Press Co., 1954.)

A Different Slant on Error Reduction

Rook[15] in his paper "Motivation and Human Error", explains that breakthrough in error-reduction demands the conceptualization of human error as the result of an "interaction of a person with a situation," rather than a mere "lapse of attention," "lack of willingness," "carelessness" or some other judgemental and therefore almost useless concept.

Blumenthal[16] points out that when an imbalance occurs between human capabilities and the system's demands, where the system's demands exceed the human's capabilities, then an accident situation is likely to occur.

In Figure 3 the lower line represents the variable demands of the system. The upper line represents the performance of the "normally competent and normally variable driver . . . at times careless, irresponsible, distracted, fatigued, ill, upset, or preoccupied" (Blumenthal, 1969). In this example, when the driver fails to react properly to the driving situation, making an incorrect decision, and performing an incorrect maneuver to counter a road hazard, an "accident" has a high probability of occurring.

A Final Note

In the process of distinguishing between error situations attributable to the human element or to the situational setting, the ball is frequently dropped. A close assessment of this problem reveals why most of the errors we hear about which are committed by workers at the lower levels of the production hierar-

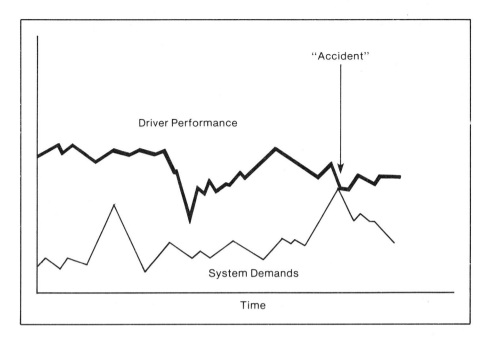

Figure 3. Hypothetical localized system failure. (From Blumenthal, 1968. Courtesy of National Safety Council.)

chy, are diagnosed by people at higher levels. Therefore, since situationally-caused errors are almost exclusively the responsibility of persons higher than the persons making the errors, most errors are diagnosed as human-caused errors, rather than the reverse.

The author's definition of "accident" on page 18 speaks of three essential variables—human, situational, and environmental aspects of the workplace. When each of these three variables interact within the context of a given job or purpose, the result is what has been traditionally referred to as a "man/machine system," defined for the purpose of this chapter as *an operating combination of human and equipment components, interacting within the constraints of a given workplace to bring about, from given inputs, some desired product or service.*

Ayoub[17] (Figure 4) conceptualizes the accident situation as emerging from a complex dynamic interaction of the human element (worker), the machine components of the workplace, and the environment in which the job takes place. Thus, any attempt to identify accident symptoms will involve a critical examination of worker, task, and environmental variables, both singulary, and as they interact in the normal operational setting.

Task Variables as characterized by the job itself contribute to overall accident potential. Within this category we can find situations such as mechanical hazards—the unguarded machinery, improper tools and equipment—poorly-maintained equipment, etc. electrical hazards—lack of or inadequately-

The Workplace and the Accident Process

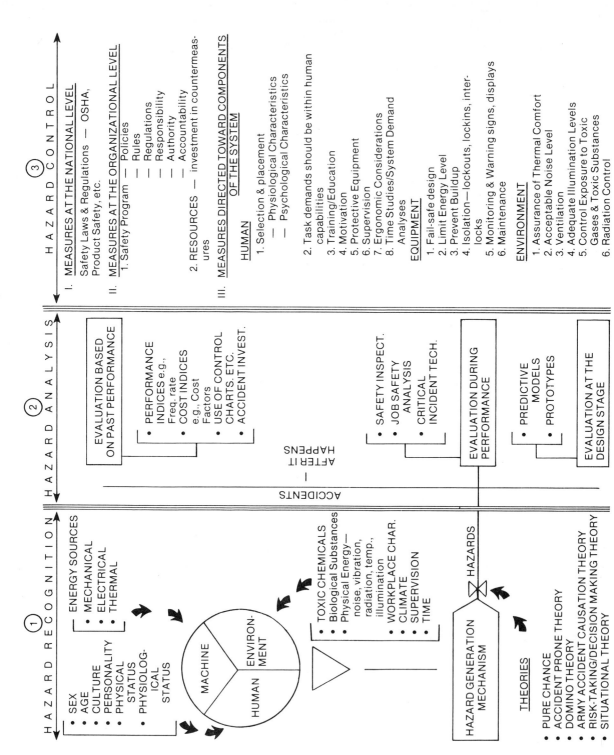

Figure 4. (With permission of the American Institute of Industrial Engineering and M. Ayoub.)

maintained grounding and bonding systems, inadequate electrical tool and equipment maintenance, etc; Thermal hazards including hot surfaces, fire produced by reaction of substances, flame contact from heat producing equipment, etc.

The machine components of the system must be looked at in terms of the demands they place on the individual worker. The hazard analyst needs to determine what speeds, what degree of accuracy, what operating conditions or hazards, what sorts of maintenance, how much weight will be involved in the use, transport or storage of the machines, tools, equipment or products. With this information under his belt the hazard analyst will assess the shape of tools, their sizes, and thicknesses. He would also consider worker comfort, along with the strength required to use or operate the tools and machinery.

In examining the *human component* of the workplace as illustrated in Figure 4 the hazard analyst must focus his efforts on a study of the worker from the standpoint of:

1. Sex. Under this variable, the analyst would be concerned about whether a worker's sex, within the job setting, could increase the workers propensity for accidents and injuries. Examples of this problem have manifested themselves time and time again in situations where a job, originally designed for a male worker has been taken over by a female who, for example, is not as physically adept at the work. Situations such as this have the potential for producing back, and other, injuries due to the excessive stress the task demands. With the increasing number of female workers taking over jobs in industry formerly held by male workers, a necessity exists to reevaluate work methods and task demands, to insure that worker capabilities are within acceptable limits of the task requirements.

2. Age. This variable is one which has been the focus of interest of safety and human factors people over the years. Many attempts have been made to draw a relationship between accidents and the age of workers who were involved in them. Although the data conflict in many regards, one point which seems to be agreed on is that younger workers have a higher potential to become involved in accidents. The reasons have been cited as the younger workers' aggressiveness, willingness to take higher risks, their need to "prove" their worth to their fellow workers. Perhaps the younger worker is often placed in higher hazard areas during the serving of his apprentice years. While the younger worker is of concern to those in hazard control, the aging worker has problems of his own. With aging, in many instances, comes the failing of eyesight, hearing, and often a loss of dexterity and strength. If these characteristics are deemed necessary for the accomplishment of a specific set of work task demands, then a mismatch could be in the making, and the worker may be exposed to a situation with higher accident and injury potential.

3. Personality. Personality factors enter the picture with respect to understanding accident causation. Schulzinger [18] proved that it was possible to assemble no fewer than 250 different personality factors which contributed to maladjustments and accidents. Among these included aggressiveness, anger, discontent, excitability, hostility, low order of judgement, and impulsiveness.

4. Physical/Physiological Status. Another set of human factors concerns the worker's capacity for work. In this regard a close evaluation needs to be made of the task demands to insure that the most effective match can be attained in light of the worker's physical state, skeletal structure, size, strength, etc. Visual acuity and depth perception might be other factors of concern.

A point to be kept in mind, when examination of the human function in a man-machine system is made, is that human considerations go beyond those which merely enable the machine components to function adequately. In allocating tasks to workers, we must be concerned with more than the immediate interface between the equipment and the worker, that is, the equipment features read or manipulated by the workers in the system. We must also concern ourselves with the selection of the right type of worker for a job, the formal training, and education he should receive, and the related training, equipment, and aids to be used in that training, to simulate real-world situations. In addition, management must be sure that the worker is provided with adequate job aids and manuals when required. Management must also be able to measure the worker's job proficiency in order to point to any inadequacies in their human factors efforts. Last, concern must be given to those motivational provisions which will insure that a worker who can do his job adequately will do it. [19]

Environmental Component

Among the environmental components of the workplace of interest from the standpoint of their influence on accidents injuries and occupational illnesses are: (1) *Atmosphere*—including such factors as the presence of toxic airborne chemical substances and particulate matter, biological agents, noise, vibration, radiation, temperature and humidity, illumination; (2) *Workplace Characteristics*—including flammable and other hazardous materials, walking and working surfaces, workplace layout and design causing excessive strain on the worker.

Environmental variables have direct influence on the amount of danger created by a particular task. These variables, depending on their level, may add to the danger level inherent in the task.

Social Factors—The people the worker works with and is supervised by are also factors to be considered when evaluating the workplace. Questions to be raised might be whether a worker's helpers, assistants, or co-workers are congenial, and whether they have common interest. It has been shown that there is a rather high correlation between the feeling of "belonging" to the group and the general level of employee morale. Another factor to consider here is the relation of the job to other jobs. An assessment needs to be made to determine how close it is, whether it requires coordinating information, materials, and human effort.[20] Take a crane operator for example, in order for him to raise a tool crib from ground level to the high steel above, he is dependent on the assistance of others to assist and guide him. The ironworker guides the hook and attaches it onto the choker of the tool crib, and then gives signals to the crane operator for lift. On the steel above, additional directions are given for proper placement of the load. On the ground, the operator depends on the fact that nobody will walk in to the swing radius at the rear of the crane cab and be crushed. Obviously, without a well-coordinated effort, without hazard controls provided in advance, the degree of risk would be excessively high, the chance of injury or death would be increased, and the productivity rate would be less than desirable.

Variables within the machine and environmental components of the workplace, separately or collectively, may act to influence the accident behavior of the worker.[21] To the extent that the hazard control specialist can, by himself or with the help of other required disciplines, discover and modify those mismatches among the components of the workplace which directly influence human error and accident causation, the more the accident-controlled work situation will be realized.

The issue that has challenged researchers as well as practitioners over the years is that of answering the question "How do accidents happen?" The challenge has produced a maze of definitions and theories of accidents and their causes. Most theories of accident causation are based on the two distinct models we have already alluded to—behavioral and situational.

Behavioral Models treat the human as being the primary, if not the only, cause of an accident. Furthermore, advocates of the behavioral models postulate that a worker's psychological and (to a lesser extent) physiological characteristics are the elements that control the accident process. From this behavioristic view emerged the celebrated and still controversial "accident-prone" theory. This theory assumes that some workers have a higher propensity for accidents than their co-workers, because of some invariant personality traits. The theory has not proved to be viable because the assumption upon which it was based has been disproved. Schulzinger[22] in his study of twenty-seven thousand consecutive industrial accidents from a wide array of industries and eight thousand nonindustrial accidents has indicated that among all accident victims, those who suffer repeated injuries year after year, over a period of three years (three to five percent), account for a relatively small percentage of all the accidents (one half of one percent). Schulzinger concluded that most accidents are due to relatively infrequent isolated experiences of large numbers of individuals.

Many people have been tagged as being "accident prone," (born with the propensity to have accidents—an inherited trait), when in fact their unfortunate involvement in accident situations was due to a psychological, physiological, or physical impairment. Consider one worker who was always getting hurt. An analysis of each of his accidents reveals the fact that almost every one of his injuries resulted from a fall. One time he fell on a flat surface, another time down the stairs, and so forth. A close examination of this worker reveals that he had a depth perception problem nobody had ever diagnosed. So then, here we have a situation with a genuine accident repeater who, unless his physical impairment is diagnosed and proper measures taken to correct it, could very well end up as a chronic injury victim or even a mortality statistic in the future.

Here is another situation involving a child whose parents had written her off as a person doomed to have accidents. The five-year-old girl was the victim of many injuries including lacerations, contusions, and fractures. Most of these injuries resulted from falls. Her parents resigned themselves to the fact that she was the "kind of kid that was always going to get hurt," thus there wasn't much they could do about it but pray that she would grow out of it.

Once again, a close analysis of the manner in which the child walked and ran revealed that, as she quickened her pace from a walk to a run, her left foot began to turn inward, causing her to actually trip over her own feet.

Here the problem is profound. In cases like this, similar to those with workers in industry, people are willing to record accidents (falls) without taking necessary time to discover the primary causes behind the accident situation. In the case of the little girl, all measures aimed at barricading her from falling into furniture or down the stairs did not solve her problem—one which needed medical expertise. In the case of our worker, measures taken by management, in the form of penalties, closer supervision, training, motivation, etc. would have been ineffective, as the worker's physiological condition could not have been altered with such intervention, so no real improvement in reducing accidents would have taken place.

Situational Models

The Situational Models, on the other hand, attempt to study the accident process by examining interactions between the worker, environment, and situation. Once such model has been derived from the epidemiological approach to accident study.[23]

The epidemiological model treats an accident situation as a system, comprised of three interacting components: man (host), machine (agency), and environment. If any one of these three components is modified, then the accident probabilities may be altered. McFarland,[24] a proponent of the epidemiological method for accident research described it as follows:

The objective of the epidemiological method is to determine the laws and inter-related factors governing the occurrence of disease or other abnormalities of health in a specific population. In any community, various factors may be at work which give rise to disease or disability. An epidemiological approach thus involves the study of influences of many kinds, including the characteristics of the host, of a variety of agents, and of the environment. This usually requires the collaboration of scientists from several fields or disciplines, and the team approach has been essential to any important advances. For example in the epidemic study of malaria, collaboration between the physicican, the entomologist, the sanitary engineer, and other specialists was necessary to secure basic data to bring about control. In industry, such a collaborative approach might include, in addition to the industrial physician, the hazard control specialist, and industrial hygienist, personnel specialists, behavioral scientists, statisticians, and equipment and methods engineers.

Risk Taking—Decision-making Model

Before this model is discussed, the concept of "risk" will be examined. Traditionally, whenever the word "risk" is used in connection with accident-reduction work, theorists cringe. Because the word carries the connotation of individual judgement, many choose not to introduce it in their "accident prevention" programs.

Webster defines *risk* several ways. First, is: "*the possibility of loss, injury, disadvantage, or destruction.*" Secondly, as "the product of the amount that may be lost and the probabilty of losing it." It is the second defintion that the author has selected for use in this text. Our chosen definition carries two significant points—how much can be lost, and what is the chance of losing it. In hazard control many members of an organization, day-in and day-out, are constantly assessing situations where risk potential is involved.

Whether it's the hazard control specialist, other members of the management team, or the workers themselves making risk assessments, the same criteria holds true. In order for a person to make sound decisions and take calculated risks, he must be aware of: (1) the job requirements; (2) his own capabilities and limitations relative to the job; (3) what will be gained if he attempts the task and succeeds; (4) the unfavorable consequences that will be suffered if the attempt fails; and (5) what will be lost if the task is not attempted at all. In each case, the worker needs information upon which to base his decisions. The better his information, the better his decision, and subsequently the more calculable the risk becomes.[25] The poorer his information, the greater the opportunity for bad decisions and bad risks—each which have the potential to influence or cause an accident situation. Before decisions are made, man seeks information that serves to remove some or all of the uncertainty involving his task. The uncertainty centers around two major areas: the requirements of the task; and the nature of the harmful consequences. If his "information bank" is adequate, the ultimate risk resulting from his decisions should be within calculable limits of risk-taking, and the chance of his failing will be lessened.

For that reason, one of the primary efforts of the hazard control program must be to equip workers with as much information as possible through training and education, so that their decision-making is facilitated, their actions made effective, and their chance of causing or being the victim of accidents minimized. A well-balanced hazard control program will, insofar as its worker population goes: (1) sensitize them to the types of hazards associated with their jobs; (2) instruct them how to mentally evaluate a hazard's potential destructive effect and how to determine which ones are worth the risk and which ones are not; (3) demonstrate the ramifications of excessive risk by virtue of destructive potential and other adverse impact.

There are however, exceptions to the rule that a worker with full knowledge of his job will always make wise, calculated decisions. Variables known as "stressors" or blocks to decision-making capability, often appear in the decision process and cloud a worker's ability to make sound, rational decisions (see Figure 6). These stressors can be of psychological, physiological, or of physical origin. They act to distort and, sometimes prevent the decision-making process from taking place. Narcotics and alcohol are examples of physiological stressors that have an effect upon the organism. Anxiety, aggressiveness, and fatigue are examples of psychological stressors. Glare, temperature extremes, and low levels of illumination are examples of physical stressors. Each type of stressor has the capacity by itself or in combination with other factors to cause otherwise safe behavior to be faulty. It is often under the influence of "stressors" that the worker makes an error. The error oftentimes is primarily responsible for an accident.

The (risk-taking)-(decision-making) points out a problem which has plagued the hazard control specialist for years. That is, when he tries to convince a worker that what the worker is doing is hazardous and likley to result in an accident the attempt is not always successful. This task becomes even more difficult when the worker, has been performing the "dangerous" procedure for many years without any mishap. Essentially then, as is illustrated in Figure 5, it is possible, due to pure chance alone, that the precise mix of failure potentials in each of the other system's components do not have to culminate in an accident situation—even though all the cards point that way. Accidents are rare events. Given all the potentials, all the little balls do not always line up in all the little holes as we might predict they will. In a situation such as this, the hazard control specialist must rely on persuasive appeal and demonstrate to the worker the degree and ramification of risk in order to acquire the cooperation required for effective control.

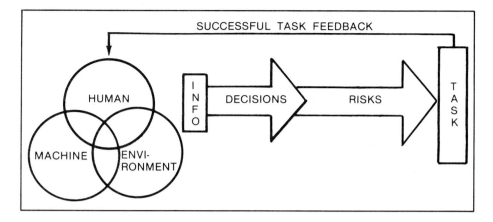
Figure 5.

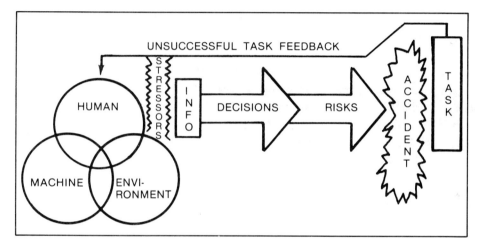
Figure 6.

During the period 1930–1948, some thirty-five thousand plus cases of accidental injury were treated in a general medical practice by Dr. M. A. Schulzinger,
M. D.[26] As a result of his analysis, Schulzinger was convinced that new directions in accident causation exploration arise out of accident syndromes. The
syndrome—(recurrent signs and/or symptoms that appear with fair regular-
ity)—as described by Schulzinger, is not entirely the usual medical usage where
pathology and symptoms are involved. Instead, it is a syndrome in the larger
sense, of any frequently recurring items in a series. The genesis of accidents is
revealed as a series of detectable recurrences that pave the way for the prediction of accident probability, wherever the essential elements of the syndrome
are encountered. Unlike many of the traditional approaches to accident
causation—particularly Heinrich's ''Domino Theory''[27] a syndrome is not the
same as an equation. Thus, it may never be stated that, of all the components
which comprise the ''accident syndrome,'' does A + B + C = an accident

The Accident
Syndrome Model

with or without an injury. Instead, Schulzinger realized that A + B + C, or some combinations such as C + D create a situation favorable to the occasion of an accident with or without injury.

Heinrich's Domino Theory of accident causation Figure 7 unlike Schulzinger's Accident Syndrome, demonstrates that a preventable accident is one of five factors in a sequence that results in an injury. Heinrich described the notion that social, environmental, and ancestral factors, coupled with faults of individuals result in either unsafe conditions or an unsafe act. These unsafe conditions or acts lead to injury-producing or non-injury-producing accidents. The Domino Theory demonstrates that an injury is invariably caused by an accident and the accident in turn is always the result of the factor that immediately precedes it. The key elements in Heinrich's Model as he saw it, is the human element. As Heinrich envisioned it, the highest areas of payoff in corrective action lies with modifying worker behavior and/or the correction of unsafe conditions.

The "accident syndrome" illustrated in Figure 8 as conceptualized by Schulzinger consists of: (1) Universal Risk; (2) Irregular additional Risk incident to physical impairment; (3) Abnormal physical Environment; (4) Maladjustment and Irresponsibility; (5) The trigger episode; (6) Behavior in the presence of the trigger mechanism; (7) The prospective accident with or without injury.

Universal Risk

Universal Risk was estimated to be associated with between ten percent and twenty percent of accidents wholly deriving from fortuitous circumstances. The research pointed up that universal risk (a stray bullet, flying particles which can impact with the eyes, etc.) becomes part of the accident syndrome because of fear of injury. Thus, the dread of an accident thus becomes a consideration in the causation of accidents.

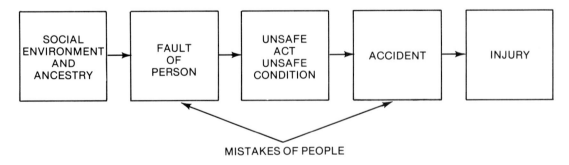

Figure 7. Heinrich model.

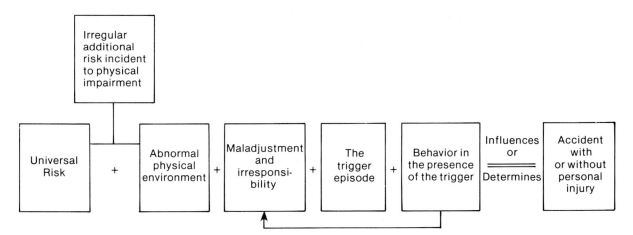

Figure 8. The Accident Syndrome. Eighty to ninety percent of all accidents present contributory human causative factors. (From Schulzinger, M. A., "The Accident Syndrome" 1956. Courtesy of Charles C. Thomas, Publisher, Springfield, Illinois.)

Irregular Additional Risk Incident to Physical Impairment

Schulzinger envisioned this element as a side issue of the influence of physical defection. "The best examples of the influence of physical impairment may be found in those persons who are diabetic and pass into a coma or near coma as a result of hyperinsulinism, or those other persons under the influence of such drugs as marijuana or benzedrine.

Abnormal Physical Environment

Although Schulzinger states that it is difficult under some circumstances to differentiate between universal risks and abnormal environments, he envisions this element in the syndrome as comprised of those factors which are usually of short duration such as: noise, static from lightning, blinding light, etc. An example would be an automobile driver, blinded by the bright lights of an oncoming vehicle, who temporarily cannot see and collides into the rear-end of a vehicle ahead.

Maladjustment and Irresponsibility

Of all the components of the "accident syndrome," mental maladjustment and irresponsibility are at the core. Schulzinger sees this area as one which holds the greatest promise in further substantial reduction in accidents given that conventional mechanical and educational devices have reached a plateau or at best a gentle slope. Among the thirty-five thousand plus accident cases studied in Schulzinger's research, it was determined that the unfortunate situation had its origin in mild and transient emotional strain which temporarily induced preoccupation, impaired perception, blunted good judgement, and improper coordination of movements. Schulzinger was able to assemble approximately two hundred and fifty factors contributing to maladjustment and accidents. Although the majority of the factors are purely mental, numerous others relate to mental states imposed by physical and environmental circumstances. Among those on the list include: aggressiveness, anger, bereavement, boredom, distraction, excitement, faulty judgement of speed and distance, frustration, preoccupation, tendency to take chances or risks, unwillingness to accept monotony or routine, etc.

The Trigger Episode

The readily discernible portion of the accident syndrome is the "trigger" event—the nail that is stepped on, airborne cinder that strikes the eye, the exploding grinding wheel. The research concluded that it was evident that the trigger episode in the majority of accidents is but the detonator of a far more powerful battery or constellation of etiologies. It is within the logic of the statement that hazard control intervention in the form of eliminating or reducing the destructive potential of physical and environmental hazards in the workplace is supported. To this end, perhaps many of our existing "safety" and "health" regulations are performing a useful function.

Behavior in the Presence of the Trigger Mechanism

Schulzinger found that the pattern of behavior of the individual when confronted with a sudden threat of danger will frequently determine whether the forces set in motion will eventuate in a near miss or in an accident. In some instances, the behavior of the person in presence of the trigger may also determine the occurence of injury as well as its severity. Schulzinger's data indicated that such behavior, at least in part, is determined not by the immediate exigencies, but by long antecedent adjustment, training or experience—conversely, faulty behavior in a measure, stems from just the opposite—maladaptations that precisely pave the way for disastrous mishaps. A good example of proper behavior in the presence of the trigger mechanism would be the worker's ability to properly flush his eyes with water in the event of having had them splashed with acid.

The Prospective Accident With or Without Injury

Considering all the circumstances which are conducive to accident causation, it does not follow that an accident with or without injury is inevitable. In this regard, Schulzinger's theory differs widely from that of Heinrich.

The Army
Accident
Causation Model

The U.S. Army Institute of Administration has developed an accident causation model, Figure 9, that attempts to depict the causes of accidents. While it is a little more complicated than Heinrich's Model, it serves to demonstrate how

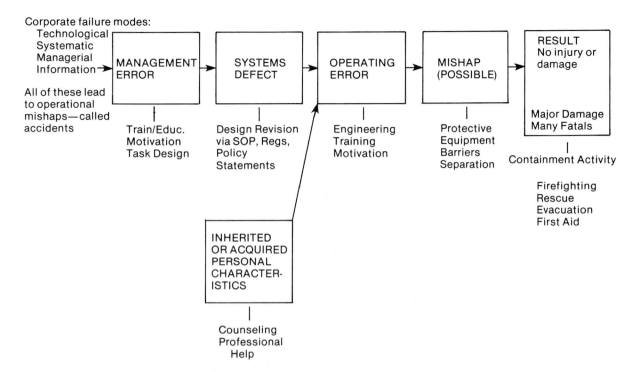

Corporate failure modes:
Technological
Systematic
Managerial
Information →

All of these lead
to operational
mishaps—called
accidents

MANAGEMENT ERROR

Train/Educ.
Motivation
Task Design

SYSTEMS DEFECT

Design Revision
via SOP, Regs,
Policy
Statements

OPERATING ERROR

Engineering
Training
Motivation

MISHAP (POSSIBLE)

Protective
Equipment
Barriers
Separation

RESULT
No injury or
damage

Major Damage
Many Fatals

Containment Activity

Firefighting
Rescue
Evacuation
First Aid

INHERITED OR ACQUIRED PERSONAL CHARACTERISTICS

Counseling
Professional
Help

accidents are caused and how these causes are corrected. What Heinrich identified in his model as "**injury**" has been renamed "**result**" by the Army, indicating that it can involve damage as well as personal injury, and that the damage could range from the very minor to the very severe. The term "**mishap**" is used in place of Heinrich's "**accident**" to avoid the popular misunderstanding that an accident necessarily involved injury or damage. Finally, the term "**operating error**" has been substituted for Heinrich's **unsafe act** and **unsafe condition**. **Operating errors** result from mistakes made by individuals; for example: taking an unsafe position; stacking supplies in unstable stacks; poor housekeeping; or removing a guard.

Figure 9. The AG School Causation Model, Countermeasure Potential. (Courtesy of the Army AG School and W. C. Pope.)

System Defects

Operating errors occur because of people's faults but more importantly they occur because of system defects. Those using the Army model feel that the addition of the recognition of system defects changes the traditional approach of identifying what needs to be done and identifies who will do it. A system defect is a weakness in the way the system is designed or operated. Typical examples of system defects include: (1) improper assignment of responsibility; (2) creation of an improper climate of motivation;(3) inadequate provisions for training and education; (4) unsuitable equipment and supplies; (5) improper procedures for selection and assignment of personnel; and (6) improper allocation of funds.

Management Error

Pursuing the development of the Army Accident Causation Model, the issue of how system defects are caused must be addressed. The Army Model conceptualizes that system defects are ultimately responsible for accident situations. The primary cause behind what the Army refers to as "management error" lies with how both staff and line management manage the system. Management errors occur when: the manager is not properly motivated, lacks specific knowledge of hazards and their control, does not assign responsiblity for hazard control, and lets the production demands of the system dictate the way the system is operated, regardless of the loss potential.

The Army Causation approach opens eight avenues through which countermeasures can be initiated. The proponents of this approach envision so many countermeasure alternatives, none of which overlap, that it becomes more of a critical problem for the hazard control specialist to select the best total combination consistent with available resources.

In comparing the Army Causation Model with that of Heinrich's traditional Domino Theory, the following differences are noted: First, the Army Model stresses the variability of results, while Heinrich's Model does not. Secondly, the Army Model identifies the possibility, as opposed to the inevitability of the accident of mishap. Thirdly, the Army Model clarifies the identities of unsafe acts and unsafe conditions, referring to both as "operating errors," Fourth, the Army Model identifies the system origin of operating errors, an aspect totally overlooked in Heinrich's Model. Fifth, the Army Model provides channels for countermeasures producing substantial system benefits in morale, efficiency, and productivity, in addition to hazard and loss reduction.

Summary   Theories of accident causation, regardless of their origin are still conceptual in nature and must be considered from that standpoint in the work of hazard control. A certain number of accidents, and hence a certain degree of safety, is characteristic of any industrial system. It is to the degree that the time, experience, and circumstances allow for hazard identification, evaluation, and control that an organization will achieve its highest levels of performance, while maximizing its utilization of human, physical, and economic resources.

Ayoub[28] states that accidents are defined and determined by the system of which they are a part. The complexity of the accident situation, as evidenced by the number of variables and their interactions, cannot be represented by a simple model containing quantifiable relationships, since the body of knowledge needed to accomplish this is deficient. Perhaps when the individual components involved in accident causation are understood, it will be possible to quantify the relationships involved in the overall process of accident causation.

As alluded to throughout this book so far, there are basically two approaches to hazard control. The **first approach** involves the investigation of accidents after they occur. Traditionally, this approach has been referred to as the Fly-Fly-Fly or operate-fix-operate approach and is after-the-fact in application. It relies primarily on the idea of trial and error. We must try out a system before we are able to locate problems of importance. When parts of the system fail, we fix the ailments and run the system again. In so doing, given sufficient time, "all" the problems that become known, are corrected, and the system is then destined for success throughout the remainder of its life. This approach relies primarily on accident investigative techniques and personal observations to determine causes before corrective or preventive countermeasures can be provided.

There are two fallacies behind this idea. First of all, the principle that *accidents are rare events* emerges again. As we already discussed in this chapter, there is no iron-clad guarantee that, though hazards exist in a system, that these hazards will culminate in an accident situation. It is possible, and is the case in many instances, that systems possessing many inherent hazards operate for very long periods before the first problem occurs. Secondly, those relying on this approach must often contend with the unwanted events of worker-injury, death and system ineffectiveness.

The **second approach** to hazard control, the systematic approach, relies on identifying and judging the nature of undesired events in a system before accidents occur. This newer approach is guiding the direction of many modern hazard control programs. What it all boils down to is that for nothing spent, we get nothing in return. The price in effort, resources, and knowledge required for an effective hazard control program is expensive. However, if the program is implemented properly, the expense will be offset by the gains to be obtained.

A critical point to keep in mind is that no matter how diligently we set out to and actually perform before-the-fact analysis, accidents will always occur. To this end, there will always be a need for accident investigation and other analysis to locate the causal factors associated with these accident situations.

In Figure 4 Ayoub[29] conceptualizes the systematic process of hazard control as consisting of three discrete processes e.g., hazard recognition, hazard evaluation, and hazard control. Chapters 4 and 6 will develop these areas further. The unique contribution made by Ayoub's Model Figure 4 is that which considers the entire process of hazard control from a comprehensive standpoint, starting out with an analysis of the system components (during the design and operation of the system as well as of the systems past performance) and ending up with the recommendation for control measures which are most effectively carried out at the organizational and national levels, and measures taken aimed at the human, equipment, and environmental components of the system.

Perhaps, each of the models examined in this chapter holds a part of the answer to the problems encountered by the hazard control specialist while carrying out his mission. The extent that he is willing to understand accident causation in his workplace and take the necessary steps to adequately reduce accident potential situations will have substantial impact on how much his hazard control program efforts will achieve.

Bibliography

Arbous, A. G., and Kerrick, J. D., "Accident Statistics and the Concept of Accident Proneness," Biometrics, V. 7: 340–342, 1951.

Ayoub, Mr., "The Problem of Occupational Safety," Industrial Engineer, April 1975.

Baker, S. P., "Injury Control—Accident Prevention and Other Approaches to Reduction of Injury," Insurance Institute for Highway Safety, Washington, D.C., 1972.

Blumenthal, M., "Dimensions of the Traffic Safety Problem," Traffic Safety Research Review, 12:17–1968.

Chapanis, A., "Research Techniques in Human Engineering," John Hopkins Press, Baltimore, MD., 1959.

Dunning, J. R., Livingston, R. T., "Frontiers of Personnel Administration," Columbia University, Industrial Report, 1952, Series No. 1

Firenze, R. J., "The Accident Process," National Safety News, Vol. 104, No. 1, August, 1971.

Fugal, G. R. "Reducing Industrial Accidents," Harvard Business Review.

Hinricks, J. R. "Psychology of Men at Work," Annual Review of Psychology, Vol. 21, 1970.

Meister, D., and Rabideau, G., "Human Factors Evaluation in System Development: John Wiley and Sons, Inc., New York, 1965.

McFarland, Ross A., "Human Engineering Aspects of Safety," Mechanical Engineering, 76:407–10, May, 1954.

McFarland, R. A., "Human Factors in Industrial Safety," ASSE Journal, 38–49, October, 1957.

Page, J. A., and O'Brien, M. W., "Bitter Wages," Grossman Publishers, New York, 1973.

Rickenbacker, E. V., "Rickenbacker," Prentice-Hall Inc., 1967.

Roethlisberger, F. J., and Dickson, W. J. "Management and the Worker," Harvard University Press, Cambridge, Mass., 1939

Rook, L. W., "Motivation and Human Error," Tech. Memorandum, SC-TM-65-135, Sandia Corporation, Albuquerque, N.M., 1965.

Ryan, T. A. and Smith, P. C., "Principles of Industrial Psychology," The Ronald Press Co., New York, 1954.

Schulzinger, M. A., M. D., "The Accident Syndrome—The Genesis of Accidental Injury," Charles C. Thoman, Springfield, Illinois, 1956.

Shapero, A., Cooper, J. I., Rappaport, M., Schaefer, K. H. Bates, C. J., "Systems Programs," WADD Technical Report 60-36, Feb., 1960.

Suchman, E. A., "A Conceptual Analysis of the Accident Phenomenon in Behavioral Approaches to Accident Research," Association for the Aid of Crippled Children, New York, 1961.

Surry, J., "Industrial Accident Research—A Human Engineering Appraisal," University of Toronto, 1969.

Swain, A. D., "System and Task Analysis, A Major Tool for Designing the Personnel Subsystem," Sandia Corporation, Reprint, January, 1962.

Tarrants, W. E., "Myths and Misconceptions About Occupational Safety," NHTSA, Washington, D.C., May 31, 1972.

Tarrants, W. E., "Applying Measurement Concepts to the Appraisal of Safety Performance," Journal of the American Society of Safety Engineers, Vol. X, No. 5, May, 1965.

Tarrants, W. E., "Utilizing the Critical Incident Technique as a Method for Identifying Potential Accident Causes."

Weschler, D., "Range of Human Capacities," Williams and Wilkens, Baltimore, MD., Second Edition, 1952.

Willis, H. R., "The Human Error Problem," Paper presented at American Psychological Association, Sept., 1962, Martin-Denver Report 6.

1. E. V. Rickenbacker, "Rickenbacker," Prentice-Hall, 1957.

2. E. A. Suchman, "A Conceptual Analysis of the Accident Phenomenon: in Behavioral Approaches to Accident Research." Reference—2240, 26–48—1961

3. A. G. Arbous, & J. D. Kerrich, "Accident Statistics and the Concept of Accident Proneness," Wat. Institute For Personnel Research, South African Coun. For Scient. & Inc. Res. Biometrics, 7:4, 1951.

4. M. A. Schulzinger, "The Accident Syndrome—A Clinical Approach," Charles C. Thomas, Pub.; Springfield, Illinois, 1956.

5. W. E. Tarrants, "Myths & Misconceptions About Occupational Safety," NHTSA, Washington D.C., May 31, 1972.

6. L. W. Rook, "Motivation & Human Error," Tech. Memo–SC–TM–65–135— September, 1965—Sandia Corporation.

7. L. W. Rook. op cit.

8. W. E. Tarrants, "Applying Measurement Concepts to the appraisal of Safety Performance, "Journal of the American Society of Safety Engineers" Vol. X No. 5, May 1965.

9. Davis Weschler, "Range of Human Capacities, Williams & Wilkens, Baltimore, MD. Second Ed., 1952.

10. F. J. Roethleisberger, and W. J. Dickson, "Management and the Worker," Cambridge Mass., Harvard Univ. Press, 1939.

11. H. R. Willis, "The Human Error Problem" paper presented at American Psychological Association, Sept., 1962—Martin—Denver Rpt. 62–72.

12. A. Shapero, J. I. Cooper, M. Rappaport, K. H. Schafer, C. J.Bates, "Systems Programs" WADD Tech. Report 60–36, Feb. 1960

13. D. Meister, G. Rabideau, "Human Factors Evaluation in System Development" John Wiley & Sons, Inc., New York/London/Sydney—1965.

14. T. A. Ryan, and P. C. Smith, "Principles of Industrial Psychology," The Ronald Press Co. New York, 1954—Chapters 14–17.

15. L. W. Rook, op cit.

16. M. Blumenthal, "Dimensions of the Traffic Safety Problem" Traffic Safety Research, Revised 12:17.

17. M. Ayoub, "The Problem of Occupational Safety" Industrial Engineering, April, 1975.

Notes

18. M. A. Schulzinger, "The Accident Syndrome," Charles C. Thomas, Publisher, 1956.
19. A. D. Swain, "System and Task Analysis, A Major Tool for Designing the Personnel Subsystem," Sandia Corp. Reprint—January 1962.
20. J. R. Dunning, R. T. Livingston, "Frontiers of Personnel Administration," Columbia University Industrial Report—1952 Series NO. 1.
21. M. Ayoub, "The Problem of Occupational Safety" Industrial Engineering April, 1975.
22. M. A. Schulzinger, op cit.
23. J. Surry, "Industrial Accident Research: A Human Engineering Appraisal," Labor Safety Council of Ontario—1969.
24. R. A. McFarland, "Human Factors in Ind. Safety" Journal of the American Society of Safety Eng. 10–57. 38–49.
25. T. H. Rockwell, F. D. Galbraith, and D. H. Centre, "Risk Acceptance Research in Man-Machine Systems," Ohio State University, Bulletin 187, 1961.
26. M. A. Schulzinger, op cit.
27. H. W. Heinrich, "Industrial Accident Prevention, 4th ed., New York, McGraw-Hill—1959.
28. M. Ayoub, "The Problem of Occupational Safety," Indus. Engr. April, 1975.
29. M. Ayoub, "The Problem of Occupational Safety," Indus. Engr., April, 1975.

The Hazard Control Process A Systems Approach 3

When we speak of systems approaches and the application of these approaches to increase organizational effectiveness, we are not speaking about revolutionary ideas. To a lesser or greater extent, the concept of systematically probing at an organizations management and operational systems to locate inefficiencies, and operational faults has been and is presently being utilized by organizational leaders throughout the world, who are interested in detecting and solving problems of importance.

Without getting caught-up in the jargon associated with systems and systems concepts, it may be helpful, at this point, to say that well-planned, methodical, analysis is most useful in helping a manager appraise his or her organization with respect to its short and long range objectives, determining the explicit need necessary to increase the organization's capacity to reach its objectives, and upon reaching them, keep the organization healthy and prosperous.

The ailments which affect most organizations are rarely the result of a single well-defined problem. Instead, a close examination of the ailment reveals groups of underlying etiologies which are instrumental in producing the undesired outcomes.

An examination of medical diagnosis helps to illustrate this point. The credence of medical practice is based on its ability to define a specific organic or systematic diseases or disorder by virtue of signs or symptoms. It then traces such a physiological disorder back through the human organism to points where the disease factors can be located, its synergistic effects understood, isolated, and either removed or stabilized to a point where the organism functions adequately again.

The process of diagnosis is not limited to the medical profession. Behavioral fields such as sociology, psychology and management science depend heavily on effective analytical/diagnostic methods to locate troublesome areas, to assess the impact of these areas, and to develop viable solution alternatives for improving the states of their systems. Most recently, the field of hazard control has been employing, with great success, analytical, systematic methods for extracting, evaluating, and offering solutions for problems existing in management and operational systems responsible for loss.

The business organization as a system functions with constant interaction among its internal components as well as the many parameters in its external environment. Among its internal components are those subsystems concerned: (1) with money, materials, products, and so forth; (2) with the flow of information; (3) with decision-making. Among those factors in a business's external system are all elements which embrace consumer relationships,—(e.g., product liability)—and community requirements,— (e.g., the environmental pollution laws). Business organizations as such do not exist in isolation but instead must, for survival, be capable of meeting the specific demands of: (1) its customers; (2) its environment; and (3) of other organizations.

During the process of upgrading the performance of any organization, one of the major tasks encountered is that of identifying problems which must be solved. A good manager knows that consideration must be given to the importance of problems in relation to their impact on overall objective attainment.

Choosing to solve problems which may occur frequently, but which are minor with respect to their ability to detract from the organizational mission, results in the expenditure of much time and good work with little or no favorable impact on the overall system effectiveness. In avoiding the pitfalls associated with addressing problems which are capable of providing low-yield results in lieu of those which can yield a higher payoff, a careful identification of organizational problems must be undertaken before such data can be sorted out and ordered on a hierarchy of importance. With such an activity accomplished, top management as well as other members of the management team are in more enlightened positions to determine the order in which problem areas will receive attention.

This Chapter is designed to introduce the hazard control specialist to the systematic integration of hazard control into the overall management process.

The Job of Management—A Preview

To the casual observer an organization is an aggregate of activities characterized by production of a product or rendition of a service. The casual observer has little awareness that, without leadership and a management game plan, an organization would be nothing more than an unorganized mass of activities, accomplishing little, rendering inefficient services, and wasting energy and other resources.

The organizational leader carries the bulk of the managerial role on his shoulders—and rightfully so. His job is to set goals and objectives for their accomplishment, to plan, organize, and coordinate the activities of personnel so that organizational objectives are realized. Finally, the manager must control the outcome of the organizational effort so that expected results are obtained within acceptable limits of the planned objective. The larger the organization, the more difficult this process becomes.

Managing an organization is one of the most interesting and deeply rewarding of all occupations. On one hand, it is a job of continuous excitement and anticipation, as something, good or bad, is always going to happen. The process of managing an entire organization, or even one of its smaller parts, always presents a challenge. For every problem identified and solved, there will be another one to take its place.

The hazard control function is a classic case-in-point. No matter how diligent an effort is expended to identify and control hazards in the operational system today, we can be sure that new ones are likely to emerge tomorrow, requiring a fresh trip back to the drawing board to come up with another solution.

In a positive light, the job of management must harness creativity and energy, while bridging differences and overcoming resistance to change. A highly dynamic job, it requires a high degree of capability and perceptiveness to bring off.

On the other hand, the job of management can entail frustrations which drain the very creativity and energy out of a job which depends on both for success. By the very nature of his role, he who is in the management position has dozens of thoughts running around in his head all the time. He must live in constant anticipation that his expected plans might not materialize, while many unexpected situations could rear their ugly heads at just the time when he would not be ready to cope with them.

He must also cope with the never-ending threat that many of his plans may never materialize. Worse, what often starts out to be a simple, logical plan of action often becomes highly confusing, inflammatory, and controversial to all involved.

The job of manager is very rewarding for most people, involving, as it does, a close interaction and a high degree of cooperation among all members of the management system. Later in this Chapter, the relationship between the hazard control specialist and the other members of the management team will be discussed in greater detail. The point will then be emphasized that the hazard control function cannot be placed on the shoulders of one person or even a select group within the organization. Instead, progress in hazard control can be realized only through the cooperative efforts of all personnel.

For centuries the managerial function was an art learned primarily from college courses, from peers, or from readings and personal experiment. No comprehensive systematic approach existed—only a set of maxims of span of control, units of command, designation of responsibility and authority, and so forth. Unfortunately, these maxims did not always produce the desired results. More often than not they fell to pieces, sometimes causing the person in the managerial function more intense problems than those he had in the first place. Perhaps one of the prime reasons behind managerial ineffectiveness has been that often new techniques and methods are introduced into the organization with little or no consideration to how these techniques and methods will interact with the already-existing organizational environment. Furthermore, there are times when little consideration is given to the question concerning what benefits the innovation is capable of producing in terms of behavioral, situational and environmental change in the organization. Thus the task of measuring improvement is often awkward and undefinitive.

Throughout the remainder of this chapter, a close examination will be made of the management process, with primary emphasis on the place of hazard control as a broad-based, integral activity. An attempt will be made to establish guidelines, concepts, and methods, by which an effective process, oriented towards hazard reduction, can be realized.

The Process of Management

If five hundred people who are serving in the management function were asked to define the term "management," we could reasonably expect to receive five hundred varied answers. Yet, a close examination would reveal that several elements could be found with a fair amount of consistency. First, *management is a purposeful activity;* it exists for a reason. Second, *management is a process or activity which expends human effort and physical resources.* Third, *it is a process which leads to a desired result—and profit,* more often than not, is the most frequent popular desired result. Back at the turn of the century Fredrick W. Taylor[1] indicated that management is knowing what you want your workers to do and getting them to do it in the cheapest and best way.

Throughout this book, the term management will be considered as *a process of accomplishing certain desired results or objectives through the intelligent utilization of human effort and physical resources.*

Is Management a Science?

The question always arises whether management is a science, or whether people performing the managerial function are merely gropers looking for solutions to problems on purely an intuitive or instinctive basis.

When this question is examined, we can see why it is so difficult to derive consistent answers. The reason quite simply is that management is not really a science, as we normally think of or define a science—a body of knowledge which has some fundamental elements and laws. Chemistry, for example qualifies as a science by this definition. However, the management of a chemistry department does not. This same analogy holds true for the hazard control effort. While many of the elements of the overall hazard control process are sciences in their own right; chemistry, physics, electronics, etc., the process by which the hazard control function operates within the organization is not.

We may not agree that the process of management can by our definition, qualify as a science. Nevertheless there are elements of the management process which are universally applicable, whether to manufacturing, construction, public service, or any other business enterprise.

Preceding any exploration of the elements of the management process, a moment spent on the subject of objectives is worthwhile. Before the mechanics of the management process can be put to work, end points must be specified. Specific objectives, or sub-objectives, leading toward the accomplishment of the overall organizational mission, must be established before planning or any other managerial activity can take place. An examination of the objective reveals that it has two basic parts. First, it must be measurable (a five percent return on an investment would be an example). Second, it must be realistic. The ability to establish realistic objectives has been and in many organizations still is a difficult process. Perhaps most managers are basically too greedy. No doubt they would like to realize more from their endeavors than is either possible or probable to obtain. A good example would be the company which sets the elimination of "all" losses as its yearly objective.

One of the major faults which has hindered hazard control programs in the past is that top management has set objectives for the operation of the hazard control system which couldn't be measured or could never realistically be achieved. In some instances top management has set up, and funded hazard control programs without any idea of what it should be getting in return for its investment. We could carry this point a step further by saying that there are many hazard control programs in business today, run by people who do not really know what objectives their programs are supposed to accomplish.

Without a well-conceived and well-administered program for action, what really needs to be accomplished is rarely, if ever achieved.

Dealing with Objectives

For years before the creation of mandatory safety and health standards and the imposition of these standards on the nations' industries, many people in hazard control positions sold their programs, among other things, on the basis of profit. Although increased profit through hazard control was a catchy phrase which intrigued organizational leaders, when the time came to demonstrate the results of the program's effort, the hazard control specialist was not always able to do so as convincingly as he would have liked.

Basing the success of a hazard control program strictly on a reduction in accidents and accident costs presents several major problems. To begin with, it

Objectives for Hazard Control Programs—The Issue of Profit

becomes very difficult for the hazard control specialist to identify all costs related to his organizations' accident experience. This includes some of the direct costs as well as a great many of those indirect of uninsured costs which were incurred during the course of and after accidents occurred. See Figure 10. The second problem of justifying a program on the basis of a savings in accident costs is that when it comes right down to the wire, even those who keep meticulous records, cannot prove with a very close degree of accuracy, that "x" dollars spent on the administration of the hazard control program were able to yield "y" dollars savings in accident costs. It becomes difficult for the hazard control specialist to convince those higher up in the organization exactly how many dollars the accidents which didn't happen would have cost the organization had they actually occurred. This situation is very frustrating to some in the hazard control function the fruits of whose efforts are not always as visible as they would like them to be.

Such logic is dangerous for another reason, and that reason is based on the fact that accidents are rare events—they do not occur at the frequency which their potential would indicate. So, it is very possible, if even for only a short time, for a company to completely disband its hazard control effort and still not be plagued with excessive costs from accident situations. This same company may erroneously deduce that the money they saved by not having a hazard control program actually put them further ahead than had they paid the price for avoiding the few nonconsequential accidents which occurred during the year.

Direct Costs
1. Medical care expenses
2. Worker's compensation costs
3. Insurance premium increase
4. Replacement costs of equipment and material damaged in accident
5. Facility repair
6. Loss of use of rental equipment damaged
7. Fees for Legal Counsel

Indirect Costs Loss
8. Slowdown in operations
9. Payment for contracted services with no work in return
10. Decrease in morale which affects production
11. Productive time lost from injured worker
12. Productive time lost by other than injured
13. Administrative work associated with accidents
14. Loss of client confidence
15. Overtime necessitated by work slowdown

Figure 10. Accident cost criteria.

We can look at another situation which, like the one previously mentioned, doesn't work out any better for the hazard control specialist. Here we see a well thought-out and administered hazard control program integrated into overall managerial activities. Adequate budget is provided for hazard control, manpower is available, and so on. Unfortunately, due to completely unexpected circumstances, lack of specific information, or problems outside the domain of the hazard control organization, the company experiences a greater number of accident situations, along with a substantial amount of associated costs. Experiences such as these may cause top management to react. They may want to start making changes in their hazard control program, changes which are not needed, and in some instances would be counter-productive. In any event, management views the problem from the standpoint of economics. They paid the price—they see nothing coming in return. Something has to be done about it.

A situation such as this one could have been averted if the hazard control specialist had taken two steps. First of all, he should have more fully acquainted top management with the purpose and benefits other than the savings in the cost of accidents alone, to be derived from a program aimed at hazard and loss reduction. Typical to most company missions is the desire to be effective, remain in business, and make a profit. The hazard control program is consistent with this mission. If the program is being administered properly, and if the hazard control specialist has documented the progress of this program's impact on overall organizational objectives over a sufficient period of time (three to five years would be a minimum baseline for comparison purposes) then he can show that a sudden rise in accidents during one year doesn't necessarily reflect a corresponding reduction in the effectiveness of the hazard control effort. The fact of the matter is, without a program, the company would run the risk of a substantial number of faults, any one of which could result in high losses, capable of detracting drastically from organizational effectiveness.

Another situation along these same lines can occur when a newly hired hazard control specialist enters an organizational situation where losses from accidents have been exceptionally high. Often, the new member of the management team offers promises of reversing the loss trend within a designated period of time—sometimes a year or less—counting on the fact that he has a good grasp on the sources of the hazards and true dollar amount the losses from these hazards are costing the company. The major problem associated with such an optimistic presumption is as follows: To begin with, the data supporting the existing loss totals may not reflect the total loss situation. Many times, only direct costs associated with accidents are calculated into a company's loss records, and sometimes these direct costs are not reflective of the true accident cost experience. In a great number of instances, the indirect costs associated with accidents are either not available or are calculated at a rate far lower than that which is actually being experienced by the organization. As a general rule, offering iron-clad guarantees with respect to reversing accident cost trends is a questionable practice.

Let us examine another hypothetical case. A hazard control specialist is hired by a company in crisis: it either has to lower its accident costs, along with other unfavorable ramifications of hazards in its workplace, or it goes out of business. The new person examines all available accident cost data, which includes worker's compensation premiums, medical and hospital costs, fines from OSHA, and the excess costs of insurance carrier penalties derived from its experience modification rates. Upon concluding his initial analysis, the new member of the management team sets out to establish a comprehensive program for effective hazard reduction. As the new system becomes operational, the new person soon discovers that the hazard data he is receiving is greater by far than what he had been told was the case. In situations like this, even the best designed and administered hazard control program may not be able to turn the tide in the immediate future. It will take a period of time—sometimes as long as a few years—to reverse the trend and bring the system under control. An analogy here would be trying to reverse the direction of a speeding freight train. Before this objective can be realized, the train needs to be either slowed down and turned around or stopped and reversed. Runaway accident cost situations in an organization are very much like the runaway train. Before the hazard control specialist is able to show a tangible favorable result from his program efforts, time will be needed to integrate his program efforts into the overall organizational system. Management must be made to understand that, instead of taking superficial actions which might appear to be providing results on the short term, their best bet is to grit their teeth, and go with a program that will yield some of their desired benefits immediately while at the same time establishing a substantial base for producing good results in the future.

In the process of setting realistic and measurable objectives and functions for a hazard control program, the hazard control specialist must make a very careful appraisal of the organization's position with respect to where it is now as well as where it wants to be going in the future. In addition, it is imperative that all members of the organization understand the purpose behind the objectives, what benefits will be accrued from them, and what their roles will be in carrying them out.

Figure 11 illustrates a set of relationships which have proven useful when attempts are made to relate specific hazard control objectives and functions to the overall objectives of the organization.

In setting up the chart in Figure 11 the hazard control specialist begins by acquiring from top management a list of specific desired objectives—both long-range and short—which the organization is striving to accomplish. With these objectives recorded for future reference, he or she acquires and lists all existing

Organizational Objectives	Deviation Detection	Intervening Factors	Necessary Immediate and Long Range Improvements
Volume of business increase over next 5 years. Product promotional plans. Physical facility expansion from 1 to 5 over next 10 years. Five-year projected increase in personnel. Approx. 15%. Need to comply with Federal and State health, safety, product safety and liability insurance through laws. To promote better labor-management relations. To portray good company image to the public. To increase profits and reduce operating expenses. To offset the cost of rising liability insurance through better cost control and management improvement.	Products produced with defects and hazards which are recognizable. Inadequate control of toxic chemicals and materials. Hazards resulting from sub standard maintenance Hazardous physical factors in the work-place. Hazardous work environment. Hazardous tools, machinery and equipment. Ineffective work-place design and layout. Excessive waste Man/machine mismatch	OSHA legislation Penalties imposed on competitors Consumer Products Safety Legislation to become more stringent over next 5 years. Increased lawsuits from consumers. Increased demands from CPSC. Competition—Projected expansion of products line and services over next 5 years. Competition is and will be installing new production techniques and plant facilities. Increasing pressure from organized labor concerning compliance with OSHA standards. Rising inflation. Competitors' products the subject of liability losses	Better control over work environment, work methods, tools, machinery and equipment. Closer evaluation of raw materials and equipment acquisition procedures. Re-evaluation of maintenance schedules and methods. In-depth noise and atmospheric studies of work-place and establish controls—immediate and long range. Re-evaluation of production purchasing and Quality Control Methods. Incorporating more safety in product performance criteria. Institute system safety evaluation techniques Perform ergonomics studies Set into motion a well integrated products liability program which will encompass design, manufacturing, inspection, purchasing, and advertising aspects of a product's life cycle.

and potential hazard and loss producing factors (deviations) which may adversely affect the accomplishment of the desired organizational objectives. When these first two important tasks are completed, the next step is to acquire and record as many factors in the environment external to the organization which have influence on the organization's survival. With these intervening factors recorded, an assessment can now be made to determine the ramifications of the interplay between the deviants, the intervening factors, and the effects on the accomplishment of organizational objectives. At this point, the hazard control specialist, working closely with other members of the management team, can begin to list the necessary immediate and long-range improvements required to foster the organization's capacity to accomplish its objectives.

Once agreement is reached on the specific organizational objectives, the hazard control specialist can begin to acquire the necessary information per-

Figure 11. Hazard control input to the organizational planning mission.

taining to those factors which can detract from the successful attainment of these objectives as well as those factors which contribute to success.

Planning

Once the hazard control specialist establishes his measurable and realistic objectives, and he has a blueprint which guides the construction of the program, his next step is to determine the course of action to be followed.

Planning, as an integral part of the management process is the function by which an organization adapts its resources to changing internal and environmental forces. As a predetermined course of action, planning has two essential characteristics: First: a plan must involve the future. Second: it must involve action.

Perhaps a prerequisite to any planning function is the perception and identification of organizational needs, and requirements. Essentially the goals or targets need to be defined before organizational activity can be focused in their direction.

During the planning process it becomes obvious that three logical steps must be taken. The first step is to appraise the future political, economic, and competitive environment in which the organization is attempting to survive. When such an appraisal is accomplished and the facts are logged, the second step is to visualize the desired role of the company in this environment. Figure 11 illustrates the results of the appraisal process by providing specific facts (intervening variables) which have direct impact on the direction which the organization has set for itself.

The results of the planning activity will provide answers to the questions concerning program requirements, courses of action which could be adopted, and how and when such actions would be taken. In addition, as a result of the planning activity, there will emerge specific policies, procedures, and methods necessary to make the plans operational, as well as ideas for overall program integration, scheduling, and a list of requirements for personnel selection and training. See Figure 12.

Organizing

Once planning has been completed and the organization has a fix on where it wants to go and what it will take to get them there, it becomes obvious that some vehicle is necessary to bring the plans to fruition. Such a vehicle is the activity known as organizing. *The organizing function provides among other things for existing and potential action in the organization.* Essentially *it provides for the intelligent and effective distribution of work among the workforce and provides the basis for the establishment of needed responsibility and authority.* In summary, organizing will determine where action takes

Question	Fundamental Function of Management Used	Results
1. What is the organization's policy toward hazard control? 2. What are the hazard control program requirements? 3. What will it take to get the job done? 4. How will an increase or decrease in performance be measured?	Planning	1. Modification in policy 2. Objectives 3. Activities, tasks, (program milestones), procedures, and methods 4. Overall program integration strategies 5. Scheduling 6. Personnel selection and training 7. Acquiring necessary resources
1. Where should actions take place? 2. What are the priorities? 3. Who in the management system will participate?	Organizing	1. Dividing work and assigning authority and responsibility 2. Coordinating the hazard control effort with other members of the organization
1. Why and how should organizational members perform their assignments? 2. How to get workers to voluntarily participate in the hazard and loss control effort?	Actuating	1. Leadership requirements 2. Communication requirements 3. Integrating the needs of people into the program 4. Incentives 5. Including workers in the training and education effort
1. Are the actions being performed? 2. What, Where, and How? 3. Are they in accordance with plans? 4. What instruments are needed to measure program effectiveness?	Control	1. Using standards to sense deviation from desired results 2. Reports of Audits 3. Modifying or Changing Procedures and methods 4. Replanning Hazard and Loss Control Effort

Figure 12. The management process. Note: The basic format for this illustration was developed by Terry, G. R., "Principles of Management," 4th Edition, 1968.

place and who does what work. The results of the organizing activity provide work division, work assignment, and authority delegation. Furthermore, they specify coordinating activities and those interrelationships necessary for harmony and effectiveness.

During the organizing activity, the manager is faced with two issues of major importance. First: to be sure that organizational productivity is maximized, and second: that the lines of responsibility and authority are clear cut and workable.

When attempts are made to maximize the productivity of an organization toward the attainment of an organizational objective, an idea introduced by Peter Drucker may be helpful. Drucker determined, that without a conscious effort to do otherwise, an organization is likely to direct 80 percent of its time and resources to issues which are capable at best of producing 20 percent of the results.[2] Of course the converse to Drucker's idea is also true. An organization could be directing 20 percent of its effort on those issues which are capable of yielding 80 percent of the desired result. The nineteenth century economist Pareto also recognized this ratio of inefficiency. He envisioned inefficient organizations spending the greatest amount of their time on what he called the "trivial many" problems while missing the "vital few" problems capable of yielding the highest payoff.[3]

A good example of such a situation might be a hazard control program which has proven ineffective. Invariably such programs fail to set specific guidelines for hazard assessment and evaluation. Where hazards are not extracted from an organizational system according to a specific plan, or where they are evaluated on a scale which does not demonstrate a clear hierarchy of importance, it then becomes easy for less important hazards, the trivial many, to attract attention, while those hazards with the most consequential impact are either overlooked or left waiting until they erupt sometime in the future. When we think about organizing a company's resources toward hazard control this becomes painfully clear.

Despite a careful plan and very definitive guidelines for development and operation, chances are that the program may, at best, be able to contend only with lower impact, less productive issues, while allowing those of higher impact to be missed.

The second major issue involves establishing responsibility and delegating authority to those in the organization who will be relied on to effect the accomplishment of the organization's objectives. This is particularly crucial in the instance of hazard control.

Among the most misunderstood terms in management, "responsibility" is right at the top of the list. The term responsibility, as it is used throughout this text is the *continuing obligation of a person or group to carry out an order, or mission to which it is assigned.* It should be understood that responsibility cannot be delegated. This means that no manager, regardless of his position in the organization, can shift responsibility to a subordinate—the buck stops with the person(s) given the obligation to get the job done.

A term which has been steadily growing in popularity among those in the field of hazard control is that of "accountability." Actually, the use of accountability, *is really just another way of stating responsibility although it pretends to indicate liability for the proper discharge of duties by the subordinate.*[4]

Authority, on the other hand, is *the necessary prerogative granted to those who are in key positions to carry out the elements which they are held responsible for.* Authority, by definition, *is the legal or rightful power granted to a person(s) to command others. Power, the result of force over time,* would suggest that those organizational personnel who are able to exert the necessary power on a continuous basis are more apt to be able to get their job done than others who have either never exerted or lost their ability to exert the prerogative needed to get the job done.

Since authority is the power to carry out assignments, and responsibility (accountability) is the obligation to accomplish them, it logically follows that the authority needed to do this must correspond to the responsibility. This parity is not mathematical but, rather, coextensive, because both relate to the same assignments.[5]

Actuating

The actuating function of the management process may be referred to as the "people" function: *that function which encourages members of the organization to carry out their prescribed tasks with enthusiasm.* When you come right down to it the actuating task is one of very skillful direction of people to achieve the objectives management wants, because the people want to. There is no stronger force to achieve success than that force created by organizational personnel who are fired up over what they are doing, who understand the purpose behind their efforts and the benefits to be accrued from the results. As great reliance is placed on members of the organization to achieve high levels of hazard control, skilled management must make a conscious effort to make people in both the line and staff organizations understand their contributions toward the overall hazard control program effort. Satisfactory participation must be rewarded. Any time we must deal with people, that task is not going to be easy. There are a million and one obstacles to be encountered along the road to shaping and aligning company member's philosophies and methods of operation toward the various organizational objectives. It is not the purpose of this chapter to delve deeply into organizational behavior, and the principles for effecting beneficial behavioral change. Wherever possible, such issues will be considered as part of the overall hazard control procedures to follow. However, there are certain particular issues which should receive some attention here.

A problem often encountered by those attempting to inspire organizational members for the task at hand is that their very methods for soliciting information and ideas from people become obstacles in their own right. A common complaint from company members is: "I gave my advice and nobody did anything with it." An analysis of this remark reveals two basic points. First, the employee was probably not fully aware of how his advice was going to be used. Second, he wasn't sure of the real reason he was asked to give it. Time and again, management has come up with new programs or reformations of existing ones, which require employee participation. Most of the time, this participation is vital to the success of the program, and without it the program has no chance of getting off the ground. Each time one of these programs appears, the natural instinct of organizational members is to tuck their heads in, roll their eyes and confide to one another how another hairbrain scheme has appeared which like those in the past will disappear if they pay no attention to it. A good example is the introduction of a new or remodeled hazard control program. For years, company members have seen "safety" and "accident prevention" endeavors come and go. For the most part, the employees didn't buy the ideas, became disillusioned, and after all was said and done, thought the whole idea of "safety" was a lot of bunk. These people had a good basis for their attitude. Seeing what happened to fellow workers who confided in management about accidents which they or their fellow workers had been party to, employees developed the stance of the three monkeys: they didn't see anything, heard even less, and said as little as possible. Imagine a new hazard control specialist coming into an organization of such people, and telling them that things will be different, that they can confide in him, that they must reveal all hazard information, which will be used to the advantage of everybody, and so on. This person had better brace himself, for he has his work cut out for him.

Another problem encountered during the actuating phase is getting organizational members to understand and appreciate the priorities for the things to be done which management has set. We can return again to the disillusioned employee who gave advice, made a good suggestion, but never saw anything changed. The reason for this outcome might have been quite legitimate, although the employee never knew it. Suppose management decided to weigh all hazards in the organization according to a one to four quantitative or qualitative scale, with the most important hazards classified in category four. It would then be logical that worst problems be corrected first. However, the employee who reports a hazard and sees nothing corrected, even though there may be a good reason for the inaction, may interpret it as an iron-clad indication that he has been given a "snow job," and that nobody really gives a damn. For all practical purposes, this employee has begun to cut off management from all future information.

There is a lesson to be learned here. If we want people in the organization to contribute information which we have no other way of obtaining on a day-to-day basis, then we must make every effort to help these people understand what we are doing, why we are doing it, why responses may not come to them as quickly as they would like, and most of all, why their continued participation and support is mandatory if the program is ever to succeed. Several years ago a case occurred which points this out very well. A hazard control consultant was contracted to conduct supervisor hazard recognition sessions for a west coast government ordinance organization. During the early part of the program, one of the participants approached the consultant and indicated his satisfaction with what had transpired during the program. To make a long story short, the consultant and participant became fairly well acquainted during the weeks to follow. The more the friendship developed, the more it became obvious the participant was one of the most knowledgeable people in the areas of explosives and explosives hazard control. This supervisor, on his own time, purchasing his own books and other materials, had become an expert in his own right. Stopping to think for a moment, the consultant realized that here, under the guise of a line supervisor of production, was someone who should have been intimately involved in the operation of the organization's hazard control program—or at the very least, included in the organization's hazard control decision network. But he wasn't. When the supervisor was asked why he didn't contribute his knowledge to management and aid them in the identification of hazard areas, his answer was classic. It went like this: "Twenty years ago, I was an eager beaver and I wanted to contribute as much as I could to the organizational mission. Unfortunately, I never received any encouragement. There were many times when I reported a problem which I knew was serious—my report was rarely responded to. What's worse, nothing constructive was ever really done. You know, a man will only be kicked so many times. When I finally realized that the rules and programs around here were basically make-believe, I decided to stop contributing. I guess I essentially cut management and those clowns in their "safety" department off from the very information they should have been getting. Worse than that, I actually started taking great satisfaction in watching things go wrong I had known would go wrong, and which management couldn't anticipate."

An analysis of this case clearly indicates that management, by their actions and omissions, destroyed the very participative behavior they solicited. However, this same situation might have occurred had the management been receptive to ideas, and had the best interest of their people in mind. Suppose the supervisor in the above case had been making recommendations which, though significant to him, fell short from the standpoint of company priorities. Others in the organization may have reported other more pressing problems which presented more of a threat to the organizational mission. These problems needed to be attended to first. Had the supervisor been informed of this fact, and had he been able to justify it in his own mind, chances are he could have understood the decision made and continuously and openly contributed ideas in the future.

When it comes right down to the wire, among all the techniques available to facilitate the actuating function, sympathetic listening to the individual employee is the most important. This is the only way to find out how people think on a day-to-day basis, and make changes in program strategies which will encourage, not limit, participation. It is the people working in an organization who know what is actually happening behind the scene. They see the errors made; perhaps they have made the same error themselves. The successful hazard control specialist will get these people to confide in him, not as a means of getting themselves or others into trouble, but because they can see how their contribution can help bring the organizational mission to the highest levels of success. This endeavor represents a challenge to today's hazard control specialist.

Control

When we speak of control as it relates to the management process, we are essentially addressing ourselves to *that activity oriented toward the prevention of bad changes—changes in operations which would be counter-productive.* Another way of visualizing the control process is as that function of the overall system which insures direction in conformity with the objectives.

The requirements of adequate controls which relate well to the hazard control mission are:[6]

1. Whatever control tools are utilized, they must be capable of sensing and reporting symptoms of inadequacy promptly, so the system can be set into action to correct the problems. If a control cannot provide such speedy efficiency, it will act as an anesthetic, lulling those involved into a false sense of security. A good example is accident, injury, and loss data which are analyzed and reported annually. Instead of being able to detect and correct deviations as they are occurring, management is shielded from these problems until the end of the year—a point in time when it is perhaps too late to take action which will yield the highest benefits.

2. A good control will be able to point out exceptions arising at critical points. The control must be able to show an aggregate of deviations while simultaneously tracing them back to those areas which are critical to the operation.

3. The control should be understood by all those in the organization affected by it. If complex mathematical formulas are used in detailed hazard analyses, or if statistical summaries carrying valuable information are too difficult to sort out and utilize for those who need them, then the necessary communication is lost, and there is a good chance that expected benefits will never occur.

4. The control should be able to point-out the path to preventive and/or corrective action. Adequate control tools for use in hazard control should be able to disclose where the failures are occurring, who is responsible for them, and what should be done to correct the inadequate situations.

5. Effective controls must coincide with (organizational) objectives. Unless every department manager, foremen, and those workers under their leadership are shown that the losses and potential losses occurring as a result of hazards in the operations under their control are disproportionate to those occurring in other company departments, it is likely that little will be done to correct them.

Figure 13 illustrates a typical feedback loop of management control demonstrating activities which are part of a continuous cycle of day-to-day activities carried out to provide an organization with some assurance that the planned objective will be realized.

One of the pitfalls management encounters when they set out to establish and implement control is that they often become victims of their own actions. That is, they become so wrapped up in the process of seeing to it that things don't go wrong that they often grow blind to the vital changes which must be sought after and effected, for the organization to prosper. Juran[7] in his book "Managerial Breakthrough," identifies this problem and offers a solution. Juran envisions that within the control process there exists another basic element known as breakthrough. *"Breakthrough is defined as the creation of necessary changes in an organization."* Both control and breakthrough, although two diverse ideas, are part of one continuing cycle of events. A good manager must conduct both of these activities simultaneously if he expects to achieve the gains necessary for organizational survival.

The role of the hazard control function is a good example of how control and breakthrough exists as part of an ongoing process. One part of the hazard control function—that part which is control oriented—involves devoting a substantial amount of energy to preventing bad changes or deviations which have loss potential capable of detracting from system objectives.

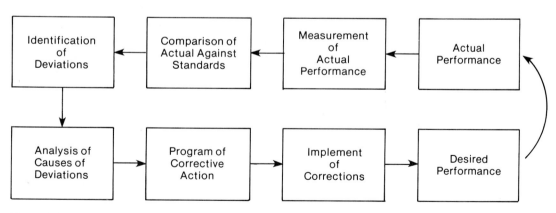

Figure 13. Feedback loop of management control. (With permission of McGraw-Hill Book Co., Inc., from "Principles of Management" Terry, George R., 4th Edition, 1968.)

On the other hand, a substantial amount of effort and energy must be devoted to creating new changes in the program which will guarantee the survival of the system. Today, probably more than any time in the history of modern-day hazard control programs, management calculates carefully the adverse effects of all areas of risk and liability. Such an analysis makes obvious the fact that merely spending all ones time watching an operational system to detect worker related injury and death potential is not enough. Pressures today dictate that the loss and liability possibilities existing in industry necessitate reaching out and establishing progressive programs to affect products, services, and the environment. Such new responsibilities will require the creation of new expertise, while at the same time flushing out the obsolete processes, techniques, methods and philosophies which are not suitably productive to meeting the new challenges.

Standards and the Control Process

When the control process is visualized in itself, basic elements emerge: Standards must exist, performance must be measured, and faults in and deviations from the planned objective must be corrected. It becomes clear that without standards, there is no logical basis for making a decision or taking action. Dalcher[8] has summed up the functions of standards in the following two points. Standards should: (a) be able to coordinate the work of several departments all working on the same problems into routine procedures which make the solution a matter of record; (b) provide a guide for all who face these problems in the future.

The main purpose of any standard should be to alert those using the standard that something is not coming off in the way it is intended. An unfortunate effect of standards however, is that the standard can make those using it blind or inattentive to any issue which is not listed as a deviation from the standard in hand. We can see this situation occurring over and over again, when the hazard control specialist sends his inspectors out to monitor a workplace, according to a set of OSHA standards. If by chance all the deviations located can be traced back to an existing standard, everything is OK. On the other hand, if a hazardous condition exists which is not contained in the standards or doesn't seem of critical importance, the inspectors are likely to miss it, unless they have been well trained to look beyond the standards to locate additional situations of hazard potential.

A general rule which can be made about standards is that they are not substitutes for vigilance and competence. Those using the standards to detect problems in the system must thoroughly understand the system's operation, must use standards along with, but not in place of, logical thinking and decision-making. Among the prime errors most commonly made by those using standards is that they don't understand the reasons behind the standards, so they try to use the standards to measure something they were never intended to, scarcely appreciating how the system, to which the standard was meant to apply actually functions. On behalf of better "safety-health" inspections, it is suggested that the inspector become intimately familiar with the process or operation, before he or she is ever allowed to go out with clipboards and inspection forms.

Since good standards, capable of sensing deviations, play an important role in the control process in general, and particularly in the hazard control process, perhaps it is worthy to examine what makes a standard good.

Characteristics of Good Standards

To begin with, *the standard must suggest something which can be attained.* The average worker or his supervisor should be able to comply with the standard under actual work conditions. When the standard demands pie-in-the-sky, utopian conditions, which are both impractical and impossible to meet, then the standard is handicapped from the outset. Soon, it will either be ignored or revised to such an extent that its original intent is lost. Second, *standards should be economically feasible.* The resources required to set and administer the standard should be proportional to the benefits to be accrued. Third, and extremely important, *the standard must be applicable to the situation in which it is going to be used.*

If the situation is one which is highly dynamic and likely to change, the standards should be flexible enough to meet the situation at hand. This point is perhaps one of the problems with some of the safety and health standards on the books today. The standards, being rigid by nature, try to bend the system to fit the standard, rather than being flexible enough themselves to fit system demands, while providing a reasonable criterion for control.

Fourth, standards should be consistent in their interpretation so that communications problems can be avoided. Should variance be made, then, the ground rules for the use of the variance must be made known to all those whom the standard will affect. Fifth, *standards must be written in such a way that the people required to use them will be capable of understanding what they mean.* Simplicity and clarity are two key characteristics of a good standard. Sixth, *a good standard is both stable and maintainable.* In addition to having a reasonably long life, to provide a basis for predictability, they should be structured in such a way that sections or sub-parts can be added or deleted without destroying the structure and intent of the entire standards package. Seventh, *it must be agreed that the standard be a fair basis for comparing what is against what ought to be.*

The following paragraph by Thomas Whiteside, excerpted from the New Yorker magazine, depicts a situation involving standards which, although amusing, arouses concern, because in one form or another, many existing safety and health standards today are inciting similar problems.

> ". . . Pondering recently the toughness of the MH-1, the tomato bred for the age of mechanical picking, and on how a particular MH-1 had remained intact after a six-foot fall to a hard tiled floor in Dr. Volin's office, I began to wonder whether America was making automobiles that would stand up as solidly to that kind of impact. Out of curiosity, I telephoned Dr. William Haddon, Jr., an auto-safety expert, who is president of the Insurance Institute for Highway Safety, and asked him if one of his technical people could compute the approximate impact speed of the Florida MH-1 in the six-foot fall I had witnessed in ratio to the minimum federal requirements for impact resistance in the bumpers of cars sold in this country. Dr. Haddon obliged, and on the basis of the figures he provided, I concluded that Dr. Bryan's MH-1 was able to survive its fall to the floor at an impact speed of 13.4 miles per hour, more than two and a half times the speed which federal auto-bumper safety standards provide for the minimum safety of current-model cars. This undoubtedly represents a great step forward in tomato safety . . ."[9]

The moral to this little episode is that if the standard is not realistic, nor sensitive to the issue it is addressing, then it will not be able to do its intended job.

Furthermore, if a standard is not designed to provide a level of acceptability in accordance with the philosophy and rationale of those to be governed by the standard, such a standard will have little impact. Should the standard not be acceptable to those to be governed by it, they will change the standard to suit their own perception of acceptability. The 55 mph speed limit imposed on the American driving public is a good example. The driving public, for the most part, feels that the speed limit is unrealistic, and interferes too much with its need for reasonably fast transportation. Furthermore, they see their tax dollars which went into safe highway construction to handle automobile speeds greater than 70 mph, wasted. Combining these reasons, with a host of others, the average driver in the nation is driving at speeds exceeding 55 mph. Perhaps their new standard is 60 mph or greater.

The control process as described in Figure 12 and all those activities necessary to carry it out will provide the manager with answers, as to whether activities are being performed, when, where, and how, and whether such activities are in conformance with plans. With such information, management can then take whatever corrective action is necessary to align procedures and methods consistent with their desired results.

Hazard Control—
An Integral Part of
the Control
Process

Hazard control is defined as *that function in an organization directed toward the recognition, evaluation, and reduction or elimination of the destructive effects of hazards emanating from human acts of commission and omission and from the physical and environmental aspects of the workplace.* The purpose of the hazard control mission is to reduce to tolerable levels, injuries, damage, production delay and other loss-producing situations, occurring as a result of problems in techniques, personnel, equipment, the environment, and from worker/machine interactions.

In summary, the hazard control mission is aimed at locating, assessing, and setting effective preventive and corrective measures for those hazardous elements that have detrimental effects on operational efficiency and effectiveness.

Hazard Control—A Failure Oriented Function

The hazard control function, as part of the overall management process could be viewed as being failure-oriented. This is not to say that those involved in the function are pessimistic about the job they are doing and are doomed to failure. The idea behind failure orientation is that the hazard control specialist spends a substantial amount of his work life looking for and responding to failure situations. It doesn't take long for a hazard control specialist to develop the philosophy that it is more advantageous to think in terms of failure, because it is easier to obtain mutual agreement on what constitutes a failure. Agreement on what constitutes success is much more difficult if not impossible to obtain, due to the fact that the people the hazard control specialist will come in contact with will be estimating success on their own set of criteria. More often than not, the criteria will not be the same from person to person. On the other hand, the same group of people who could not come to mutual agreement on the issue of success are more readily able to see and understand the consequences of failure, thus facilitating the communication process. Another argument for failure-orientation might be the fact that in any system, there are fewer failures occurring than successes. Simply stated, more things are going right with most organization's operations than are going wrong. Those in the hazard control function can benefit from this relationship by more clearly focusing the most substantial amount of their efforts on things which have the potential to cause undesirable effects on organizational operations. The last factor to substantiate the philosophy of failure-orientation is the psychological one. Quite frankly, it is more challenging and fulfilling for a person to find "holes" in something while at the same time being able to offer effective solutions. This psychological fulfillment gained by the hazard control specialist, as a result of his work, may be the only reward he or she ever gets, and may be the strongest compensation for a basically difficult, and many times frustrating, job.

The Production Process and Hazard Control

In the production process model Figures 14 and 15, a mixture of workers, equipment and materials interact within the plant setting or other workplace environment, to accomplish a particular product or service. Added to these elements is the additional vital element of "time, for without it the process could not take place."[10] Furthermore, when something happens to extend the allotted time, the system has to pay the price. Sometimes, when the system is accelerated and employee work hours increased, to make up for lost time, a condition is created which is conducive to increasing rather than reducing the

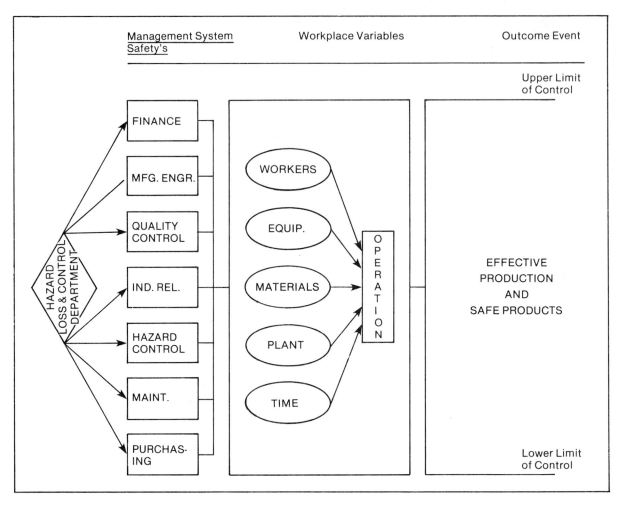

Management System Safety's	Workplace Variables	Outcome Event

Upper Limit of Control

HAZARD LOSS & CONTROL DEPARTMENT

FINANCE

MFG. ENGR.

QUALITY CONTROL

IND. REL.

HAZARD CONTROL

MAINT.

PURCHAS-ING

WORKERS

EQUIP.

MATERIALS

PLANT

TIME

OPERATION

EFFECTIVE PRODUCTION AND SAFE PRODUCTS

Lower Limit of Control

Figure 14. Production model.

losses which management is trying to avoid. An accident, whether or not it culminates in an injury, property damage, material waste, or any number of other undesired events, interrupts the productive process to some degree, and this interruption carries a price tag. Each interruption increases the time needed to complete the job, often reducing the efficiency and effectiveness of the overall operation, and raising the costs of production. In some cases, numerous or sustained interruptions prevent production schedules from being kept—sometimes costing the company future business.

Time loss is of particular concern to the production manager or those charged with seeing to it that the job comes off on time according to plan. Such people readily equate "downtime," with materials waste, property damage, death or injury to people inside and outside the organization, and damage to the workplace, with increased operational costs and decreased operational effectiveness.

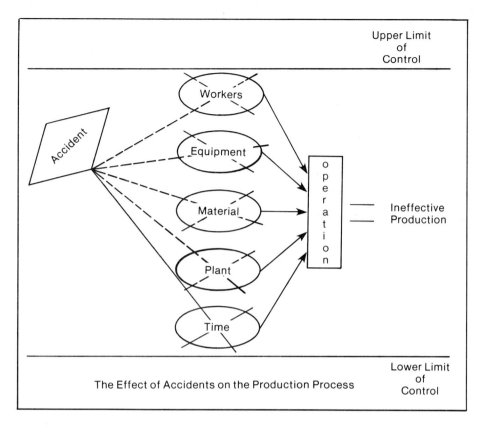

Upper Limit
of
Control

Workers

Equipment

Accident

Material

o
p
e
r
a
t
i
o
n

Ineffective
Production

Plant

Time

The Effect of Accidents on the Production Process

Lower Limit
of
Control

Figure 15. The production
process out of control.

An example of an accident which carried a high price-tag due to the time and production loss it created is described as follows. A construction company had rented a crane for a very critical phase of the construction process. During a lift, the crane's outriggers, which were set on soft ground without mud mats to support them, punched through the ground, causing the crane to fall over on its side thus dropping its load. The accident severely damaged the crane buckling the boom sections beyond repair, to say nothing of the material damage which was incurred. As a result of this episode, the entire project came to a standstill. Before the job could continue as planned, the crane had to be carted away and the damaged boiler which was being lifted replaced by a new one. In addition to the time and cost involved with the clean-up and equipment and material replacement, the workers which would have normally been doing their jobs were left idle. As a result, in addition to the costs involved, the job fell behind schedule. Here, an avoidable situation has detracted from the expected construction time schedule and has diminished the efficiency of the job.

The Effect of Hazards on the Production Mission

The production process indicates that control is the necessary ingredient by which operational efficiency and effectiveness are maintained. As has already been explained, control allows within allowable limits, for the introduction of variations from system procedures.

Management builds into each of its production systems standards of acceptability and unacceptability, which in fact provide direction and leeway for the system's operation. An example of these control limits which have impact on a production operation can be understood by the following: An Ordinance manufacturing company is granted a contract to produce ten thousand 500 pound bombs for an agency within the Department of Defense. Assuming that the company's workforce is able to perform its task without interruption, equipment and machinery do not break down, materials and the finished product meet standards, the physical plant is not damaged, and the production schedule runs along with minimum time loss—the production goal will be met, and the operation will be under control. That is, it will come off according to plan with a minimum of loss and interruption. On the other hand, suppose a worker is injured in an accident due to either a human, machine, or environmental failure. What happens? Obviously, time is lost, production may be slowed down, the cost of the operation may increase, and to some degree the efficiency of the operation will be lessened. Suppose a problem occurs in one of the explosives mixing kettles that results in a mass detonation. What happens this time? Again, the operation is interrupted, severe injury or death to personnel, equipment loss, and damage to the physical plant may occur. In addition, the product might not be available on time.

Comparing the second situation with the definition of control, it is clear that the latter operation is "out-of-control," and production was not accomplished within the acceptable limits of the planned objective.

An examination of the production process also suggests the implications of "success" and "failure," as they relate to effective production. Figure 16 indicates that the result of any operation can be categorized theoretically as a "total success" or "total failure." If the person in charge of an operation is

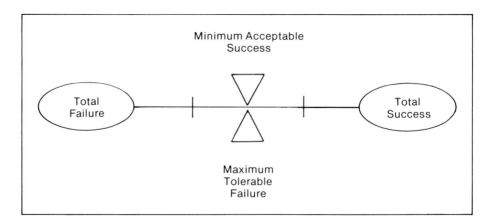

Figure 16.

able to complete the job without a failure of any kind, maximize on the productive effort of the workforce, keep the maintenance of equipment to a minimum, and make a profit, he can deem the operation as being totally successful. On the other hand, suppose that during this same operation, numerous mistakes are made, many of which account for prolonged interruptions, equipment and plant damage, personal injury, poor quality control, etc. This time the person in charge can't deliver an acceptable product on time, and has incurred additional costs for repair, replacement, and compensation. This time he has lost. He is wiped out. Things couldn't have gone worse. Fortunately, operations are not usually total failures. On the other hand, total success, although strived for, is rarely achieved. Usually there is a compromise. A point somewhere between total success and total failure is designated as the break-even point which can be referred to as "minimum acceptable success" or "maximum tolerable failure." That is, the point where, although the job doesn't come off totally successfully, processes are accomplished with a tolerable number of losses and interruptions, thus maintaining the efficiency and effectiveness of the company's operations.

Management must carefully consider that error-free performance is a goal that is rarely ever reached. To counter this problem, it must concentrate its efforts on eliminating, or at least reducing the major accident causative factors within the company's operations responsible for failure situations. In order for management to be successful in eliminating major failures within the production processes, it must first determine where they can occur, how important they are, and what their potential effect is. Only then can they provide the necessary defense mechanism to counter these problems. This hazard evaluation can be done informally, or it can take the shape of recorded, detailed analysis. Regardless of the methods used, the output must be valid data for informed management decisions. Corrective measures based on accurate hazard data may prompt a production innovation, personnel change, or the guarding of a tool or machine. In addition to locating the hazards and providing effective controls, management must institute a monitoring function capable of continuously assessing the effectiveness of its corrective actions. Indeed, there have been instances where a corrective measure caused more problems than it was designed to eliminate or where an operation was altered to such a degree that the control was no longer functional. The concept, "minimum acceptable success," will set direction for further thinking in hazard control programming, as all efforts will be oriented towards guaranteeing minimum acceptability before additional efforts are made to establish further refinements aimed at bringing organizational output to the highest levels of productivity. In so doing, we have a greater chance of reaching and maintaining higher levels of operational effectiveness. The process of keeping operations within acceptable limits gives credence to the concept of hazard control. The usefulness of the hazard control process is to pinpoint hazards before they culminate in failure situations which may detract from productive operations. In essence, hazard control programming plays a crucial part in maintaining an organization's mission capability.

The Role of Management Systems in the Hazard Control Process

As was inferred earlier in this chapter, the hazard control function is one which cannot be placed on the shoulders of a single person or department within an organization, if that organization expects to realize a decrease in the losses resulting from hazards in the workplace. An analysis of many safety programs classified as less than effective reveals a common trait. These programs were designed with the idea in mind that the "safety director" and his staff would handle all safety matters of concern to the organization. Under such an arrangement, the line organization was actually cut loose from the burden of integrating hazard control into their operations and having to account for losses occurring under their control. A situation such as this encourages line officers to call in the "safety person" when their back is up against the wall or at times blame the "safety person" for accidents which occurred in their operations.

Hazard control as a well-designed integrated activity in an organization depends heavily on an interchange of ideas and a cooperation and collaboration between the staff and line organization and the hazard control department. Quite simply each group has something to offer the other.

The successful hazard control specialist has recognized that he cannot realize the company's hazard control objectives all by himself. He soon learns that a cooperative effort between his office and those of other key people in his organization is necessary if headway is ever going to be made. Of course, recognizing what needs to be done and doing it are two different things. It is no secret that the history of the safety function in many companies has left a bad taste in the mouths of the line organization. Perhaps the fellow running the safety department didn't have the abilities or characteristics needed to add significant inputs to the operations of those in design and manufacturing, and thus established a credibility gap. Maybe, the safety person really knew his stuff but was afraid to take the initiative to disturb those in powerful positions in the line organization or, equally bad, perhaps he thought that he could shape the system to conform with his ideas for hazard control, instead of orienting his strategies to fit into the existing system and slowly but ever so consistently bring about the favorable change he desired.

What it all boils down to is that there is no substitute for competency. The hazard control specialist has to know what he is doing and has to gain the confidence of everybody in the organization—from the workers up through those in top managerial positions. Credibility is not something which comes with a position—it has to be earned.

The hazard control specialist will find himself halfway home towards establishing a viable hazard control program within his organization, if he very carefully interweaves his hazard control effort into all aspects of organizational activity—even if he loses some personal credit for some of the benefits which are accrued from his efforts.

The hazard control effort, to be effective, will require very close relationships among each of the organizations' management departments and between these management departments and the hazard control department.

Sensitizing those in key management positions to the true extent of the hazard control problem is one of the most important steps in the development and maintenance of any effective hazard control effort.

In the author's experience of speaking to management groups on the subject of hazard control, the design, manufacturing, engineering, purchasing, quality control, and other organizational groups are concerned with the ramifications of federal safety and health legislation as it affects the survival of their individual universes. Leaders of these groups rarely understand that they have the capacity to alleviate or at the least reduce many of the hazards occurring in their operations. They usually express the opinion that safety problems should be handled by the "safety department." Of course this has been proven to be false. In fact, if the people running these departments were to examine their designated functions carefully, it would be quite obvious that many of their duties dove-tail with those of the "safety" department, and that to a certain extent they are responsible for part of the hazard control effort.

A fact of life existing in many organizations is that each management system artificially limits itself to its designated responsibilities and functional requirements. Only when necessary, do the people in these systems attempt to do "someone else's job!" even if by so doing ,they will increase the effectiveness and efficiency of their own operation. This problem manifests itself time and time again when we attempt to acquire support for the hazard control effort. The old cliche that "hazard control is everyone's responsibility but no one's job" is especially applicable here. Rarely do the leaders of other departments actually add concrete contributions to the hazard control effort, though organizational policy nominally requires as much. There are, however, many justifiable reasons for this. First, department managers may have limited manpower to accomplish their essential operational roles; thus they feel that they cannot take on additional work assignments. Secondly, their resources may be limited. Finally, no one may have pointed out just exactly what their contribution is to the total hazard control effort and, conversely, how they can benefit from the hazard control department. Although the previously mentioned points can be valid reasons which impede various departments active participation in "someone else's job," the point made here is that these same department leaders can give significant support to the hazard control effort while simultaneously providing their assigned operational task—often more effectively and efficiently. Without additional expenditures in time and resources, they can simply become aware of, look for, and report those suspected factors which are responsible for accidents, and maximize on the inputs from the hazard control system.

Figure 17 illustrates this point quite clearly. For instance, while the manufacturing engineering department is making regular plant audits to assure that processes are in conformity with established performance standards, it should at the same time be viewing the conformance of these same processes with established safety, health, and environmental standards. Deficiencies should be reported to management.

Another example of a management system that plays an essential role in hazard control is the purchasing department. Over the years this department may have unintentionally brought countless hazards into the organization in the form of unsafe tools, machines, materials, substances, etc. The prime reason for this situation is that purchasing people most often acquire resources for the organization without being aware of the hazard ramifications of their purchases. This situation is indeed not entirely the fault of the purchasing department per se. Top management has rarely considered that purchasing should be attuned to the minimum, necessary, and sufficient safeguards to protect against inherent hazards in their acquisitions, and, consequently, it hasn't taken the time to establish this awareness.

Attuning each interfacing management department to its role in organizational hazard control requires several steps. First, top management must define its hazard control objectives. Secondly, the functions of each management system must be viewed to determine exactly what contributions it can make to the hazard control effort. Finally, the hazard control department must be aware of the technical support that it must provide the other departments in the organization. Figure 17 represents a suggested format for developing this relationship.

The information listed in Figure 17 serves several functions. It provides suggestions concerning what the hazard control department should offer each of the other departments. It lets each department know what it can expect from the hazard control department and vice versa. It allows the hazard control department to solve one of its most difficult problems—finding a way to incorporate its expertise into the activities of other organizational departments, while at the same time developing an effective information and communication system necessary for breakthrough in reducing accident/injury experience.

Department	Typical Management System Functions	Typical Hazard Control System Inputs
Manufacturing Engineering	Analyzing new and existing production models to determine logical sequences and recommending design changes to effectively reduce labor cost and material cost consistent with product quality. Improving utilization of labor through advanced tool design, changes in procedures, lay-out and equipment, and assuring the implementation of these changes at the most opportune time in the production schedule. Making regular audits to assure conformance to established safety, health and environmental standards. Engaging in research and development on advanced manufacturing techniques for future application in company production systems. Coordinating and scheduling the implementation of new methods in order to effect the greatest production savings while maintaining maximum production output. Investigating material handling problems and related practices to determine the most effective handling methods, improve production, facilities handling and increase production of product. Assisting in plant layout. Coordinating with Finance Department in preparing cost estimates for new installations.	Providing hazard analysis of new and current production systems to locate failures that have detrimental effect on production system operation. Pinpointing hazards at man/machine interfaces during functions of scheduling, planning, routing, etc., and recommending necessary safeguards, design revisions, personnel requirements, etc. Providing information on new hazard recognition methods for manufacturing engineers. Reporting hazards and failure modes uncovered in materials handling, and other man/machine interactions that would improve production, conform with established standards, and increase total system performance. Recommending tool and equipment design modifications that become evident as the result of hazard evaluations during the design and production phases of the system's life and as a result of accident investigation. Aid in attaining optimum man/machine relationships by considering the factors of man's capabilities and limitations, reliability, maintainability, etc. Assuring that purchased production machinery introduces minimum hazard potential.
Quality Control	Examining, testing, and inspecting all materials and finished products. Recommending to Purchasing Department corrective action such as the reduction or elimination of purchased materials from vendors with poor performance records in terms of material quality. Conducting studies of components, etc., to determine whether alternate design, material, and method of manufacture could improve quality of the product. Analyzing new engineering models and pre-production samples in order to establish quality standards and to determine quality problems to be overcome. Assuring that manufactured product meets product liability standards.	Assuring that product is equipped with fail-safe devices, is not delivered to consumer with known hazards improperly controlled or not carrying proper instructions for us. Providing hazard standard data to be included in the development of quality standards. Offering ideas for improving the quality of the product that were discovered during hazard studies. Keeping Quality Control informed of new developments in product liability laws and standards. Providing data on failure rates of materials uncovered during analysis.

Figure 17.

Figure 17. *Continued.*

Department	Typical Management System Functions	Typical Hazard Control System Inputs
Purchasing	Providing for development of reliable, economic sources of supply. Providing for placement of orders at the lowest price consistent with quality requirements. Interpreting and assuring that materials to be purchased are within established standards. Determination of materials and parts requirements based upon orders received. Integrating the material orders from various departments.	Assuring that equipment, materials, machines, tools, protective devices, etc., are purchased with adequate knowledge of inherent hazards, conform with established standards, are equipped with adequate hazard controls, and are of the quality that will assure adequate wear and that won't require excessive replacement.*
Maintenance	Installing, constructing and maintaining plant buildings, facilities, grounds, equipment and machinery. Providing utility services of heat, light, power, compressed air, etc., for plant operations. Providing planned preventive maintenance on all buildings, electrical systems, facilities, machinery, and equipment to prevent abnormal deterioration or loss of service. Touring plant to ascertain condition of all buildings, equipment, and machinery. Providing for deposit of scrap material and waste. Coordinating with hazard control inspectors.	Assuring that plant layout, (including walking and working surfaces, floor and wall openings, stairs, fixed ladders, etc.) conform with established safety standards. Informing Maintenance of required safety inspection regulations and test requirements for equipment, tools, machinery, etc. Informing Maintenance about toxicity, hazard, flammability, etc., characteristics of materials and substances including information on storage and compatibility. This also includes hazardous materials identification, safe methods of transporting, handling and using cryogenics and compressed gases; providing information on proper methods of scrap and waste disposal. Providing back-up support in detecting equipment, machinery and plant deterioration and malfunction. Providing hazard information on electrical and fire systems including assurance that each conforms with established safety, heath and environmental standards.
Industrial Relations	Acquiring a competent reliable work force. Assigning personnel according to physical and mental abilities. Increasing individual productivity. Providing medical facilities. Maintaining plant security and protection. Administering employee suggestion programs.	Assuring the proper selection, training and re-training of personnel with respect to proper work techniques, hazard awareness, etc. By indicating human error resulting from hazard analysis that requires personnel action. Processing and implementing employee safety suggestions. Designing and conducting hazard training sessions.

*These inputs will apply to other management systems as well.

Figure 17. *Continued.*

Department	Typical Hazard Control System Inputs	Typical Management System Functions
	Ascertain training needs and develop training programs including sourcing and preparation of instructors, providing proper training aids and facilities, and developing new training techniques, methods, etc.	Keeping Industrial Relations aware of environmental hazards in the workplace that effect the health and safety of personnel.
	Establishing and maintaining minimum personnel attribute requirements.	By initiating medical studies of personnel that are suspected of occupational illnesses.
	Developing motivational techniques that will secure "good" individual and group attitudes.	
	Acting as coordinator between management and labor organizations.	
	Handling grievances and other labor/management discrepancies.	
Finance	Preparing, adjusting, reporting, and controlling the inventory of all raw materials, work-in-process, and finished products.	By assuring that expenditures for equipment, materials, tools, etc., are the best investments on a cost-effectiveness basis (from a hazard control standpoint) and are of a quality that will last and that won't require excessive replacement.
	Preparing variable and fixed operating expense budgets for all functions.	By keeping Finance appraised of accident costs including Workers' Compensation and other insurance costs as well as the cost of property damage resulting from accidents.
	Coordinating the various accounting functions with all intra-plant functions and with corresponding staff functions.	
	Reviewing and recommending changes in proposed expenditures for equipment, materials, etc.	Informing Finance of fines for violation of federal safety, health and environmental standards (OSHA, EPA, etc.).
	Responsible for assuring that plant facilities, equipment, and inventory are adequately covered by insurance.	Informing Finance of costs resulting from product liabilities.

Bibliography

Barnard, C. I., "The Functions of the Executive," Harvard University Press, Cambridge, Mass., 1938 and 1968.

Dalcher, L. M., "The Role of Administrative Standards in Business and Industry," American Management Association, 1951.

Drucker, P. F., "The Practice of Management," Harper and Brothers, New York, N.Y., 1954.

Juran, J. M., "Managerial Breakthrough, A New Concept of the Manager's Job," McGraw-Hill Book Company, N.Y., 1968.

Koontz, H., and O'Donnell, C., "Principles of Management," 4th edition, McGraw-Hill Book Company, New York, 1968.

Newman, W. H., Summer, E., Warren, K. E., "The Process of Management," 2nd edition, Prentice-Hall, Inc.

Taylor, F. W., "The Principles of Scientific Management," Harper Row Publishers, Inc., New York, 1947, pg. 7.

Notes

1. Frederick W. Taylor, "The Principles of Scientific Management," Harper & Row, Publishers, Incorporated, New York, 1947, p. 7.
2. P. F. Drucker, "The Practice of Management," Harper and Bros., New York, 1954.
3. J. M. Juran, "Managerial Breakthrough," McGraw-Hill, New York, 1968.
4. H. Koontz, C. O'Donnell, "Principles of Management," McGraw-Hill, 1968.
5. Ibid.
6. H. Koontz, and C. O'Donnell, "Principles of Management," 4th edition. McGraw-Hill, 1968.
7. J. M. Juran, "Managerial Breakthrough," McGraw-Hill Book Company, New York, 1964.
8. L. M. Dalcher, "The Role of Administrative Standards in Business and Industry" American Management Association, 1951.
9. From the article, "Tomatoes," by Thomas Whitesides in the *New Yorker* Magazine January 24, 1977, New Yorker Magazine, Inc.
10. D. Haasl, From a lecture on Systems Safety at the University of Washington, 1969.

Fundamental Elements of Effective Hazard Control Programming 4

Programs designed to curb the loss of human, material, and environmental resources don't just happen by themselves. Instead, such programs are the result of a careful planning and mixing of the right elements necessary to achieve an organizations designed objectives. This chapter will deal with those elements of the hazard control process which have proven themselves capable of reducing hazards and unwanted losses in organizations.

Before getting into a detailed discussion of the design of an effective hazard control program, a general explanation of the elements of such a program will be undertaken.

The Fundamental Elements—An Examination

Over the years, the author's experience has shown that there has been controversy coupled with gross misunderstanding of how and why hazard control programs should be operated. Much of this confusion stems from the fact that some programs were established without prior analysis of organizational hazard and loss producing situations and the ingredients necessary to eliminate or reduce them. Consequently, many hours and dollars were invested in systems which failed to reverse losses from deaths, injuries, illness, and damage.

Before any program designed to reduce or eliminate hazards in the workplace becomes operational, care must be taken to assure that the program addresses itself to the issues of the highest importance. Thus, the first activity in a comprehensive hazard control program, as illustrated in Figure 18 is the establishment of a program arm which has as its primary objective to identify and evaluate hazard in the workplace.

Element One—Hazard Identification and Evaluation

Element	Process	Expected Result
1. Hazard Identification and Evaluation	Acquiring information via experience, testing, and analysis	Accurate data for informed management decisionmaking
	Assessing a hazard's potential destructive effect	
	Sorting gross hazard data by importance ranking	
2. Management Decision-making	Deciding not to implement any change	Strategies for selection and implementation of effective controls including training and education, process change, equipment upgrading, etc.
	Deciding to modify system Deciding to redesign system	
3. Selection and Implementation of Controls	Selection of countermeasures which are capable of coping with hazardous energy	Effective solutions for elimination or reduction of workplace hazards
4. Monitoring	Inspection and other surveillance procedures directed toward work operations and products	a. Assurance that controls are functioning as specified
		b. Assurance that workplace changes have not nullified the effectiveness of controls
		c. Assurance that new problems have not entered the workplace or product system
5. Measuring Program Effectiveness	Establishing program evaluation criteria and measuring instruments	Assessment of cost/benefit of hazard control program effort
	Measuring existing performance against desired performance	Determining degree of participative effort

Figure 18. Fundamental elements of hazard control programming.

For clarification purposes, a *hazard is defined as any existing or potential condition in the workplace which, by itself or in combination with other variables, has the capacity to result in the unwanted effects of deaths, injuries, diseases, damage and mission loss.* This defintion carries with it two significant points—First, that a condition doesn't always have to exist at the moment to be classified as a hazard. Potential condition defects are also considered in the total hazard assessment. Second, hazards may not result from independent failure of workplace components, but instead by the result generated as the result of one workplace component acting or influencing another—such as gasoline and sulfuric acid interacting with each other to produce sufficient heat for combustion along with toxic smoke and fumes. In order to understand the phenomenon of "hazard" more fully it may be helpful to refine it further. Hazards are normally couched into two broad categories—those dealing with "safety" issues and those falling into the health area. When it comes right down to it, there is no basic difference between the two classes. However, for ease of communication in certain instances the broad hazard category will be subdivided. A safety hazard evloves from a situation in which workers may be injured or killed from such problems as faulty electrical wiring, platforms without railings, unguarded gears or cutting devices, etc. A health hazard, on the other hand, is defined as a work situation that has the potential to cause sickness by chemicals or other harmful agents such as heat, noise, x-rays, dust, fumes, and so forth.

One of the aims of a viable hazard control program will thus be to seek information about the worker/machine/environmental components of the system, and at the interfaces among these system components in order to determine what specific hazards exist, capable of resulting in accidents; how these hazards are occurring; the frequency of their occurrence; and then, finally, the impact of their potential destructive effect.

Rule: During these hazard recognition activities, both those hazards associated with the worker/task relationship as well as those pertaining to existing processes, proposed processes, manufactured goods, and services will receive attention. In addition, those factors in both the workplace environment as well as that external to it will be examined.

The methods available to the hazard control specialist to help him accomplish the task of locating hazards in the workplace under his jurisdiction are:

1. By experience: To find out exactly how an operation would fail as the result of the hazards associated with it, a very reliable form of information would come from those who have worked with the operation, who understand all its complexities and problems, who have discovered the hazards and failure modes themselves, or are close to others who have either corrected the problem themselves or have been party to the correction by others. Although data acquired via direct experience is highly desirable, it is often difficult to obtain, especially when information is wanted on a system in its design phase, or on one that has not been operated according to its intended usage long enough for sufficient data on its inherent hazards to have become known. Because those with direct past experience concerning hazards pertinent to a particular system of interest are not always available, an alternative can be followed: those with related experience—those who have worked with systems similar to, although not exactly like the one of interest.

Although philosophers may tell us that these data acquired through experience are the most valid of all data for informed decision-making, and in some instances this idea is correct—the hazard analyst must always keep in mind the fact that the data he is getting from others may be incorrect. Thus, the actions he takes could be wrong. There is a popular adage which here applies: most things work out right for all the wrong reasons. If someone we are relying on for accurate data is measuring the successful performance of his system on its lack of system failures incurred during use, without any positive assurance that this successful outcome was not the result of chance, then information from such a person could lead us down the rosy path to disaster. We will then make decisions and take action, for all the wrong reasons. So there is a lesson here which needs to be considered. Before any data are plugged into the decision-making process, such data must be verified or at the very least viewed along with other data inputs, before decisions are frozen, and action gets underway.

Among the empirical sources which the hazard control specialist has at his disposal, to acquire specific hazard information pertaining to his area of interest, include but are not limited to: insurance company surveys and audits; accident investigation data; safety inspections; interviews with foremen—the example of the interview with the foreman on page 55 is a good example; communication with hazard control specialists in other organizations working with the same type of product or operation.

2. *By virtue of testing*—Test data serves to provide answers concerning many problem situations. If a test program is set up and conducted properly, it will yield valuable data for hazard control decisions. A common fault of many organizational leaders is to look toward testing and the results of test data as the only means of assuring themselves that what they are doing is acceptable. Although testing may be the only way to acquire desired information on certain occasions more often than not, it may not be producing the information desired. To begin with, the data may not pertain to the particular system configuration under scrutiny. Second, a testing program is both expensive and time-consuming, thus such constraints may limit how far the test program can go. Third, there are political and economic factors involved which act to limit the breadth and scope of a test program. Finally, and ever so important, is the fact that the major drawback to any testing program and its resultant data is that there is a good chance the system to be tested was not tested in every possible mode to which it would be subjected during its normal life cycle. As it often turns out, it is usually the failure mode which is not entered into the test program which undoubtedly is the one which becomes the host for the hazards which present problems in the future.

The purpose of this discussion is not to downgrade the results of test data; there are times when such data will be absolutely necessary to have and use. Nevertheless, caution is given to use test information with a full knowledge of its capabilities and limitations, and to understand that more times than not, other forms of information will be necessary before final conclusions are drawn and actions are taken.

3. *By virtue of analysis*—When we think about analysis, we visualize it as an orderly process to acquire specific hazard information which is pertinent to a given system. In the context of hazard control, it represents a very careful probing of operational and management systems in an effort to detect problems; understand the relationship between the problem and the system of

which it is a part; obtain a grasp of the destructive potential of the deficiency, and acquire an awareness of what needs to be done to upgrade the overall effectiveness of the system. The hazard control specialist has at his disposal many hazard analytical techniques which are capable of aiding in the identification and evaluation of hazards in the workplace. An examination of these hazard analytical techniques will be undertaken in Chapter 6 when we examine the hazard identification process in greater detail.

To summarize what has previously been stated, when a company decides to establish a program to attend to hazard and loss potential it becomes obvious that before anything happens in the way of establishing specific functions, the full nature and scope of the hazard and potential loss problem must be identified and evaluated. Much like any other situation, before anyone can approach a problem to solve it, a full understanding of the problem becomes a prerequisite. While this statement may seem very basic and simplistic, it is nevertheless a fact that a lack of true problem identification has hindered the progress of all sorts of technical and management programs by either causing issues with profound impact on operations to be missed, or by calling for controls which were either ineffective or not required at all. Sometimes the corrective action did more harm than if it had been omitted altogether.

When the hazard control specialist sets out to acquire an accurate picture of his company's problem he finds that his inquiry will confront him with three major dimensions of the hazard and loss problem—human error, situational faults, and environmental stressors.

Human Error

For years, the worker has been looked upon as the major contributor to accident and loss situations. A familiar term—"unsafe act"—has been coined to describe the situation where the worker by either his act of commission or omission has been tagged as the primary factor responsible for the loss. If management tries hard enough, it is certainly easy enough to find a worker at fault for close perusal invariably shows that the worker was associated with the problem in one form or another. As we learned in Chapter 2, a great many accident cases are written off as caused by human error over which management "had little control over." By its very sound the phrase "unsafe act" connotes independent humanly committed error with little reference to anything someone else could have done to have prevented the unfavorable situation from happening.

Words are often used without time spent thinking out the ramification of their definitions. "Unsafe act" is is a classic example. Normally, when we think of the word "act," we visualize a voluntary, thought-out, premeditated process which involves rational decision-making. If this interpretation is applied to the millions of accident cases where the worker is declared at fault, it becomes clear that, in many cases, the worker was placed in a situation beyond his control, which forced him to commit an error resulting in the accident situation. On the other hand, there have been and will continue to be cases where "unsafe acts" (clearly worker-controlled errors) actually are responsible for accident situations.

Is it important to differentiate between worker acts of commission and omission and the effect these acts have on the success of a hazard control program? The answer is a definite yes, and with good reason. Perhaps the following example will be of value: suppose management recognized specific hazards associated with a particular job, and went through the effort of defining the hazard, evaluating its effect, and providing controls which would reduce worker risk. In addition, assessing the fact that such counter measures would slightly impede production, management modified the job demands in terms of speed and quantity, to conform with a revised standard of productivity. Suppose, furthermore, that management provided ample instruction to the worker, hired supervisors who had knowledge of both the hazards capacity to cause harm and of the capabilities and limitations of the hazard controls, and by every reasonable avenue open to it, did its best to prevent the marshalling agent from injuring the worker. Yet, suppose the worker removed the control and was subsequently injured. Is this an—"unsafe act?"—No question about it. The idea demonstrated here is: the buck has to stop somewhere. In this instance, the worker violated the responsibility vested in him by his company, for he knew what to do and chose not to do it. He had control over the situation and decided not to exercise it. He acted in a manner contributing to his own injury, and perhaps to the injury of others.

On the other hand, suppose management did a half fast job of assessing the job hazard and selecting a control measure. Suppose management selected a control which actually impeded work flow and productivity, only this time no modification to the production standard was undertaken. The only instructions the worker received concerning the hazard and the control came in the form of a brief explanation by his foreman, two days after the control was provided. The worker, forced to achieve a production quota demanded by management removed the control to get his work done. Hazard or not, the worker wasn't going to risk his job by not producing what was expected of him. Unfortunately, in the process of removing the control, the worker injured himself. Can we classify this case as an "unsafe act?" Not in this case. The reason is that management, by the very nature of the manner by which it tried to correct its problem, caused additional problems. In this instance, if error were assigned to anybody it would have to be assigned to management itself. They committed a cardinal sin. They, by a lack of knowledge of the problem, provided countermeasures which not only didn't work but, worse, fostered the very undesirable situation they were trying to avoid in the first place.

The amount of real improvement which an organization can realize in hazard control is a function of three factors: (1) modifying human behavior through training, movtivation, and supervision; (2) modifying the work situation; (3) modifying general management practices to assure a proper focus on safety and health matters.

A major prejudice in industry concerning the nature of worker-error-caused accidents is that such accidents are due to the result of a "lapse of attention" on the part of the worker. The same people who have voiced this philosophy feel that if people would try harder, performance would be error-free. Those involved with federal "zero-defects" programs in the past know that such a philosophy doesn't work. A more rational view contends that worker errors are the result of an interaction of a person with a situation in an environment. Subsequently, the major responsibility for reducing errors lies with management rather than with workers performing the tasks in which errors occur as discussed in Chapter 2. A viable program must not rely solely on motivating people to avoid accidents. There is an upper limit to the amount of improvement realized by only motivation efforts. A well-conceived program will use motivational efforts within their limits, but will also concentrate on identifying error-likely situations and either eliminating or modifying them.[1]

Identifying the nature and scope of his company's hazard control problem, differentiating between human error and or situational or management error is a critically important function of the hazard control specialist. Corrections applied when contending with human error problems, where the worker is the controlling factor, are drastically different than those countermeasures employed when management itself is at fault.

Having completed a gross hazard assessment of hazards in the workplace, (by whatever means available), the hazard control specialist finds himself having to sort out worse problems first, on a hazard-importance hierarchy. See Figure 19. On the basis of either a qualitative or quantitative scale, he is able to justify, which problems warrant immediate action, which ones can take second priority, and which ones can be addressed at some point in the future. Without such a system the hazard control specialist has no justification for corrective action and, worse, could be directing his efforts and resources to problems of lower consequential impact while high impact, high consequential issues are allowed to exist in the system without anything being done about them.

Many attempts have been made to establish quantitative scales which weigh the relative importance of hazards. Unfortunately, without experience data pertaining specifically to a hazard in a specific failure mode, such a quantitative scheme is difficult to design. Where such experience data exists, quantification of hazard data is to be sought after. Without a quantitative scale to weigh the importance of hazards, the only alternative is to use the qualitative hazard assessment schemes. Several commonly used qualitative hazard assess-

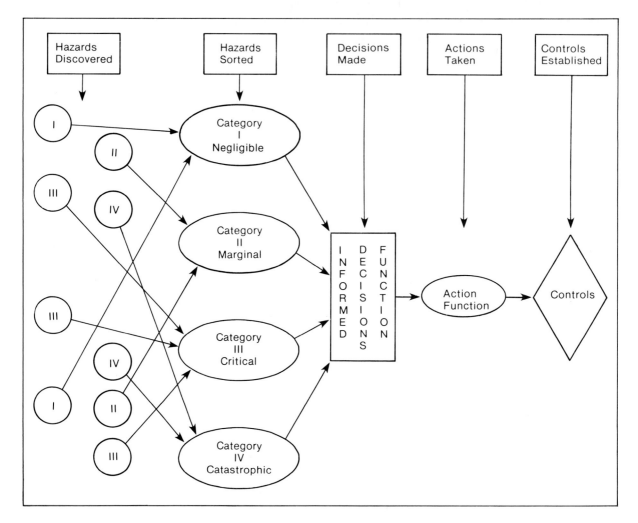

Figure 19. Specifications for controls.

ment schemes appear in Figure 20. It is interesting to note the variations from category to category in each of the various schemes.

Although qualitative hazard assessment schemes are most often selected, since more quantitative alternatives are not available, such schemes still have several shortcomings which should be noted. To begin with, they are often made without prior experience with a particular work process, so workers are left vulnerable. As it often turns out, these workers become the instruments for gaining such vital experience data day by day, as they go about their work activity. Often, these data are costly in lives, productivity, and dollars. Second, if alterations or modifications are made arbitrarily in processes, on the speculation that changes will improve the system, even though data does not exist to support this action, we are still operating in a blind.

Given the fact that all hazard assessment schemes have some basic faults, they nevertheless represent the only practical way to establish a system for hazard correction on a daily basis. If the law of consistency is applied—and the same system is used all the time—eventually everybody in the organization will learn to understand it. If attempts are made to change the system, or modify its language too often, chaos will result, as members of the organization become confused, misguided, and eventually distrustful of the competence of he who is administering the hazard control program. In his attempt to establish a hazard evaluation scheme, the hazard control specialist may find himself killing two birds with one stone. If he recruits the aid of those organizational personnel who will have to live with the established evaluation scheme, who then form a consortium for the sole purpose of listing specific criteria for whatever hazard categories are decided upon, two accomplishments are likely to result. First, those governed by the standard will be more apt to live with it, primarily because they had a part in its creation. Second, when all organizational personnel are fully aware of the details of hazard evaluation, and where emphasis for correction must go, then the

---

SCHEME A

Category I—Negligible

Hazard will not result in an injury/illness

The most that could happen would be a first-aid case

The chance of hazard causing other damage is extremely remote

Category II—Marginal

Hazard can cause injury/illness and equipment damage under some circumstances **but** injury/illness would not be serious (compensable)

The chance of death is remote but not entirely impossible

Category III—Critical

If hazard is not corrected as soon as possible it has a high probability in resulting in

serious injury/illness

property and equipment damage

job delay

death

substantial and permanent reduction of worker efficiency on and off the job

Category IV—Catastrophic

If hazard is not corrected immediately it has high probability to cause

deaths—possibly multiple deaths

widespread occupational illnesses

loss of facilities

RISK PROBABILITY

1—Probable

2—Reasonably Probable

3—Remote

4—Extremely Remote

Figure 20. Hazard ranking systems.

Figure 20. *Continued.*

SCHEME B

Category I—Catastrophic

May cause death or loss of facility

Category II—Critical

May cause severe injury, severe occupational illness, or major property damage

Category III—Marginal

May cause minor injury, minor occupational illness, or minor property damage.

Category IV—Negligible

Probably would not affect presonnel safety or health, but is nevertheless in violation of specific criteria

Mishap Probability

The probability that a hazard will result in a mishap, based on an assessment of such factors as location, exposure in terms of cycles or hours of operation, and affected population. Mishap probability shall be assigned an Arabic letter according to the following criteria:

   a. Subcategory A
      Likely to occur immediately or within a short period of time

   b. Subcategory B
      Probably will occur in time

   c. Subcategory C
      May occur in time

   d. Subcategory D
      Unlikely to occur

SCHEME C

Category I—Imminent Danger

Imminent danger exists when there is a reasonable certainty that the hazard will cause death or serious physical harm immediately or within a short period of time

Category II—Serious Violation

Serious violation exists when in a place of employment if there is a substantial probability that death or serious physical harm could result from one or more practices, means, methods, operations, or processes which have been adopted or are in use in such place of employment unless the employer did not and could not with the exercise of reasonable diligence, know of the presence of the violation.

Category III—Nonserious Violation

Nonserious violation would be an accident or occupational illness that could result from a violation of a standard, but probably no death or serious irreversible physical harm would result from the violation.

Category IV—De minimous

De minimous violations which would probably not be related to affecting employee safety or health, but are nevertheless in violation of a specific OSHA standard in terms of a total accident prevention program

likelihood of their becoming distrustful of the hazard control program is minimized.

In summary, the first element of an effective hazard control program: that of identifying and evaluating hazards must produce accurate, meaningful, and reliable data which will be used to foster informed decisions. This first element, as is illustrated in Figure 18, essentially allows us to assess the full destructive potential of a hazard before decision-making is carried out and recommendations are made to introduce preventive and corrective measures into the workplace.

At this stage in the program, assuming that those involved in the activity of identifying and evaluating hazards did a credible job, the next logical step will be for those in command to do whatever is required to either eliminate the problems entirely, or reduce them to at least tolerable levels. So then, *the second key activity in a viable hazard control program is the actual specification of alternatives* for hazard reduction or elimination. Essentially, information must be presented to top management in such a form that it provides the basis for short and long-term solutions for the improvement of hazardous situations.

Element Two— Specification of Alternatives for Informed Decision-making

What it all boils down to is that when the hazard control organization presents top management with the hazard problems along with the decision-making alternatives, those in top management will normally have three alternatives to guide their actions. The first alternative is to take the data presented to them, review it, and then do nothing about it. More than one hazard control specialist has had this happen to him at least once in his career. An examination of the choice of this alternative by top management reveals three underlying factors which played a role in the decision. First, the hazard data with recommendations fell upon an unsympathetic ear—a management which didn't really understand the loss ramifications associated with the hazards, or one which understood the benefits but didn't want to commit themselves to a full action plan for hazard correction. It is sad to admit it that one could find safety programs existing throughout this nation today, in organizations where management no more intended to make significant improvements in hazard reduction than the man in the moon. Such programs are kept around for the image they reflect, and their value from a public relations standpoint. But when push comes to a shove, management rejects any recommendation for "safety" when such recommendation carries too stiff a price tag, it is politically controversial, or shows a seemingly adverse effect on the production effort.

The second reason behind the "do nothing" alternative lies in the fact that management often has good justification for not acting on the hazard control specialist's recommendations. Although the decision-maker has full knowledge and appreciation of the hazards and the risks involved, it may well be that the ramifications of the hazard, compared to the immediate constraints in the form of finances, crucial production schedules, or even the fact that a plan for revamping the operation and thus eliminating the hazard may be scheduled to take place in the near future.

No matter what the reason, legitimate or not, no immediate corrective action takes place. The buck stops here, however, as the decision-maker has been apprised of the danger, but has chosen to act on other priorities first. What is important for the hazard control specialist to remember is: just because the decision to do what he recommends is not carried out, it doesn't mean that he should give up. It is a very sad commentary that so many "safety people" have, upon repeated rejection of their ideas, actually stopped making the suggestions and recommendations for which they were hired. A good hazard control specialist will continue to strive to have management act on his recommendations, even if it means approaching the solution from a different viewpoint with a different set of strategies. We must keep in mind that those in the hazard control function are or should be members of the staff organization. The primary purpose behind their job activites is to give advice to the chief decision makers. Even though such advice may or may not ever be used to effect change, their staff role is not altered. When the hazard control specialist's frustrations reaches critical proportions, because "no one will listen to his ideas," then he had better examine the quality and utility of the information he is providing, before he decides who is to blame

The third reason why favorable decisions are not always made when it comes to correcting hazards in the workplace, is that the information presented by the hazard control specialist is structured in a manner that perhaps only one—and maybe the most expensive one—problem solving alternative is given. In instances like this and there have been many—those in the hazard control organization had not provided the decision-maker with ample alternatives— from "band-aid" approaches which would guarantee at least a modicum of shortrange protection to those which reflect more permanent solutions. In this day and age, with the pressures brought to bear on organizational leaders continually mounting, there is a limit to how much can be spent on operational improvement. With this in mind, the hazard control specialist is forced more than ever to push his imagination and creativity to the maximum, in order to arrive at solution alternatives which will guarantee at least minimal protections.

The second alternative involves taking action to modify the work system. The philosophy behind this alternative is that most systems or operations are not totally beyond repair, even though such systems and operations may be hosting faults which take their toll in reduced system performance. With this in mind, the hazard control specialist's most common alternatives will involve adding to or subtracting from the existing system in order to bring it to a higher level of acceptability and reliability. As illustrated in Figure 21, the introduction of a machine guard, a process change, the installation of a ventilation system all fall into the system modification alternatives.

The third alternative made available to the decision-maker is that of redesign. When this option is chosen, its promoter has concluded that the existing system is beyond repair. No further good will come from additional modifications. The only way out is to design a better mouse-trap. Of course,

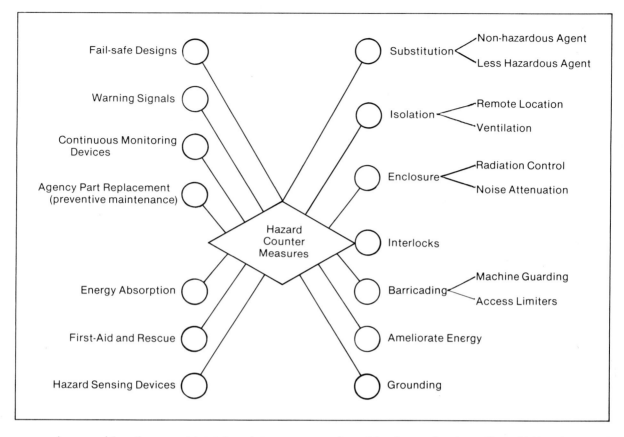

Fail-safe Designs

Warning Signals

Continuous Monitoring Devices

Agency Part Replacement (preventive maintenance)

Energy Absorption

First-Aid and Rescue

Hazard Sensing Devices

Hazard Counter Measures

Substitution — Non-hazardous Agent / Less Hazardous Agent

Isolation — Remote Location / Ventilation

Enclosure — Radiation Control / Noise Attenuation

Interlocks

Barricading — Machine Guarding / Access Limiters

Ameliorate Energy

Grounding

Figure 21. Hazard counter-measures

one major consideration must be taken into account when this alternative is suggested: there are no iron clad guarantees that the new system design will not present new hazards. So then, whenever a redesigned system is selected, the onus of responsibility is placed squarely on the shoulders of the hazard control specialist to anticipate as many of its problems as possible so that these problems can be countered early in their life cycle. In Chapter 6, this idea will be expanded further, when the role of hazard analysis is discussed as a tool utilized to extract hazard data from a system during the conceptual design and operational phases of its life cycle.

Figure 22 summary hazard evaluation report illustrates a way in which hazard data can be displayed for management decisions. By seeing what the problem is, its severity by hazard class, and recommendations for its improvement, those in the decision-making function are able to understand the hazardous situation and its ramifications. When this same decision-maker reviews the corresponding suggested corrective action report Figure 23, which not only tells what needs to be done to correct the hazard but how much it will cost, he is in a fully enlightened position to make the most effective decision.

A final note is offered here concerning problem solving and the offering of solution alternatives. One of the major shortcomings of decision-makers in

Department
Building
Location
Date _____

SUMMARY HAZARD EVALUATION

VIO NO	Description	Specific Location	Standard Violated	Hazard Class.	No. People Exposed	Remarks
MA-2	Guarding on all lathes in machine shop area. 4) unguarded drill press in Electric Shop 5) pulley belts exposed on Shaper, both vertical and horizontal milling machines, a surface grinder and the 13 inch horizontal lathe, all in the Machine Shop Area 6) Inadequate point of operation guarding on 14 inch cut-off saw, band saw and drill press in basement.	As indicated	OSHA Subpart 0 Section 1910.212, 1910.213 and 1910.219	III	40	See Recommendations under Violation Number P-8
MA-3	A 10 ft. high Dake Hydraulic Press, when in the up position is unstable and could easily fall over.	In the middle of the Maintenance Shop Area	OSHA General Duty Provision	IV	40	Short Term: this press should be secured to the floor.
MA-4	Fire extinguishers are not properly located, identified checked and recharged.	At various locations in the Maintenance Shop	OSHA Subpart LL Section 1910.157	III	40 (See note 1)	See General Recommendations Number 1
MA-5	Oxygen and acetylene piping is routed through the Paint Shop (a fire hazard area) and where it runs between buildings, it is exposed to the elements and has become badly rusted.	Between Paint Shop and Maintenance Shop	OSHA Subpart Q Section 1910.252	III	40 (See note 1)	Short Term: the piping outside should be painted with suitable materials to protect against further corrosion. Piping should also be identified in accordance with ANSI 13.1 — 1956

Figure 22.

PXI NO	VIO NO & PG	VIO TYPE	HAZ CL	Short term (This Year) — SUGGESTED CORRECTIVE ACTION							Long Term (Two or More Years)				Scheduling		
				ISSUE/ ENFORC REG	TRAIN EDUC	SUPER	R & D IN HOUSE	SAFETY EQUIP PURCH	ENGR/MOD & CONSTRUCT	ESTIMATED COST	TRAIN/ EDUC	SUPER	R & D	MTLS ACQUIS	IN-HOUSE	OTHER SOURCES	ESTIMATED COST
1	MA–1	Unapproved electrical Installation	IV	X		X			X	$ 250		X		X	X		$ 500
2	MA–2	Inadequate guarding of machinery	III	X		X		X	X	$ 600		X					
1	MA–3	Unstable hydraulic press	IV	X		X			X	$ 300							
2	MA–4	Improper fire extinguishers	III	X								X			X		$ 700
2	MA–5	Corroded welding gas piping	III	X		X			X	$ 100							
2	MA–6	Improper storage of flammables	III	X		X		X		$ 300							
2	MA–7	Unapproved ladders in use	III	X		X						X		X			$ 20
2	MA–8	Improper storage of combustibles	III	X		X					X						
1	MA–9	No inspection or maintenance of hoists	IV	X		X			X	$ 400		X					$ 500

Figure 23.

general is their inability to see the problem at hand from various viewpoints. This type of decision-making has been coined vertical thinking. In his book "New Think" Edward de Bono[2] discusses vertical thinking as well as its converse—lateral thinking. Vertical thinking begins with a single concept and then proceeds with that concept until a solution is reached. On the other hand, lateral thinking refers to thinking that generates alternative ways of seeing a problem before seeking a solution. As all solutions affect people other than the problem solver, these other people's concerns must be considered. Hazard control decisions are a perfect case in point. The hazard control specialist must view the utility of his recommended controls from the standpoint not only of the workers who must use the control but also of their supervisors, production control, and maintenance organizations, local and federal safety inspectors, and others which the control will have impact on.

A summary of the decision flow for hazard corrections appears in Figure 24. This model is designed to depict the decision-making process from the initial sensitivity to the hazard issue on through what is necessary for both short and long-term corrective measures.

Element Three— Installation of Effective Preventive and Corrective Methods

The third activity in an effective hazard control program involves the actual installation of effective preventive and corrective measures to assure that existing and potential hazards are kept at an acceptable level.

During this activity, after the hazardous agent has been identified, the energy transfer must be assessed. Surry[3] suggests that, in many cases, the energy which can result in the unwanted deaths, injuries and damage, is the same energy which is harnessed to carry out a task, that is to turn a taper on a machine lathe is desirable, but to cut a hand on the same lathe in precisely the same action, is undesired and is classified as an accident. In another situational

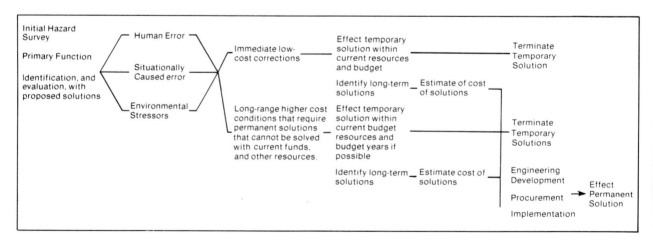

Figure 24. Decision flow for hazard correction.

configuration, the "dangerous" feature is an unnecessary by-product of some other desired property, i.e., a worker who receives lung damage while degreasing a part with a solvent is the victim of vapors which would not have caused problems, if another suitable less toxic substance had been used to do the job.

When attempts are made to control hazards in the workplace, there are several strategies to choose from. These strategies may be used singularly or in combination, depending on the nature and scope of the hazard to be dealt with, and the degree of back-up protection desired.

Strategies for Hazard Control

Before any attempt is made to prescribe a suitable measure to control a particular hazard, an examination of the hazardous situation is in order. Figure 25 illustrates in diagram form a condition which exists when a hazardous energy form, in this case the chemical Benzene is used in a work operation without adequate controls to safeguard the workers' safety and health. The uninterrupted hazardous energy, in this instance, Benzene vapors above acceptable threshold and used for long periods of time, have the capacity to cause occupational illnesses among the worker population. If the hazardous condition is allowed to exist, without any intervention, the outcome events are predictable. Faced with this situation the hazard control specialist has several options at his disposal to rectify the problem.

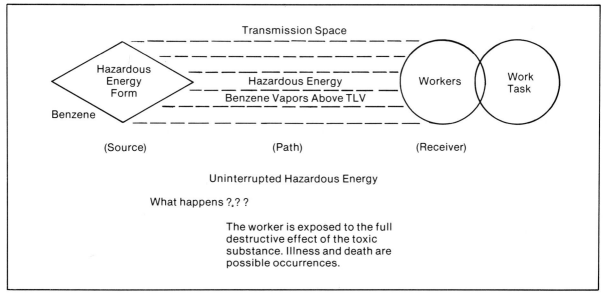

Figure 25.

Option 1—Remove the worker from the operation via remote processing or automation. Figure 26 demonstrates this option. The decisionmaker recognizes that nothing has been accomplished to reduce or diminish the toxic fumes problem. It still exists as it did before the process change. However, the removal of the worker from contact with the hazardous energy (vapors) has sufficed in solving the problem

Option 2—Remove the hazardous energy form by substituting a less harmful agent for the one causing the problem. In Figure 27, having substituted the toxic substance, the threat of worker illness is reduced to an acceptable level.

Option 3—Erect a physical barrier which will intercept the hazardous energy at a point before it reaches the worker (Figure 28). When substitution of a nonhazardous agent is not feasible, or when an agent of lesser hazard potential is selected, the selection of a mechanism which will intercept the hazard may prove to be an effective solution alternative. The barricading principle may take the form of a local exhaust ventilation system used to vent toxic vapors, a sound absorbing panel to attenuate noise levels, or the erection of a fire resistant wall to prevent fire spread. Figure 29 demonstrates how, once management recognized that their workers were being exposed during testing operations to materials which were capable of causing death and destruction, the test operation was modified. Based on the hazard control department's recommendations, two control strategies were utilized—using a remote monitoring process which kept the workers away from the hazardous procedure, and erecting substantial barricading walls to protect the workers should a failure occur.

Option 4—Ameliorate (slow down) the energy impact by providing for a wider distribution of the hazardous energy to the workers.
This option is chosen with the idea in mind that full injury prevention will not be realized. Such an injury reduction system has its primary objective to provide the worker with a protective medium which will, under most circumstances, reduce the probability of injury occurrence. The proposed "airbag" system for automobiles fits into this category.

Option 5—Incorporation of Personal Protective Equipment. When all options have been exhausted, and it is determined that the urgency of the problem or the particular configuration of the work process does not lend itself to correction by virtue of engineering upgrade, a last resort is to institute a program of personal protective equipment. See Figure 30. No matter what justification is provided for selecting protective equipment, the decisionmaker must be fully cognizant that the selection of such a control measure has one major shortcoming: nothing has been done to reduce or eliminate the hazardous energy. The control has been moved to the point closest to the worker. Should the protective membrane (the glove, ear protector, eye shield, etc.) fail, the worker is subjected to the full destructive effects of the hazardous energy. When such a situation occurs, injury or perhaps even death are distinct outcome possibilities.

Before any control strategy is selected, the full destructive effect of the hazard must be understood, and the control must be capable of handling it. With this theme in mind, coupled with the fact that many variables could alter original assessments of hazard potential, it is of critical importance that those in the hazard control decision-making role be very cautious of recommending

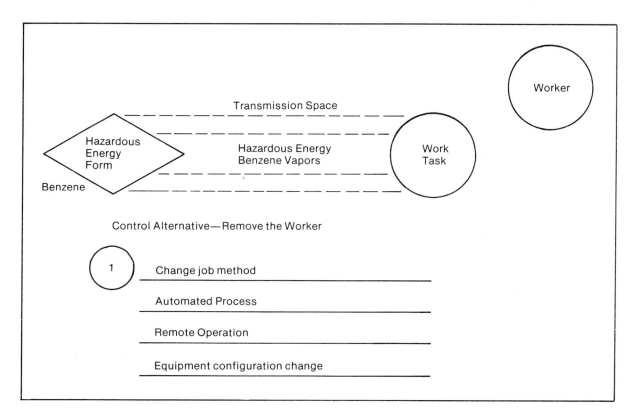

Figure 26.

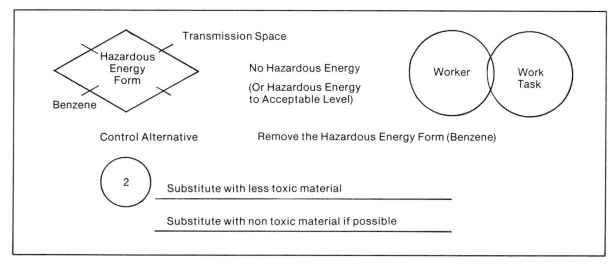

Figure 27.

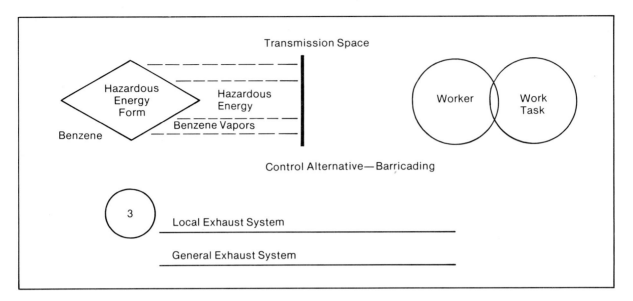

Transmission Space

Hazardous
Energy
Form

Benzene

Hazardous
Energy

Benzene Vapors

Control Alternative—Barricading

Worker

Work
Task

3   Local Exhaust System

General Exhaust System

Figure 28.

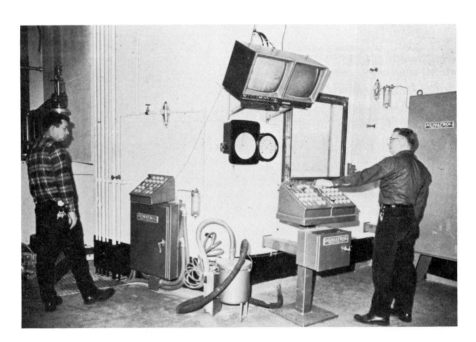

Figure 29. Hazard controlled test operation.

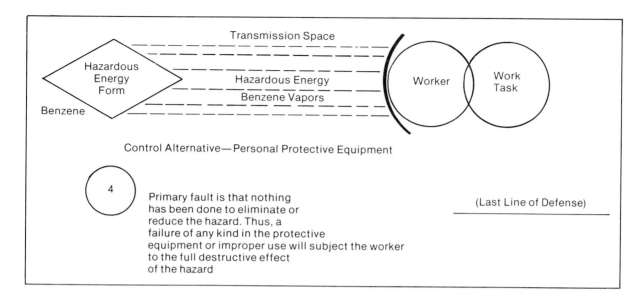

Transmission Space

Hazardous Energy Form

Benzene

Hazardous Energy
Benzene Vapors

Worker

Work Task

Control Alternative—Personal Protective Equipment

4 Primary fault is that nothing has been done to eliminate or reduce the hazard. Thus, a failure of any kind in the protective equipment or improper use will subject the worker to the full destructive effect of the hazard

(Last Line of Defense)

controls which will not only fail to function as intended but could add to the very injury which the control is attempting to reduce. Figure 31 illustrates what happened to a pair of safety spectacles when a worker was exposed to the forces of impact of pieces of carborundum while working with a bench grinder. The lenses were shattered when a grinding wheel degraded during use, causing the worker to lose sight in one eye. This situation was the direct result of a bad decision on somebody's part. A control was selected without ever considering the fact that the high speed particles from a degraded grinding wheel would create energy forces far greater than the protective lens could withstand. Even had a lens material been chosen which could have withstood the impact, other parts of the worker's face and neck would still have been exposed to injury. This example illustrates two common problems. First, the intended protective medium was not capable of providing its intended protective function. Second, once the protective medium was integrated into work operations, nothing was done to assure that the grinding wheel was maintained to reduce the possibilities of higher energy impact threats. To further complicate the matter, management was expecting protection for which they had never been entitled to receive. In this case, their choice was the wrong one.

In summary, the installation of controls into a work situation, to eliminate or minimize worker exposure to a hazard, are provided either at the source of the problem (the hazardous agent), somewhere along its path, or as a last

Figure 30.

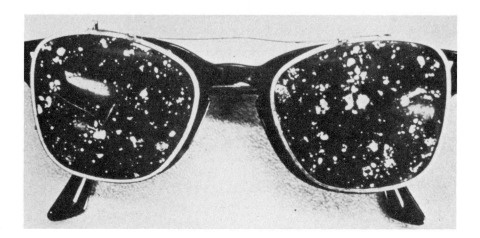

Figure 31.

resort at the receiver (worker). The most desirable alternative is to engineer the problem out of the system. When this is impossible due to the circumstances or as an interim measure while engineering procedures are underway, protective equipment may prove to be of value.

Figure 32 demonstrates various control measures employed to counter various hazardous energy forms.

Steps in Establishing Controls

Once the most effective and practical strategy is selected, it is crucial to the future success of the control as a viable injury reducer, that those involved with its use and maintenance be aware of the reasons for the control, along with its limitations and special requirements. Figure 33 demonstrates how such information can be prepared for those in the line organization. Such information will help assure that the control is used properly, and inspected by those who have a full knowledge of the control's capabilities and limitations.

Element Four— The Monitoring Function

The fourth activity in a viable hazard control program deals with monitoring or continuously evaluating the effectiveness of the established controls, as well as staying abreast of new conditions in the workplace which may contribute potential hazards.

The monitoring aspect of any program designed to curb the number of losses from accidents is extremely important. It tells us what is going on and how effective our controls are.

In essence, we monitor to insure that the controls are functioning as intended, that workplace modifications have not been altered to such an extent that the controls no longer function effectively, or that new problems have not

Hazard	Control Measures			References
	Source	Path	Receiver	
Mechanical Energy	1. Enclosure guards (fixed or adjustable) 2. Interlocking guards (mechanical or electrical) 3. Reduction in speed 4. Limitation of stroke	1. Guarding by location (rope off area, etc.) 2. Remote control	1. Education 2. Rules and regulations regarding clothing, etc. 3. Pull away devices 4. Aids for placement, feeding, ejecting of work pieces 5. Two hand-trip switch buttons	U.S. Department of Labor, 1973
Noise	1. Enclosure 2. Surface treatment 3. Reduction of impact forces	1. Building layout 2. Increase distance 3. Channel away acoustic filters mufflers path deflectors	1. Protective equipment earmuffs earplugs 2. Limiting exposure time 3. Education	National Safety Council, 1969
Electrical	1. Low voltage instrumentation 2. Fuses, circuit breakers 3. Insulation 4. Lock outs 5. Labeling and test points	1. Grounding 2. Use of ground fault detectors	1. Protective equipment 2. Education	National Safety Council, 1969
Thermal Stress	1. Shielding 2. Insulation 3. Painting 4. Ventilation 5. Limiting physical demands of the job	1. General ventilation	1. Section and placement 2. Acclimitization program 3. Adequate supply of water and salt 4. Special clothing (ventilated suits) 5. Proper work-rest schedules 6. Limiting exposure time	Leithead and Lind, 1964
Chemical Hazards	1. Isolation 2. Substitution 3. Change in process	1. Ventilation	1. Protective equipment respirators, etc.	Stellman and Daum, 1973

crept into the workplace since the most recent controls were introduced. A discussion of the monitoring function will be taken up again in Chapter 9.

The monitoring function is only one of five other important activities. Many organizations in the United States today devote more of their hazard control efforts to the monitoring or inspection function, to the neglect of other needed activities. The point made here is that without efforts made and resources

Figure 32. (Courtesy of the American Institute of Industrial Engineering and M. Ayuub.)

Rules:

1. List the principle behind the control selected
2. List the logic of your choice
3. List the applicable standard if there is one
4. List the limitations of your choice of control measures
5. List the special requirements necessary to assure workability of selected control

Example:

Type	Principle	Logic	Standard	Limitations	Requirements
Provide metal hood above resaw	Barricading	Only practical solution to assure that worker's body parts or clothing doesn't come into contact with saw blade	OSHA 1910.213 (e) (1)	Saw must not be used with guard in up position Worker cannot use chocks to hold hood in up position when saw is in cutting mode	Hood must be adjusted properly Hood must be maintained properly Hood must be in position at all times

Figure 33. Steps in establishing control measures.

allocated to identify and sort out hazards in the workplace, without top management's sensitivity to the hazard reduction issue, and without the resources allocated to provide necessary controls, the monitoring activity by itself is unable to carry the whole program.

Element Five—Evaluating Program Effectiveness

Without some indicator which points out whether the amount spent on the hazard control program has had favorable impact on increasing overall organizational performance, the hazard control specialist's job of demonstrating his programs worth becomes extremely difficult.

The Role of Evaluation

Evaluation suggests various meanings to workers and organizational managers. Simply stated, evaluation is defined as a process for making decisions. It should produce then, accurate and meaningful data for informed management decisions. Unfortunately, a misconception of evaluation is that it is something done at the end of a specific period, to justify efforts and monies spent. Evaluations of this kind exist in great quantity. Seldom are they meaningful, because they do not produce information useful for program upgrading and organizational decisions at points in time when such information could be utilized most beneficially to upgrade the overall program effort.

Meaninful Evaluation

Evaluation consists of two essential phases: assessment and judgment.[4] Assessment is simply measurement—measurement of activities or products related to the program effort. Usually assessment is directed to conditions or changes in an organization, its services or its clientele. "What . . . ?" and "How much . . . ?" are issues central to assessment. (For example, what was the effect of a particular machine guard on punch press operations? How much fewer accidents did the workers have since the experimental hazard recognition training began?) Assessment, in order to be meaningful, must reflect the objectives of the program.

Once measures of change or conditions have been taken, judgments may be made about the adequacy or quality of those matters. "How significant. . .?" and "Is the change enough?" are the focal questions at this point. (For example, did the workers change enough to warrant adopting the new training program?) Judgment requires attention to values—values of the organization, the workers, and the community. Thus, meaningful evaluation for management decision entails a careful integration of program objectives, measurement approaches, and values of the organization. This view may be expressed in the following questions: "What did we intend to do?," "How close did we come to accomplishing our intentions?" and "Did we come close enough?" Such a set of questions implies cohesion throughout an entire program effort. Meaningful evaluation does not start at the end of a program; it starts in the planning stages.

Types of Evaluation

Evaluation may have two broad points of focus: *program* and *impact*. *Program evaluation* is an examination of activities, events and procedures in the context of the project or plan of operation. *Impact* evaluation is a study of the immediate and long-term effects and consequences of the program.

Evaluation may occur at either the end of a project or program period, or over the course of the project. The first form is *summative* evaluation, and is the more frequently-used approach. The second is *formative* evaluation. The two types serve different purposes; which approach to use depends entirely upon the aims of the program, the needs of the organization, and quite often the needs of the funding source or parent agency.

Summative evaluation provides information about total program efforts: that is, about changes that occurred in the status of a program *at its conclusion*. This type of evaluation is especially suited to established, continuing programs for which annual examination or accounting is necessary. Information gathered would provide a base for decisions about program continuation or termination. It would provide a data base for major program modifications for the future. Because a summative evaluation can do nothing to upgrade the program in which it takes place, it is principally a method for demonstrating the achievement of goals and the accounting for funds, energies, and materials spent in accomplishing the program effort.

Formative evaluation, in contrast with the summative type, provides information for program managers and decision-makers while the program is developing. This approach produces data by which mid-course adjustments may be made in order to strengthen positive, goal-achieving parts of a program effort and to correct weaker parts. Because periodic inspections and assessments enable development in its fullest sense, formative evaluation benefits programs aimed at hazard and loss control.

Impact Evaluation

Every program yields effects and consequences beyond its context. Training a supervisor to sharpen his leadership skills, with respect to hazard control, for example, may produce the intended improvement in his group management skills and affect his communication skills with others outside of his leadership role.

The effects accompanying program changes are the interest of impact evaluation. The assessment of impact requires considerable sensitivity to human, social and organizational conditions, because obvious changes intended and produced by a program may result in numerous other changes, some obvious, some masked. Still more important, the changes outside of the program effort may produce consequences contrary to program objectives.

Impact evaluation is especially important in human and social dimensions of business, industry, health, education and public service. Properly conducted it produces information not only on attitudes held by worker groups effected by a program, but about the behavioral and social consequences as well.

Criteria of Hazard Control Performance

When a good criterion of hazard control performance is sought, it becomes obvious to the hazard control specialist that the more such a criterion can be quantified, the closer the performance measurement he will obtain. Over the years, accident and injury frequency and severity rates have been used with some success. Accident cost figures which show damage, material waste, and so on have also been useful in some situations. The safety performance chart in Figure 34 is illustrative of the Questor Corporation's design of a format which not only quantifies accident costs by virtue of man-hours worked, but also places accountability for accident reduction squarely on the shoulders of its division managers.

Over the years, the hazard control specialist attempted various forms of qualitative evaluation of his program efforts. Rockwell[5] contends that qualitative evaluation of safety performance prohibits statistical inference and opens the way for individual interpretation. So, whenever and wherever the hazard control specialist can establish criteria such as those under the direct cost category in Figure 10, the better he will be able to measure results and communicate more quantifiably, these results to those who are responsible for a change in performance.

Figure 34. (Courtesy of the Questor Corporation.)

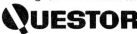

QUESTOR

Safety Performance Chart

THIRD QUARTER - 1977

AWARDS

Awards have been presented to the following locations during the third quarter, 1977

Certificate of Award - Kantwet, Milford

Award of Merit - Spalding Sales, Foster City

Questor Safety Award - Spalding Sales, Foster City
                       Leslie-Locke, Tucker

President's Award -

Questor Juvenile/Home Products	Spalding Sales, Foster City
AP Parts D.C., Pinola Ravenna	Spalding Sales, Edison
Spalding Sales, Newport Beach	Spalding Sales, Bedford

Plaque Bar -

AP Parts Print Shop, Toledo	Spalding D.C., Grand Prairie
AP Parts D.C., Carson	Leslie-Locke, Akron
Spalding D.C., Atlanta	Leslie-Locke, Mount Carroll

* *

COMPRESSED GAS CYLINDERS

Compressed gas cylinders, if mistreated, can become lethal weapons. It is important that an assigned storage area be located where cylinders will not be knocked over or struck by a passing or falling object. Pick a well-ventilated area away from heat in excess of 125°F. Your cylinder storage area should be posted with the names of the individual gases stocked, and a warning posted against tampering by an unauthorized employee.

Oxygen cylinders must be stored at least 20 feet from fuel gas cylinders or any highly combustible material. Cylinders, whether full or empty, in storage areas must have the cap connected in place. Acetylene or liquefied gas cylinders shall not be placed on their sides but shall be stood valve end up. Most important, a chain, bracket, or other restraining device shall be used at all times to prevent cylinders from falling.

Additional details regarding the use and care of compressed gas cylinders can be found in your State or the Federal Standards for welding and cutting.

LOCATIONS WITH NO CLOSED CLAIM COSTS DURING QUARTER	MAN HOURS WORKED WITHOUT CLAIM COSTS
1-Q.E.P. - Wood-Ridge	249,104
2-Spalding D.C. - Atlanta	202,246
3-Spalding D.C. - Chicopee	119,944
4-Spalding Ski - Westfield	114,660
5-AP Parts Rec. C. - Dowagiac	90,183
6-Spalding D.C. - Indianapolis	72,088
7-Spalding D.C. - Grand Prairie	48,760
8-AP Parts D.C. - Detroit	43,550
9-Leslie-Locke - Mt. Carroll	41,679
10-AP Parts D.C. - Needham	41,117
11-AP Parts D.C. - Carson	34,814
12-Spalding D.C. - Honolulu	28,100
13-Leslie-Locke - Tifton	27,777
14-Spalding D.C. - Sparks	24,680
15-Kantwet - Jasper	19,949
16-Contract - Oil City	18,855
17-Kantwet - Milford	12,205
18-AP Parts D.C. - Atlanta	5,159

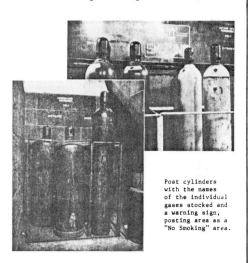

Post cylinders with the names of the individual gases stocked and a warning sign, posting area as a "No Smoking" area.

LOCATIONS WITH CLOSED CLAIM COSTS DURING QUARTER	$ COST/MAN HOUR WORKED
1-Fischer - California	.0015
2-Infanseat - Eldora	.0050
3-AP Parts - Pinconning	.0058
4-AP Parts D.C. - Chicago	.0066
5-Spalding Mfg. - Chicopee	.0074
6-AP Parts D.C. - Arlington	.0075
7-Spalding D.C. - Hollywood	.0079
8-AP Parts D.C. - Hayward	.0093
9-Leslie-Locke - Fr. Park (Melrose St.)	.0096
10-AP Parts D.C. - Pinola	.0104
11-Fischer - Tipton	.0120
12-Q.E.P. - Bronx	.0137
13-AP Parts - Dyersburg	.0154
14-Leslie-Locke - Ft. Worth	.0175
15-MPR - Wausau	.0255
16-Q.J.F.D.-West - Los Angeles	.0262
17-MPR - Muskegon	.0338
18-MPR - Sparta	.0517
19-AP Parts - Grand Haven	.0638
20-AP Parts D.C. - Dayton	.1042
21-AP Parts - Goldsboro	.1202
22-Crator Mfg. - Tionesta	.1214
23-Lullabye - Stevens Point	.1855
24-Leslie-Locke - Fr. Park (King St.)	.1930
25-Leslie-Locke - Tucker	.2190
26-Leslie-Locke - Madera	1.2978

The above article and photographs are supplied by AP Parts Grand Haven Division.

OHIO LOCATIONS WITH NO CLAIM COSTS DURING QUARTER	MAN HOURS WORKED WITHOUT CLAIM COSTS
1-Leslie-Locke -Akron	93,424
2-Questor Hangar - Swanton	41,909
3-AP Parts Print Shop - Toledo	23,639

OHIO LOCATIONS WITH CLAIM COSTS DURING QUARTER	$ COST/MAN HOUR WORKED
1-Q.J.P.-Ravenna	.0027
2-AP Parts R & D - Toledo	.0036
3-AP Parts General Office - Toledo	.0160
4-Kantwet - Piqua	.0289
5-Harcort - Ravennal	.0316
6-Questor General Office - Toledo	.0795
7-AP Parts-Toledo Division	.2310
8-Evenflo Mfg. - Ravenna	.2581
9-Leslie-Locke - Lodi	.2808

The following are postulated characteristics of a good measuring technique without regard to their relative importance:

1. The first characteristic of a perfect measuring instrument is administrative feasibility. We must be able to construct and use it. The necessity for careful consideration of this characteristic is easily recognized. The personnel resources available for use in implementing a measurement system may strongly influence the type of instrument to be used. In some cases, the urgent need for immediate results will predetermine that the type of instrument must produce practical answers in the shortest period of time.

2. The second attribute of a good measuring instrument is that it be adapted to the range of the characteristics to be evaluated. For example, a test of simple addition and subtraction is not a suitable instrument for evaluating relative skill in arithmetic possessed by college students. We would expect all of them to have this skill. Similarly, a test on which all students received 100 percent or zero would not be indicative of the range of the group's abilities.

3. The third characteristic is that the unit of measure should be constant throughout the range to be evaluated. In other words, it should yield readings which may be graduated into equal units. This means that the difference between successive points at the lower end of the scale should be the same as the difference between successive points at the upper. For example, the difference between 12 inches and 13 inches is exactly the same as the difference between one mile and one inch and one mile and two inches on a linear scale. Constrast this with the results obtained from an examination. There is no proof that the difference between a score of 30 and 31 is the same as the difference between a score of 60 and 61.

4. Of crucial importance is the necessity for the measurement criterion to be quantifiable. A qualitative evaluation of hazard control program performance limits statistical inference and opens the way for individual interpretation. The ideal criterion of hazard control program performance should permit statistical inference procedures to be applied because, like most other measurable quantities dealing with human behavior, hazard control performance will necessarily be subject to statistical variation.

5. Another characteristic of a good measuring technique is sensitivity. It must be sensitive enough to detect differences and to serve as a criterion for evaluation. No one would attempt to weigh a diamond on a cattle scale, since cattle scales obviously are not sensitive enough for that purpose. Similarly, we wouldn't judge the effectiveness of a hazard control program by looking at a death rate alone. The ideal measure of hazard control program performance must be sensitive to changes in environmental and behavioral conditions. This characteristic of a good criterion is significantly lacking in present-day measurement of hazard control program efforts. With insensitive measure of performance, the proper evaluation of hazard control methods becomes extremely difficult.

6. The technique should be capable of duplication with the same results obtained from the same items measured. In other words, it should be consistent or reliable over time. An ideal measure of hazard control program performance should be reliable to the extent that it provides minimum variability when measuring the same condition. The repeatability of a measure is related to the accuracy or precision of the measurement itself. In hazard control, this involves the notion of reporting. First-aid frequency, for example, has always had dubious reliability since under identical situations some workers will report to a dispensary for first-aid treatment while others will self-administer minor injuries. Similarly a criterion must be stable. This involves the maintenance of a given range of values under repeated measures of worker behavior and environmental conditions.

7. There is a need for the technique to be "valid," or representative of what is to be measured. In our pursuit of improved measures of hazard control program effectiveness, the question of what is to be measured is a critical one. Does "safety" involve the minimization of disabling injuries and first-aid cases or the minimization of all consequences of unsafe behavior and unsafe conditions? Near-injury or no-injury accidents constitute a dilemma in this regard, since their occurrence may result in a definite loss to the company and serve as indicators of future disabling injuries. In the absence of property damage or injury, moreover, the effect of unsafe behavior on production efficiency may constitute a considerable cost to the orgainzation, and yet go unmeasured. Thus, despite the fact that there is injury or property damage, unsafe behavior in itself requires the attention of the hazard control specialist and line managers.

8. Another characteristic of a perfect measuring instrument is that it yield error-free results. There is no perfect instrument in this respect as the type and magnitude of errors differs with different techniques. Certain kinds of errors creep into the readings or results which are obtained from all types of instruments. Errors may be classified into two types: compensating errors and biased errors. Compensating errors tend to cancel out, when readings are made an infinite number of times. For example, if you toss a coin six times the most probable number of heads and tails in these six attempts will be three each. There are likely to be errors from this expected one-to-one ratio in any sample of six tosses. However, as the number of throws increases, the ratio of heads to tails will approach unity. If a biased error exists, no amount of replication will eliminate the error. If the coin used happens to be loaded in such a way that it will fall tails more than heads, no amount of tossing will produce a ratio of unity between the number of heads and the number of tails.

The satisfactoriness of our measures of hazard control program effectiveness may be evaluated in the light of these two types of errors. Compensating errors in hazard control program performance measures will tend to disappear as the number of accidents included in the rate computation is increased, and as the number of instruments used to identify the same disabling injury information is increased. When both of these factors are increased to infinity, compensating errors will tend to disappear. No increase in such factors, however, will eliminate the biased errors.

Four types of biased errors prevail in our present measures of hazard control program performance. The first type arises from the accident investigator's failure to identify all of the causal factors associated with the accident. Perhaps this is due to weaknesses in his own problem perception capabilities, or perhaps because he has fallen into the trap of using sterotyped, general terms such as "inattention" or "carelessness" which provide little or no usable information as "causes" of accidents. At this point, the investigator's problem consists of making sure that his appraisal of the accident situation yields the type of evidence which leads to the identification of all associated problem areas.

The second type of biased error derives from the accident analyst's failure to break down to relatively homogeneous levels these causal factors to be evaluated. The classification of accident causes according to ANSI-Z 16 standards, for example, results in a lack of homogeneity in the intraclass identifications, since the categories included in the standard are too broad for a precise identification of the problem.

A third type of biased error prevailing in measures of hazard control program performance arises from the accident analysis's failure to consider all behaviors and conditions which show the potential for producing future disabling injury losses. A good cross-section of all unsafe acts and conditions which show this injury potential should be identified, for appraising the true accident state of the entire system within which control is desired.

The fourth type of biased error arises from the accident investigator's failure to report all accidents. In reaching for an Award of Honor, there may be a temptation to stretch a point here and there to avoid reporting an injury which might blemish the record.

9. Finally, a good measurement technique should be both efficient and understandable. Efficiency requires that the cost of obtaining and using the instrument be consistent with the benefit gained. Understandability suggests that the criterion be of such a nature that it can be comprehended by those charged with the responsibility of using or approving it. Statistical measures are often confusing to the uninitiated, yet terms such as "emotional instability, neurotic, accident prone, etc.," in addition to possessing inherent problems of guantification, have little meaning to the average manager.

These characteristics of a good criterion of measure are rarely achieved by any one instrument of evaluation. Often, only a combination of measures can provide a reasonable compromise. In the field of hazard control, presently used measures of program performance are inadequate in many of the characteristics cited. New measures are needed which will enhance our ability to predict and control accidents. Most probably a combination of several measurement techniques will be required in order for us to achieve our ultimate control objectives.

We have identifed what we would like to get, if we could wave our magic wand and create a perfect measuring instrument. These items, taken collectively, represent the zenith toward which we should direct our attempts to improve our hazard control measures. We have seen where we would like to be. The next step is to examine briefly where we are now, and then quickly move in a direction which will take us out from under the cloud into the light, and perhaps move us along the path to the star of measurement perfection.

Several indexes of hazard control program performance are now in use: Number of disabling injuries, the previously mentioned injury frequency, and severity rates, accident costs, number of deaths, number of first-aid cases, the ratio of severity to frequency, and the "serious injury index" which includes information about accidents resulting in major injuries, regardless of the degree of disability or lost time involved.

Indexes of Hazard Control Performance

A close examination of these presently used methods of evaluating hazard control program performance reveals a number of major difficulties. A review of a few of these difficulties will serve to highlight our problem:

1. The standard method of evaluation based on injury frequency and severity rates is not sensitive enough to serve as an accurate indicator of program effectiveness. Only those accidents with a relatively high injury severity are included in the rate computations. See Figures 35 and 36.

2. The smaller the work force, the less reliable is the frequency and severity rate as an indicator of hazard control program performance, particularly when less than the base number of 1,000,000 man-hours is worked during the period. In fact, with exposure below 1,000,000 man-hours, the frequency rate is technically a meaningless, hypothetical figure.

3. Lost-time accidents, deaths, and other reportable injuries are relatively rare events. Small units may go for a long period without a reportable accident under the present system of measurement.

4. A single severe injury or death will drastically alter the severity rate in smaller organizations, and thus this index may not accurately reflect overall accident prevention accomplishments. The problem of chance influences also attends frequency rate measure. In this case, chance determines whether or not an injury is of sufficient severity to be included in the "reportable" classification in the first place. If by chance a period of less than 24 hours lost time is involved, the injury does not appear in our frequency rate measure.

5. Comparisons are made among accidents occurring in various types of environments involving nonparallel hazard categories. We lump the exposure and accident experiences of material handlers with office workers, and combine milling machine operators with stockroom clerks.

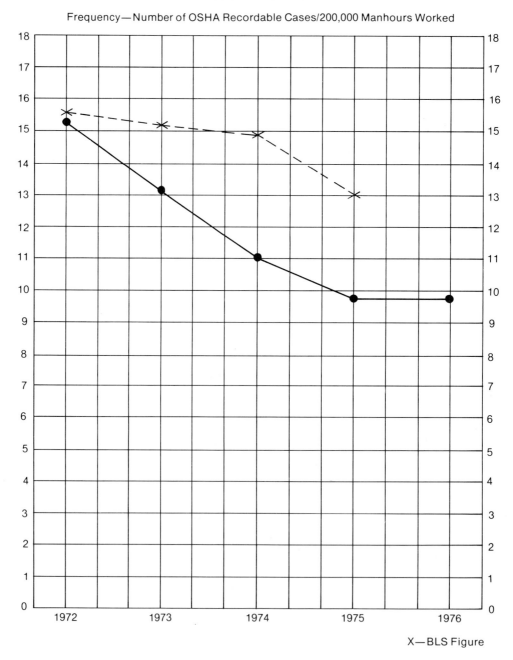

Questor Corporation

Frequency—Number of OSHA Recordable Cases/200,000 Manhours Worked

X—BLS Figure

Figure 35. (Courtesy of the Questor Corporation.)

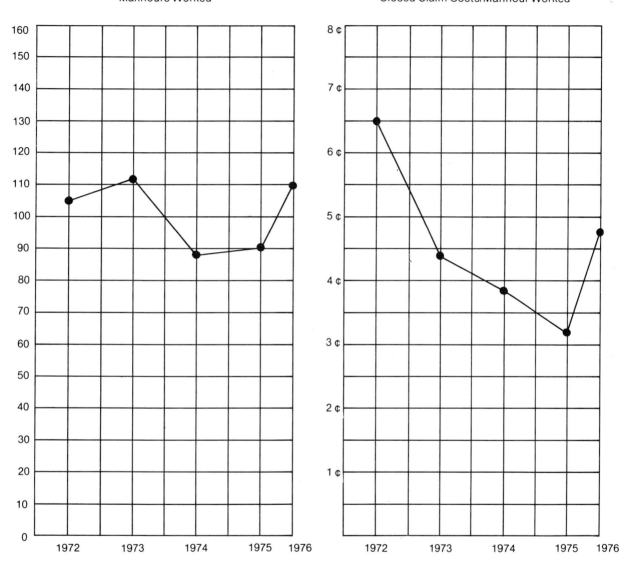

Severity—Number of Lost Workdays/200,000 Manhours Worked

Closed Claim Costs/Manhour Worked

Figure 36. (Couresty of the Questor Corporation.)

6. The measurement techniques presently in use are only remotely related to the behavioral and environmental changes which our hazard control programming activities are designed to bring about. How long does it take for a new safety training program to be reflected in a reduced frequency rate? In most cases, we must wait a considerable period of time to allow sufficient exposure to accumulate so that adequate data can be collected for a realistic frequency rate appraisal. There may be serious discrepancies between the frequency rate measure of a problem and the direct appraisal of the behavioral malfunctions that safety programs are designed to influence.

7. Most of our present indexes of hazard control program performance are based on hindsight appraisal of injury-producing or property-damaging accidents. Some loss must be involved with a certain degree of severity before an accident appears on a report form. In most cases, our accident causal information is derived solely from an examination of causal factors associated with loss-type accidents. What is needed is some way to examine accidents at the no-injury stage, where the potential for loss is involved but where the loss has not yet actually occurred.

8. And finally, many accidents, particularly the less severe ones, are never reported. Information valuable for analysis and control purposes is thus not included in the presently used evaluation system. This problem may become especially acute when there is strong competition to show a reduction in the frequency rate number, as the basis for winning a contest or coming out on top in a safety award program. No doubt the most reliable index we have is the number of deaths. We simply cannot hide the body under the rug and forget about it. As the injury decreases in severity, it becomes progressively easier to ignore it or to remove it from the "reportable" category. For example, when we put pressure on the supervisor to cut down on this first-aid cases, he may tell his men not to report their injuries to the dispensary, but to see him for a little antiseptic and band-aid. In a multi-plant operation, we may put pressure on a particular plant to reduce its frequency rate, and the plant manager may decide to pick up all of his injured workers by ambulance each morning and transport them to work at so-called "regularly established jobs." Often these jobs are never filled except by an injured employee who is unable to return to the job he normally performs.

These items represent a few of the major difficulties associated with our currently used measures of hazard control program performance.

Accident and Injury Reporting Systems—An Analysis

A critical element in any management system is accurate, meaningful, valid, and reliable information upon which to base decisions. Without such data, the hazard control specialist is unable to direct his program effectively and has a nearly impossible task of trying to demonstrate his program's accomplishments.

In order to assist the hazard control specialist in setting-up or revising an accident and injury data system capable of producing quality data for informed decisions, the following section has been included. The thoughts which follow are arranged to provide the reader with an overview of the most perplexing problems associated with accident and injury information systems with suggestions aimed at areas where improvements can be made. Accident and injury systems will be studied from the standpoint of (1) how data flows into the system, from the time of an accident to the preparation of information for entry into the data system; (2) preparation of report information; (3) definitions and interpretations; (4) data system characteristics.

Data Flow

It is essential that the person tasked with the job of filling out the accident report understand the necessity for the task and have the necessary skills required to be able to perceive, acquire, and report data which accurately portrays the accident situation and its causal factors. Among the key problems associated with accident report preparation is the general lack of consistency within organizations over who actually acquires and reports accident data. In some cases, the injured records the facts, in others a supervisor may do the job. In still other cases, a department head or "safety" supervisor may be the one assigned to the task. Current research has demonstrated that a more thorough and reliable accounting of an accident or injury situation is made when the immediate supervisor, knowledgeable of the accident, confers with the injured to ascertain the accuracy of the facts.

Variation Among Accident and Injury Report Forms

There exist many and varied types of report forms used through industry to collect and report accident and injury data. These report forms vary in both their comprehensiveness and format. Report styles cover the range from totally narrative, standard check-list type, to those which combine both the check-list with a narrative section. When attempts are made to draw correlations among data reported in the three styles, often data of specific interest becomes obscure or are lacking entirely.

While check-list type report forms do not always address every area of concern, they are useful vehicles for recording and conveying information. If constructed properly they serve to remove some of the threat associated with accident-reporting the threat that someone has to be made to "look bad," or that the trust established between the workers and supervision has to be strained.

Perhaps an accident/injury report should be developed, which provides a smaller amount of narrative information but which is easier to use. Rather than using a reporting format which is complex and lengthy, a form may be designed which will limit the amount of interpretative data recorded, in lieu of obtaining the data critical to decision-making.

Variations Among Methods of Verifying and Classifying Data From Accident/Injury Reports

Generally speaking, there exist wide differences among the methods and schemes which are used to verify and classify the data taken from report forms. Many existing classification schemes appear to yield descriptive data obscuring interrelationships among worker actions, environmental factors, and situational events. Such schemes make it very difficult to pinpoint accident factors contributing to injury, disease, or mortality situations. Furthermore, an examination of industry's reporting systems indicates that once inquiry is made for information which goes beyond that contained in the original report, few systems are capable of providing it. The reason behind this problem is that the systems are not designed in such a way that a case-by-case relationship may be drawn between a given accident and a resulting injury.

Preparation of Report Information

Variation Among Accident Classification Systems

Perhaps the most restricting factor which prevents the acquisition of desirable detailed information is the wide variation among the methods by which accident/injury data are classified. Organizations throughout the nation utilize many different schemes to classify their data, from the ANSI Z16.2 Standard in tact, to a host of modified Z16.2 systems, to many in-house schemes. The major limitation associated with a wide variety of classification schemes and the data produced by such schemes is that it is extremely difficult, if not impossible, to draw direct correlations among data from many organizations. The hazard control specialist may be forced to opt to design a system that will work best for his organization, though the data will be difficult to compare with those of other organizations—even those within the same standard industrial classification (SIC). The point to keep in mind is that data must be primarily useful to the organization which is acquiring it to reduce injuries, diseases and losses. If the data doesn't serve this purpose, then it is of little value even though it may meet federal requirements or other demands outside the organization.

Describing Relationships Between Accidents and Resulting Injuries When attempts are made to trace injury—producing accidents to their root causes, it becomes essential that a one-to-one relationship be drawn between a given accident and a resulting injury. With such data available, the accident data analyst is better able to draw conclusions with a higher degree of accuracy than, if such data are not available and conjecture remains the only source of arriving at conclusions. Common to most organizations is the fact that their data are not able to show such relationships, while other can produce such information only when an injury involves time lost.

Injury Distribution by Worker Activity Codes Of interest to the designer of an effective accident/injury information system should be the categorization of accident and injury data by worker activity. Such a system would allow the organization to pinpoint those areas of work activity where the highest degree of threat exists, and thus be able to organize its resources and talent to modify either the work situation or the workers performance, accordingly. Under many of the present schemes, particularly those which depend upon the OSHA reporting system, difficulty is encountered when accurate appraisals are attempted. In those organizations where worker activity codes are treated casually, more often than not, false impressions of problems are portrayed, and the organization ends up placing more emphasis on what it thinks are "target areas", than spending the time trying to solve the real problems at hand.

Management Contribution to Accident and Injury Situations A well-designed accident/injury information system should be capable of indicating management contributions to a particular accident or injury situation—e.g., their decisionmaking errors, failures to train or educate adequately, failure to supervise properly, problems they built into their operations, etc. Data on managements' contribution to accident and injury situations is of high value in the overall struggle for hazard and loss control. If the hazard control specialist could from the reported data, differentiate between worker error, and acts of omission or comission of management which were directly or indirectly responsbile for the accident situations, such data could foster recommendations for most effective corrective action and to reduce or eliminate future accident-causing situations. While these data are most desirable, one should keep in mind that sometimes things are more easily said then done. Some organizations may be reluctant to demonstrate inadequacies in their management system. Such an admission may open them up to ridicule and persecution. The hazard control specialist in such an organization must diligently attempt to convince his top management that the gains from a system where such data are acquired far outweight the limitations, and overall will provided the type and caliber of data which will be cost—effective as well as exceptionally valuable in locating and assessing organizational problems of vital importance.

Variation Among Situational, Human, and Environmental Factor Categories In many current accident/injury information systems, there appears to be scant systematic conceptualization of salient variables related to accidents and injuries. Human, physical, and situational factors associated with accidents and injuries occurrences are inconsistently recorded across many organizations existing schemes.

Examples:

Human Factor
1. Failure to use personal protective equipment
2. Improper body position

Situational
1. Slippery work surfaces
2. Defective tool or equipment

Environmental
1. Toxic gas in work place atmosphere
2. Low levels of illumination

This system causes two major problems. First, accurate data comparisons from organization to organization becomes very difficult if not impossible. Secondly, each individual organization is not getting as good a fix on their own problems as they might have. As part of the total design criteria for a workable information system, the hazard control specialist must take special care to design his accident causal factor categories in such a manner that they will be representative of the type of work and operations of his own organization. In so doing, the organization stands a better chance of obtaining meaningful data on which to base decisions and take action. Current examinations of accident and injury information systems reveal that the total lack of, or absence of classification of, schemes appropriate to an organization's specific characteristics, either seriously reduces or eliminates its capability to produce useful descriptive information. Consequently, organizations end up with no adequate data base on which to inquire into safety and health hazards, and the relationship between these hazards, as they pertain to the actual conditions in which their workers must work.

A final point to consider is that a well designed and functioning system will be capable of demonstrating the *Interactions Among the Situational, Human, and Environmental Factors* associated with an accident's occurrence. It is often only through such associations that the hazard control specialist is able to gain the insight needed to define the primary causal factor(s) associated with any given accident situation.

Definitions and Interpretations

A pervasive problem, common to many accident and injury information systems, is the diversity of definitions and interpretations among organizational personnel of terms like "accident," "injury," and "occupational disease or illness." Examples of the diversity among definitions in the three categories are:

"Accident"
1. Any situation involving personal injury or property damage
2. Any incident that causes damage to persons or property
3. Any disruption of normal activity

"Injury"
1. Any accident requiring an injury report
2. Any bodily harm which is reported
3. Any bodily hurt which prevents the worker from performing his regular work or job assignment at least one working day following the injury

"Occupational Disease"
1. Any abnormal condition or disorder, other than in injury
2. Any abnormal condition or disorder, other than one resulting from an occupational injury, caused by exposure to environmental factors associated with employment. Included are acute and chronic illnesses or diseases.

The variations among the definitions of terms creates problems when comparisons are attempted from organization to organization. In the process of designing a new system or revamping an existing one, the designer must be careful to define the terms that will set the direction for all the data to be acquired, make sure that all organizational personnel understand the definitions, and apply the defintions consistently, day after day.

Data System Characteristics

Variation Among Coding Methods   Critical to a data system is the person(s) in charge of coding the raw data from the accident report form into a format which is suitable for data handling purposes. An examination of many data systems reveals that in those organizations where a person with experience in the organizations' operation and what goes on in the workplace, classifies the injury data and assists in the data analysis, a higher degree of accuracy is obtained. In instances where adminstrative people, hampered by the lack of personal experience in the various facets of organizational procedures and methods, handle the data classification function, meaningful insights necessary for accurate accident appraisals are often not realized.

Variation Among Expectations from Data System   Generally speaking, it may be said that organizations keep accident and injury data for one of three reasons. First, to satisfy state or federal requirements. Second, to be able to validate workmen's compensation claims, or for other administrative reasons. Third, to determine what accidents occur, what variables contribute to accident situations, how frequently specific accident types take place and, finally the consequences of the accident situation.

No doubt, management's lack of motivation to know the specifics of their accident and loss picture has been the major drawback to the establishment of adequate accident/injury information systems in many organizations. The hazard control specialist's job therefore, is to be able to demonstrate to his management the need for and benefits of acquiring information which has direct favorable impact on the total organizational system. Without adequate data, management is shooting in the dark when it comes to establishing changes and instituting effective preventive and corrective measures designed to decrease loss and increase productivity.

Utilization of Accident and Injury Data by an Organization's Staff and Line Organization   When it comes right down to the basic issue of what accident data are all about, it would be hard to find agreement that the data are only a means to an end, that they are only valuable if indeed some useful change takes place because of their existence. One of the key faults associated with many accident and injury information systems is that the data rarely end up where they will do the most good—in the hands of those key staff and line officers who are at critical controlling positions within the organization and who, if they had the data, could enact the changes necessary to counter accident problems. An examination of many data systems reveals the fact that most of these systems exist solely for the purpose of meeting the organization's administrative or legal requirements e.g., Workmen's Compensation, OSHA, etc., rather than maximizing the use of the data to upgrade organizational performance. A well-administered accident and injury information system will be assured, when those in manufacturing, quality control, purchasing, maintenance, industrial relations, finance, and other key management positions receive relevant accident and injury data in a form that can be used to upgrade system performance. If the data do not reach this level of the organization, it is likely that top management either does not understand the benefits of the data or are not willing to have them readily known throughout their organization.

Intervals When Data Are Summarized and Reported

Collecting accurate, meaningful, and reliable accident and injury information is only part of the problem. That is, once the data are collected, they must be disseminated in such a fashion that necessary changes can be instituted at a point in time when they can do the most good. It is amazing how many organizations do not attempt to analyze and distribute their accident and injury data until the end of their fiscal or calendar years.

Under this system, a problem which may manifest itself early in the year, during a specific time frame, process, etc., will often not be realized by an organization until many months have passed. Such an organization has, by not utilizing its data properly, been cheated of its full value as an error and fault detector and, consequently has not reaped the rewards from the information system for which it is paying.

Reliablility of Report Data

The reliability of accident and injury information can only be estimated by the degree to which verification procedures confirm the detail in an original report filled out by those in management and supervision or by the injured himself. Among many organizations, verfication procedures are lacking. Instead of verifying the information, the organization is content with merely certifying that the accident and injury report contains all the necessary information, regardless of the accuracy of that information. When verification procedures concur with the data in the initial report, it may be assumed that the information given has higher reliability. Reliability undoubtedly increases when the accident/injury situation has been investigated properly by immediate supervision, department heads, and hazard control personnel. The importance of acquiring and using reliable hazard information will be studied in Chapter 8 where the process of accident investigation is explored in detail.

Checklist for Evaluating the Effectiveness of an Accident and Injury Data Information System

The following checklist is provided to assist those who may wish to assess the effectiveness of their organization's accident and injury information system. Each of the questions are aimed at a different level of the system and are designed to provide a total picture of the system, its operation, and its results.

I. *Definitions*
1. How is "accident" defined?
2. How is "vehicular accident" defined?
3. How is "injury" defined?

4. How is "occupational disease/illness" defined?
5. How well known are the definitions within the organization?

II. *Flow of Information from Time of Injury to Preparation of Information for Entry into Data System*
1. Who initiates and files the original report?
2. Type of report: Narrative _____; Checklist _____; Combination _____.
3. What documents are generated by the injury report?
4. Is an investigation conducted of the accident which produced the injury? By whom?
5. Are vehicle accidents investigated? By whom?
6. How are no-time-lost injury reports handled compared to time-lost injury reports?
7. Who classifies the injury and specific details in the original report?
8. Who verifies the report? What is their verification procedure?

III. *Preparation of Report Information for Entry into Data System*
1. Who classifies the information to be coded and recorded in the information system?
2. What happens to the original report and its associated documents?
3. Which information from the original report and associated documents is recorded in the information system? Which is not?
4. Is the identity of the injured lost in the data system?
5. Are accident data gathered when injuries do not occur?
6. What accident classification scheme is used?
7. Can a case-by-case relationship be drawn between a given accident and a resulting injury?
8. Can types of accidents be related to types of injuries?
9. Can types of work activities be related to accident and injury events?
10. What type of human-factors classification system is used?
11. Is the system able to classify management contributions to injury by decision-making variables by education or training?
12. How sensitive is the system to worker use, misuse, or nonuse of protective and safety equipment?
13. Is a situational factors classification system being used? What are its elements?
14. Is an environmental factors classification scheme being used. What are its elements?
15. Are the human, situational, and environmental factors schemes able to show interactions among human, physical, situational and environmental contributors to accidents?
16. What body parts classification system is being used?

17. Can injuries be related directly to specific equipment, machinery, locations, etc?
18. Are injuries related to equipment and machinery categorized by:
    a. worker using equipment beyond specified parameters
    b. improper maintenance
    c. using equipment for purposes not intended
    d. not using equipment as prescribed by circumstances, instructions, etc.
    e. inadequate design
    f. component or part failure
    g. component or part degradation (although used within design parameters)
19. How is the severity of an accident or injury determined? Is a standard system used in placing importance on specific injuries?
20. How are accident severity (or importance) rates determined? What formula is used?
21. How are severity data used?
22. Are accident frequency rates determined? By what formula?
23. How are frequency data used?

IV. *Entering Information into the Data System*
    1. Who codes the information to be entered into the data system?
    2. Are injury report classifications directly translated into information codes? If not, what transformation from injury report to information system takes place?
    3. How frequently are data entered into the information system?

V. *The Data System*
    1. What kind of data system is employed? Manual or machine?
    2. Is the system capable of adequately meeting the informational requirements posed on it?
    3. Do written objectives exist for the system?
    4. What is expected of the system?
    5. What purposes do members of the management system and others have for the accident/injury data?
    6. Are these objectives being adequately met?
    7. How suitable is the information generated by the system for worker "safety" and health objectives?
    8. How suitable is the system for administrative objectives?
    9. How long are original reports retained?
    10. At what interval are injury data summarized?

VI. *Analyses and Reports*
    1. Are regular periodic reports of accident/injury data made?
    2. How often is trend information calculated and distributed?

3. What actions or decisions are expected of those who receive injury reports regarding injury and illness control? Who oversees this matter?
4. How useful are the periodic reports for the needs of those in the organization who need them?
5. Is the information in reports sufficiently detailed to enable pinpointing of problem areas?
6. Who receives data in the management decision-making tree?

VII. *Gaining Access to the Data*
1. Who can authorize access to the data system?
2. How long does it take between request for access and access entry decision?
3. Is the time delay related to the complexity of information request?
4. What does it cost to use the system per access and complexity of information need?
5. Are there declared guidelines or confidentiality of data?

VIII. *Products and Effects of the Data System*
1. How long does it take to detect trends in accidents and injuries via the present system?
2. What are the criteria used for estimating accident direct and indirect costs?
3. How do data become converted from report to recommendation?
4. Is management and labor willing to commit themselves to action or innovation based on information produced by the data system?

Computers in Hazard Control

The computer has made its impact known in hazard and loss control. Some major industries and federal agencies are using the computer effectively to improve their management as well as their operational systems.

Electronic data processing (EDP) is being used not only to isolate situations of human error and condition defects, but also to highlight those correctable situations found closely related to management's policies, practices, procedures, and so forth.[7]

"Many legitimate questions are still to be resolved about management information systems. These questions, however, should not obscure the fact that integrated information systems are already here and being used," says Robert Beyer.[8] Required first is a mind open to change and willing to understand what the computer is and how to use it. A move in this direction requires that the hazard and loss control specialist have a solid understanding of the management process.

Many professional magazine articles and papers treat the subject of management information systems well and in great depth. One of the better is a brief report of McKinsey and Company, management consultants. It is based on a recent survey of 36 large U.S. and European companies and their practical experience with computers. It is titled, *Unlocking the Computer's Profit Potential* and is well worth reading.[9] Here are two points raised in this report important to the hazard control specialist.

1. In devloping computer programs, don't try to work alone. The establishment of a management information system requires a joint effort by the data processing specialist, the hazard and loss control specialist and a host of other functional managers.

2. Ultimate success of a management-oriented information system will rest largely on the meaningful participation of line (operating) managers and the staff (planning and controlling) specialists, especially those in the functional areas at which the information is to be directed. If the organization has information needs which require and justify it, EDP will do in seconds what it takes weeks, or even months, to do using conventional clerical means of data compilation.

A computer data-depository will permanently store all pertinent data about accidents for instant recall. Time is no limit. Geographical location is no handicap. Information, which is compressed into coded form to conserve storage, can be just as easily translated back into English language equivalents on paper coming out of the machine (printout).

But the computer is more than a mechanical accounting device. Given proper instruction, it can perform any information retrieval, data manipulation, and logical analysis of the information. This can be done through standard stored program routines, or through instructions generated as need by ad hoc inquiries. These instructions must be fitted to the specific and well-defined demands of the user. Under these conditions, the computer can become a cost reduction servant to any hazard control specialist who chooses to be its master.

Use of the computer is one of the several new approaches to successful hazard control programs today. Programs of this nature demand radical change in both theory and practice by those in the hazard control business. Computer users will find that much that is held sacred in traditional hazard control work will be subject to revision.

For example, a computer based information system will demand strong central control of hazard control programs. Loose direction and shifting generalization will wreck the system. The use of EDP to improve management control will require that the hazard control specialist embrace a systems concept in his method of operation. This concept is primarily a way of thinking about the job of managing that will provide a framework for visualizing internal and external elements of management as a whole, not as fragments.

The computer will go far beyond the setting of accident rates. It will encourage users to speed up research, improve the ability to diagnose problems, help set priorities, identify cost-to-benefit situations, and predict results.

Hazard control specialists who choose to use data processing will immediately be faced with the need to revise their accident report forms. The duplication of data must be removed from each kind of report in use and be consolidated into as few source documents as possible. However, the report must be comprehensive enough to foster a complete understanding of the accident, injury, and loss picture.

Once the hazard control specialist has outlined his "need-to-know" items (why, who, what, when, where, how, and cost), his next step is to develop a dictionary of cause-codes. Coded items are used computer systems because they reduce the storage requirements and because they are easier to program. Codes tend also to be less ambiguous than free-form English language statements. While the use of codes does cause loss of some information, it generally forces information into categories that are more susceptible to quantification and statistical analysis—both important in hazard control.

Each industry will have its won unique pattern of accident problems with different sets of opportunities for profitable correction. There will always be a danger in trying to apply generalized code dictionaries to specific work conditions. What works for one program may not work for another. Creating a set of cause codes for management improvement is like buying a new suit of clothes—the final fitting is quite personal, and the tailor had better know what he is doing.

There is a general impression among many working in hazard control that a supervisor must be fully responsible for each of his employee's accidents. This idea must be fully responsible for each of his employee's accidents. This idea must be modified. The supervisor is but one of many member in a total management system and, as such, cannot be expected to accept any more or less responsiblity for performance errors reported as accidents than any other line or staff person in the organizational hierarchy.

Causes of imperfect performance are a concern of all managers, especially the functional managers in areas in personnel, operations finance, and law. Line supervisors, because they are closest to the scene of trouble, should not be made to feel that they alone could have prevented an accident. Furthermore, in making a report, line supervisors should not be made to feel that they are being asked to testify against themselves in their responses. This is not a practical reporting procedure. Two actions are recommended to correct this:

1. Design the source document (accident report) so that it will not be highly critical of anyone involved in the accident—especially the reporting manager.

2. Train all managers (line and staff) to think of the report as a way to improve management and to avoid cost—not just to correct employee mistakes. Everyone involved must be encouraged to find ways that will improve the system. Blaming people adds little to the improvement of management.

The custom of sending accident reports directly from the supervisor to the hazard control office must be broken. Involve different managers, at different levels of the organization in the review process. If statements about weaknesses in specific functions of management are going into the computer memory bank, it will become apparent quickly that the managers of those functions will want, even demand, to be given the chance to reveiw the actions first.

The end result of this change is an organized system for identifying improvement projects as shown in the following examples:

1. Computer identification of unacceptably high operational losses involving personnel, material, and machines that demand corrective attention in the form of a formal project. Object: To reduce general and administrative expenses and cost-of-goods produced by avoiding manpower waste and excessive property damage.

2. Tabular details of causes and costs of specific product and equipment failures, maintenance breakdown, and misuse of tools and machinery. Object: To initiate action that will raise quality requirements, improve operating efficiency, and upgrade maintenance standards.

3. Machine-processed facts about where and why repetitive tort claims arise because of accidents involving the general public, contract personnel, etc. Object: To find solutions to problems that harm industry and public relations and to counter excessive cash outlay for situations caused or aggravated by employee negligence.

4. Critical occupation profile listing the specific work categories found to be contributing the highest numbers of imperfect performances causing accidents. Object: To improve employement practices, reduce fitness-for-duty problems, and make employee training more effective.

5. Tabular listings of a wide range of operating failure modes, using computer programs that produce decisionmaking data about cause/cost shortcomings related to work performance and management within specific organizational units (regions, districts, areas, office buildings, plants, etc.) The solution to problems is not provided by a computer program. This is part of the experienced, analytical service of the hazard control specialist. No computer can decide for itself what questions to ask of the data it uses. And no computer can be asked to evaluate the data it produces. The value of EDP to the hazard control specialist lies in the fact that it vastly reduces the time between the generation of a question and the delivery of the information from which the anlaysis can be made.

It has long been possible for the hazard control specialist to use the accident report document for his analysis without resorting to a computer at all. But if he wants to expand to a **total** accident reporting system, the information to be handled for cost/cause analysis will icnrease a hundred-fold. those who are now dealing with the limited information that disabling work injuries provide, may be seriously hurting their hazard control programming potential.

Those who are fortunate enough to be using any computerized report program "generator," will find themselves no longer tied down to a cyclical timetable in order to collate and issue valuable accident facts for the standard monthly reviews, quarterly summaries, and annual reports. Computer systems have a build-in ad hoc capability that goes deep into the past or will pick up details of last week's report. Neither timespan nor quantity of data used need bother the analyst.

Cost of computerization can be a major issue when considering a new management information system. Experience shows that speed and selectivity offered by the computer are enhanced by a per-question cost often substantially lower than that of card-based methods.

Any hazard control program employing at least one full-time statistician would be well advised to consider the establishment of a machine-operated accident/injury information system. Computer application in the hazard control process shows promise of returning much more dollar value in the reduction of operating errors than its use-cost. Much will depend, however, on the time it takes top-level administrators to understand, accept, and actively support the system and the new concepts it introduces about management improvement. But it can be done.

In summary, experience has shown that line managers will conceive of accident reporting as beneficial and will be happy to cooperate when they are assured that the system works for them-not against them. The accident reports, properly used, open a new system for rapid communication of line problems to the planning and programming managers who must read what is being said in them. A key to the hazard control process is the full appreciation and understanding that any accident is an indicator, a warning to the management team that something has gone wrong with the system. "If the hazard control specialist can make it clear to the other members of his organization that he has a positive role in the organization from the standpoint of isolating mistakes in policy, practices and procedures, he will become a full participating member of the management team, not a social worker operating in an organizational vacuum.

For the businessman, a low-cost system for honest assessment of where he is losing money because of ineffective management has always been high on his list of needs. "Business management in the United States," said Elmer B. Statts, today is looking increasingly to formalized systems to produce the information necessary to offer alternate choices as basis for decision-making, and to plan the future.[10] Hazard control people have had this capabilitiy inherent in their work for years. It has taken the computer to awaken us and make it a practical reality. A computer-based management information system could well be the modern hazard control specialist's dream come true. It produces facts, not suppositions. It backs these facts up with economic consideration, not just with rates. It presents loss prevention in a manner that cannot help but impress the hard-nosed, profit minded executive.

Important benefits to accident loss prevention are tangible. The computer reduced lengthy time loss in hand-produced statistics. And, most important, it demands the attention and respect of management as a tool for its own improvement and for cost avoidance.

Data Processing Systems For Hazard Control Information

For those who, after an analysis of their organization's accident and injury information requirements, determine that an Electronic Data Processing system is an advantage, it is imperative that they consult with someone who is knowledgeable of data systems and computer programs which are capable, on a cost-effective basis of producing desired information. The following information has been added to this section to enable those unfamiliar with data processing systems to obtain a grasp of the basics.

A data processing system is more readily described by separating it into the major data processing functions of input, processing, and output.

Input   Basic input to any system will be the individual accident report submitted for any accident involving organizational personnel. This report is to be initiated by the injured worker's immediate supervisor or department head so as to best describe the accident and the effects to person and property. Policy and procedures regarding reporting of accidents must be developed and distributed by management and understood by all organizational personnel. It is imperative that the report be so designed to provide the information desired including the ability to allow for various causal relationships to be drawn, as well as being reasonably simple to use by those responsible for the reporting function.

Processing   The basic data processing function must contain the capabilities of data input editing, updating, and file, processing and output. See Figure 37.

1. *Edit* All data input to the system must be validated within the acceptable range of values. Null conditions must be tested alone and in various combinations of data elements. The determination of edit criteria is one of the prime tasks of the system definition phase.

2. Update of files should be designed to provide for efficient processing of the file maintenance function (element level addition, change or deletion) either in a sequential or random update mode. As a general condition, design of all processing functions whould be conducted to favor sequential processing

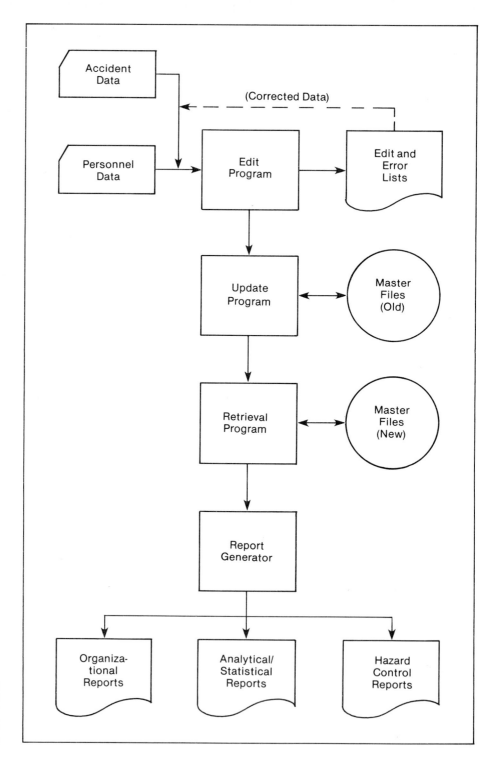

Figure 37. Functional flow—data processing system for hazard problems. (Designed by H. Davis, Consultant, RJF Associates, Inc.)

in the initial batch orientated application, and allow for transition to an indexed sequential, or data base handling function for future, more sophisticated applications, including on the inquiry and retrieval.

The two basic file sections (Personal and Accident) must be cross-referenced through internal or external tables and/or pointers to allow for complex conditional retrieval. This retrieval may be part of the normal report processing or a special ad hoc analysis for management purposes.

Output   Initially, system implementation does not require the use of on-line reporting capabilities. However, such consideration should be part of the analysis and design to allow for on-line update and/or retrieval. The reports, as previously outlined, will be formatted to allow hardcopy, or computer output microfilm (COM) report production. Because many copies of individual reports may be produced, COM would be cost efficient, pending suitable viewing equipment's availability.

The criteria utilized in recommending a computerized information system, as previously outlined are the following:

Criteria for Computer System Recommendation

1. *Data volume*—If manually maintained, the data rates and record lengths are large enough to present a sizable problem in accuracy and reliability. This is in addition to the higher personnel costs which are a direct cost avoidance with the computer system

2. *Accuracy and consistency*—The requirement imposed by an automated system with regard to standard fields and codes greatly enhances system performance over manual data preparation and maintenance. More stringent data editing and more complete error recording and possibility of correction also are factors in favor of computerization.

3. *Retrievability*—This is undoubtedly the single strongest factor which necessitates the choice of a computerized system. There is no other way to provide the capability of near instant processing of data and preparation of reports. Even with unexpected growth in file size and/or historical retention e.g., 5 years—10 years—20 years, the computerized system remains capable of producing a full spectrum of summary data. As an option, these data files could be made accessible on an as-required basis through the use of on-line computer programs and hardware devices. Even though this capability is left as a future option in this recommendation, it would be impossible without the initial construction of machine processable data files.

Bibliography

"A Comprehensive Study of Fire Fighter Injuries and Injury Reporting Systems," A Final Report—International Association of Fire Fighters and National Fire Prevention and Control Administration, October, 1977.

Ayoub, M., "The Problem of Occupational Industrial Engineering," April, 1975.

Beyer, R., "A Positive Look at Management Information Systems," Financial Management, Mt. Kisco, N.Y., June, 1968.

de Bono, E., "New Think," Basic Books, New York, 1967.

Elmer, B., "Information Systems in an Era of Change," Financial Executive, New York, 1967.

Payne, C. L., "APEX—A system for rating accident prevention effort," National Safety News, Sept., 1966.

Rickenbacker, E. V., "Rickenbacker," Prentice-Hall, 1967.

Rockwell, T. H., "Measuring Safety Performance," Journal of Industrial Engineering, No. 1, Jan.-Feb., 1959.

Rook, K. W., "Motivation and Human Error," Technical Memorandum, SC-TM-65-135, Sandia Corporation, Albuquerque, N. M., 1965.

Surry, J., "Industrial Accident Research—A Human Engineering Appraisal," University of Toronto, 1969.

Tarrants, W. E., "Applying Measurement Concepts to the Appraisal of Safety Performance," ASSE Journal, May, 1965.

Tarrants, W. E., "The Evaluation of Safety Program Effectiveness," "Unlocking the Computer's Profit Potential" (A Research Report to Management) McKinsay and Company, Inc., New York, 1968.

Notes

1. L. W. Rook. "Motivation and Human Error," Tech. Memo. SC-TM-65-135, Sandsor Corp., Albuq. N.M., 1965.
2. Edward de Bono, "New Think," Basic Books, New York, 1967.
3. J. Surry, "Industrial Accident Research, A Human Engineering Appraisal, Univ. of Toronto, 1967.
4. With the permission of Dr. Ronald D. Baker, RJF Associates, Inc., 1977.
5. T. H. Rockwell, "Measuring Safety Performance," Journal of Industrial Engineering, Jan.-Feb. 1959.
6. W. E. Tarrants, "Measurement of Safety Performance" Park Ridge Illinois: American Society of Safety Engineers, 850 Busse Hwy., 60068, 1978.
7. Reprinted with permission of "National Safety News," 1970 and W. C. Pope.
8 "A Positive Look at Management Information Systems," Robert Beyer. *Financial Management,* Mt. Kisco, N.Y. 10549. June 1968, p. 56.
9. Unlocking the Computer's Profit Potential, (A research report to Management) 1968, McKinsey and Company, Inc. 245 Park Ave., N.Y. 10017.
10. "Information Systems in an Era of Change," B. Elmer, *Financial Executive,* 50 W. 44th St., New York 10036. 1967. p. 39.

Analysis of Operational and Management Systems for Loss Potential

5

In Chapter 3, the diagnostic process was explored from the standpoint of its role in the overall management process. This chapter will extend the diagnostic process a step further to enable the hazard control specialist to locate and assess problems in an organization's capability to counter hazards and losses. The chapter is designed to provide further discussion of the process of diagnosis, in addition to establishing specific areas of inquiry which the hazard control specialist may use in an attempt to assess any organization for hazard and loss potential. The criteria included here have been successfully used in the conduct of many organizational analyses. Perhaps these criteria will be of value to the reader during the course of his or her work in hazard control.

The term *"diagnosis," as it will be used exclusively throughout this chapter, is the systematic process for determining the cause and nature of specific organization problems responsible for hazards and their resultant losses, identifying alternative courses of action, and promoting action for favorable change.*

The diagnostic process, as demonstrated in Figure 38, starts out with a goal and specific objectives. *A goal, for our usage here, is defined as the endpoint—the ultimately-desired plateau. Objectives, on the other hand, are the steps leading to the accomplishment of that goal. Objectives are measurable and must be measured if a fix on organizational change is ever to be accomplished. Secondly, the analyst must define the desired results he wants to achieve.*

Objectives commonly set for organizational hazard and loss studies are:

1. To produce more complete data concerning those management systems, jobs, job tasks, equipment, machinery, and man/machine

The Process of Diagnosis

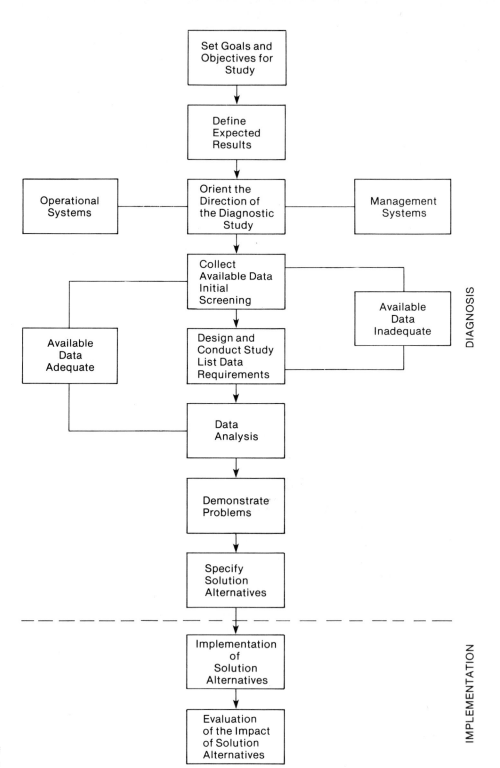

Figure 38. Outline of
diagnostic study.

mismatches that have the capacity to cause the undesired events of injuries, deaths, damage, and other factors and the losses accompanying these.

2. To pinpoint weak areas in management systems responsible for accident losses and recommend steps to alleviate the problem areas.
3. To define the managerial and operational constraints having an adverse effect on providing effective hazard control measures for employees.
4. To indicate both short and long term corrective measures for hazards and OSHA non-compliance situations.
5. To determine methods of employee instruction in hazard recognition and to make recommendations for implementing them into existing organization training programs.
6. To revise administrative requirements for the hazard control program to include staffing recommendations.
7. To determine the effectiveness of current accident data compilation and information retrieval.
8. To review current methods of purchasing products and materials.
9. To review the procedures of each of organieation's departments from the standpoint of hazard control practices.
10. To determine the effectiveness of current practices for the inclusion of hazard recognition into supervisor training and work procedure design.

Thirdly, based on the adequacy of information available, a determination will be made concerning where the analyst will orient his initial efforts—at segments of the organization's operational system, within the components of the management system, or a combination of both. Fourthly, available information is collected and analyzed to assess its accuracy, sufficiency, and reliability in order to determine whether it is adequate enough to define problems or whether additional information is required, and the analyst needs to probe further to obtain sufficient data to meet his data requirements.

Fifthly, assuming that available data are insufficient for informed decisions, an in-depth study will be launched to acquire additional information, to demonstrate problem areas, which will form the basis for solution alternatives. Sixthly, a plan is required to assure that system changes, resulting from the diagnostic process, are phased into the organization (implemented) according to specified intervals required for optimum situational change. Seventh, and last in the process is the implementation of a plan for on-going evaluation of the new system improvements on overall organizational effectiveness.

The cost of conducting any study, particularly one which is concerned with organizational hazard and loss potential, can vary with the size of the organization, the number of problems encountered, cooperation received, and so forth. But the single factor which carries the highest price tag is: time. The

Preliminary Considerations— How Much Will It Cost?

more time spent, the more costly the job becomes. It behooves the analyst at the onset of the diagnostic process to establish a limit of resolution before setting out to gather information. This limit will be determined by how much information is needed plus how much time he has to acquire it. A point to keep in mind is that time is always a limiting factor. We never seem to have enough time to do what needs to be done. We have all heard this statement from somebody else or have spoken it ourselves. Actually, if we are organized properly, have our directions clear, and use our time to the best advantage, it is amazing what can be accomplished. Before the hazard control specialist sets out to perform a diagnostic study of an organization he must take a long, hard look at his time constraints, and make the available time work to his advantage.

The Locus of Effort

Although the areas for inquiry will usually be similar for large and small organizations, a large parent organization, with many subdivisions spaced far apart, will usually be more time-consuming to analyze. In such a situation, the hazard control specialist may be wise to set his sights on an analysis of the parent organization, first, in order not to spread himself too thin. Actually, efforts spent to acquire a small amount of useful information will be more productive than efforts taken to accumulate a great deal of superficial information from many parts of the organization in a short period of time. Once the parent organization has been completed, then action can be taken to acquire information on the various organizational subdivisions. There is no magical solution to this problem. You only get what you are willing to pay for. Put the time in, do a thorough job, and the results will have a high pay-off. On the other hand, do a fast and superficial job, and the results are likely to be inadequate and worst of all, can be misleading in defining problems and forming the bases for workable solution alternatives.

Procedures

Preparation for the Diagnostic Process

1. Determine (a) Time available; (b) The names and titles of those organizational members who will be interviewed.
2. Acquire a preliminary rough estimate of interviewee's attitudes on hazard reduction in their areas of jurisdiction.
3. Prepare a list of subject areas which will guide your inquiry (See Areas of Inquiry, beginning on Page 132)
4. Study the interview criteria thoroughly until you know the major topical areas without having to refer to a written document. Situations may occur when you would rather not have to keep referring to your papers.

5. Start the diagnostic process by interviewing those in the highest management positions first.
6. Give each interviewee a brief outline of your project, including your objectives, general areas of inquiry, and the ultimate benefits to be derived from the information acquired.
7. Notify those to be interviewed a minimum of two weeks prior to the interview date, and follow-up with a telephone call or memorandum three days before the interview takes place.
8. Acquire a commitment from top management guaranteeing anonymity to any interviewee who wants it.
9. Before the study begins, arrange a briefing meeting with top management. At this meeting explain the overall purpose of the study, pitfalls expected, what can be done to minimize them, what is required of each organizational member selected for interview, the plan for inquiry, and the expected results and benefits of the results from the diagnostic activity.

Recording Information

1. Put the interviewee at ease during the interview process by describing what you are trying to do, the benefits to be realized, and that, without the interviewee's cooperation, critical data will be lost, and the cooperation of those under his command will be difficult to get. Furthermore, and ever so important, never indicate that the interviewee or the interviewee's operation is under scrutiny. Should the threat of *evaluation* exist, the interviewee is likely to offer only the information which he determines to be nonthreatening or potentially harmful to himself, his personnel, or his operation, holding back data which may be very useful.
2. Show the interview form to the interviewee and let him see what you are recording. At the end of the interview, review the data you obtained with the interviewee for accuracy.
3. Be certain that the correct names of the interviewees be listed with the information acquired at each interview.
4. Attach all supplemental information to each survey format.
5. Transcribe the rough notes into typewritten form as soon after the interview as possible, to avoid forgetting the relevance of certain thoughts as well as to keep relatively "clean" data which will be invaluable when the time comes to write the final report.
6. Promise those in management position a copy of the final survey results and recommendations.

Debriefing

When all data have been acquired, analyzed, and put into final form, a meeting should be arranged with top management to discuss what has been learned, your recommendations, etc. Furthermore, this session will provide the opportunity for each of those in attendance to interact and offer ideas which may be valuable in upgrading the study recommendations, in implementing new ideas for hazard and loss control, and in gaining necessary support and cooperation.

Major Areas of Consideration

During the process of conducting a hazard control diagnosis of an organization's operational and management system, the analyst will concentrate his efforts on the following broad areas:

- Organizational Characteristics
- Physical Work Environment
- Tools, Machinery and Equipment
- Individual/Job Compatibility

A brief description of the rationale underlying the items contained in each category appears below.

Organizational Characteristics

The items in this section are designed to reflect the operation and policy of the organization, with regard to the communication of hazard control information to workers and the extent of contact between the hazard control department and other organizational subsystems that can impact on the safety and health of the individual worker. These items were chosen to analyze specific organizational practices that have ramifications on hazard control as an organizational goal.

In addition, this section will deal with the analysis of characteristics of existing training programs with respect to their ability to promote positive transfer to the actual job setting. Finally, supervisor practices and work group characteristics will be examined to determine how they affect worker performance.

The Physical Work Environment

This section includes items dealing with: hazardous conditions in the physical work environment; hazard control methods the organization has used in the past to deal with hazardous situations; and conditions in the workplace that may contribute to errors, accidents, illness, or injury. The physical hazard items provide an indication of conditions on the job that have been a factor in previous accidents or incidents. The items on hazard control mechanisms provide an indication of the organizational philosophy in dealing with hazards. For example, reliance on personal protective equipment to the exclusion of all other control methods suggests that the organization tends to place the burden of protection on the worker rather than attempting to adopt alternate (although perhaps more costly) engineering or work process solutions. Use of a number of different approaches indicates a more flexible organizational philosophy. The third set of items deals with situations in the immediate work area that may increase the likelihood of accidents. These items pertain especially to the lay-out of the workplace as a potential contributor to poor hazard control program performance.

Tools, Machinery and Equipment

The first group of items in this section attempts to define the extent to which the job under study involves interaction with tools, machinery, and equipment, and to what extent these factors have been involved in previous hazard control problems. These items are designed for overall screening. If the job under study involves no contact with tools, machinery, and equipment, it is not necessary to complete the remaining items in this section. The next group of items deals with potential problems associated with guarding devices for equipment and equipment maintenance. Failure to use guarding devices is a frequently taken shortcut that can promote accidental injury to equipment operators, thus it is especially important.

Other items deal with the social consequences of operating a piece of equipment improperly and of improperly maintaining equipment. The awareness of these acts and their consequences are important influences on worker behavior. Thus, these items reflect this awareness and so provide some indication of the extent to which the social climate of the work setting works to promote good hazard control practices.

Consideration is also given to specific indicators of improper or unsafe control-display design. A frequently-cited contributing factor in equipment-related accidents is some improper control movement, or an improper interpretation of some information on a display. Items in this category are designed to help the hazard control specialist pinpoint such deficiencies.

The final set of items in this section deals with: the personal protective equipment required and the extent to which it is used when required; some reasons why the equipment is not used when it is supposed to be used; and some of the consequences of not wearing personal protective equipment when it is required. Since failure of workers to wear required personal protective equipment when required is a persistent problem, this item should be studied to not only identify the existence of a problem, but also in providing some clues to potential solutions.

Individual/Job Compatibility

This set of items is designed to assess from a different point of view the "match" between individual workers and their jobs. There is an underlying assumption which affected the choice of these items. This assumption is that to the extent that individuals and jobs are not "matched" in terms of human abilities, experience, interests, and needs, their work motivation and work performance, including safe work performance, will be adversely affected.

Particular groups of items in this section deal with individual/job compatibility in terms of factors affecting job stress, goal setting, and use of incentives to motivate workers to work in a more hazard controlled manner. Finally, the last set of items relates to an evaluation of the degree of individual/job compatibility by assessing the level of worker safe work performance.

Areas for Inquiry

I. The Management System

Organizational Characteristics

Major Area
The Organization
General Analysis

Extent Scale

0. Does not apply
1. To a very small extent
2. To a limited extent
3. To a moderate extent
4. To a considerable extent
5. To a great extent

Note: Extent Scale is to be used to answer questions where a numerical estimate is best.

Questions

1. *Has the organization established a goal for its hazard control program?*
   a. Is it written? _____
   b. Do all organizational personnel know about it? _____
   c. Is it realistic? _____
   d. Does it indicate the true intent of top management behind its hazard control mission? _____

2. Using the extent scale, indicate the extent to which *new workers* are made aware of; or become acquainted with:
   a. written company hazard control goals _____
   b. written hazard control goals at the department or section level ____
   c. federal, state, and local safety and health laws and regulations ____
   d. accident reporting procedures _____
   e. members of the safety committee _____
   f. members of the hazard control department _____

3. *Has the organization established specific objectives for hazard control?*
   a. Does top management understand the full scope of its hazard problem and the costs incurred? _____

b. Is top management being fully appraised of accident and loss trends? _____

c. Do all organizational personnel understand the objectives? _____

d. Has the organization specified the roles of the staff and line organization in the attainment of organizational objectives? _____

e. Has top management recognized the importance of hazard control as a contributing factor toward the accomplishment of the organizational objectives? _____

4. *Are the organizational goals and objectives for hazard reduction compatible with those of the hazard control department?*

a. Does top management perceive its hazard control program as a means for doing only those things which are good for public relations while the hazard control department is operating with a different set of objectives—perhaps incompatible with top management's desires? _____

b. Is management interested in using its hazard control program to only handle OSHA related issues? _____

c. Does management understand the full benefits to be accrued from comprehensive hazard control effort? _____

5. *Does an organizational chart exist?*

a. Where is the hazard control department located in relation to other organizational units? Explain: _____

b. Is the hazard control department set up as a staff unit, or does it report to one of the line officers? See Note #1 _____

c. Does the hazard control department seem to be functioning adequately where it is? What indicators exist to support your assessment? _____

d. Is information flow between the hazard control department and top management impeded by the position of the hazard control department in the organization? _____

e. Has the hazard control department been located in the organization on the basis of its ability to gain access to top management? What would happen to the hazard control department's effectiveness if the head of the unit to which it reports should change? _____

f. Is hazard control decision-making and action hampered under the present organizational scheme? _____

g. How much power does the individual to whom the hazard control director reports have to make decisions and take direct actions?

h. Can the informally powerful organizational members be located? Do these individuals have a positive or negative attitude toward the organizations hazard control mission? _____

Extent Scale

0. Does not apply
1. To a very small extent
2. To a limited extent
3. To a moderate extent
4. To a considerable extent
5. To a great extent

i. What re-positioning would be necessary to increase the effectiveness and efficiency or the hazard control department? _____

j. Does organizational policy call for the establishment of linkages between the hazard control department and other organizational management systems e.g., hazard control and purchasing; hazard control and production, etc.? See Note 2 and Figure 17 page 69 and 70. _____

k. Further inquiry into the operation of the hazard control departments is on page 144. Using the extent scale, to what extent is there direct and frequent contact between the hazard control staff and the following functions?

Extent Scale
0. Does not apply
1. To a very small extent
2. To a limited extent
3. To a moderate extent
4. To a considerable extent
5. To a great extent

(1) Research _____
(2) Engineering _____
(3) Production _____
(4) Legal _____
(5) Marketing _____
(6) Medical _____
(7) Purchasing _____
(8) Insurance _____
(9) Corporate Management _____

l. How many layers of supervision exist? _____

5. *Do the functional descriptions for each of the organizations management subsystems indicate responsibility for hazard control?*

a. Does the functional description clearly state what is to be done? OR

b. Does the functional description show hazard reduction responsibilities casually implied or not mentioned at all? _____

c. See Chapter 3—pages 69–71 for additional information on functional responsibilities of management systems.

6. *Does written policy for Hazard Control Exist?*

a. Does the policy statement indicate management's intent, delegate responsibility, and establish authority for carrying out the hazard control mission? _____
(See note 3 p. 158)

b. Does the policy statement place appropriate importance on accident and injury reduction? _____

c. Does it specify that hazard control be integrated into all organizational operations? _____

d. Does it spell out requirements for active leadership and direct participation? _____

e. Does it specify who will be held accountable, and how accountability for hazard control will be measured? _____

Leadership Roles in Hazard Control

The relationships suggested below are examples of leadership relationships within a viable hazard control program.

Hazard Control Program Prerequisites	Management Systems Leadership Roles	Leadership Functions of the Hazard Control Specialist
• policy • sound objectives • hazards defined and evaluated • an integrated plan for corrective action • communications • training • education • funding • monitoring • measuring	• knowing safety and health standards and regulations. • Providing directions and enforcement • Establishing liason with hazard control department. • Implementing hazard control procedures into their functional area.	• Recognizing and evaluating potential and existing hazards. • Determining importance of hazards. • Developing methods, strategies and procedures to effect hazard control. • Understanding company operations and particular operational situations which require safety and health considerations and tradeoffs. • Coordinating with other management organizations. • Effectively measuring company hazard control effectiveness.

7. *How is hazard control information communicated throughout the organization?*
   a. Is it done informally via the "grapevine"? If yes, consideration should be given to the fact that the "grapevine," although a speedy form of information transmittal, can distort information.

   Studies conducted to find out the relative effectiveness of various media reveal that the "grapevine" was mentioned by 38 percent of those surveyed, as the means by which the employees would most likely get the word first.[1]

b. *Formally*
  i. *Through the Supervisor?*
     In the same study[1] the supervisor was mentioned by 27 percent of the group as the means by which they got the word.
  ii. *Official Memos*
     This technique is estimated by 17 percent effective among those in the study.
  iii. *Bulletin Boards*
     Bulletin boards were estimated by 4 percent of those interviewed as the way they got the word.
  iv. *Approximately 14 percent estimated that they got the word through Newsletters, Company Magazines or Posters.*
c. *Note:*
   Communication is lost as it is distributed downward in the organization. Terry[2] indicates that in a limited study among approximately one hundred companies, the flow of communication downward from the top to the bottom indicates that a considerable alteration in the communicative message takes place. See Figure 39. It is also ironic that the nonmanagement members (the workforce) who are relied upon to produce the organization's product or service operate with far less data than they should have. This inadequacy caused by data dilution as they pass through the upper levels to the worker, is worsened by what additional information (factual or not) the worker receives through the grapevine.

Extent Scale
0. Does not apply
1. To a very small extent
2. To a limited extent
3. To a moderate extent
4. To a considerable extent
5. To a great extent

8. *To what extent are each of the following methods used to communicate hazard control goals, policies and procedures to the worker?*
   a. Pre-employment interview _____
   b. Orientation at the time of hiring _____
   c. Formal classroom training _____
   d. On-the-job training _____
   e. Introduction of new workers to experienced, safe-working employees _____
   f. Special safety campaigns and promotions _____
   g. Continuing safety programs and reminders _____
   h. Counseling programs _____
   i. Workplace talks by foreman and supervisors _____
   j. Encouraging foreman and supervisors to "set the example" _____
   k. Use of safety records in rating worker job performance _____

Management Interest
1. Does top management demonstrate an active interest in hazard control? Specify _____

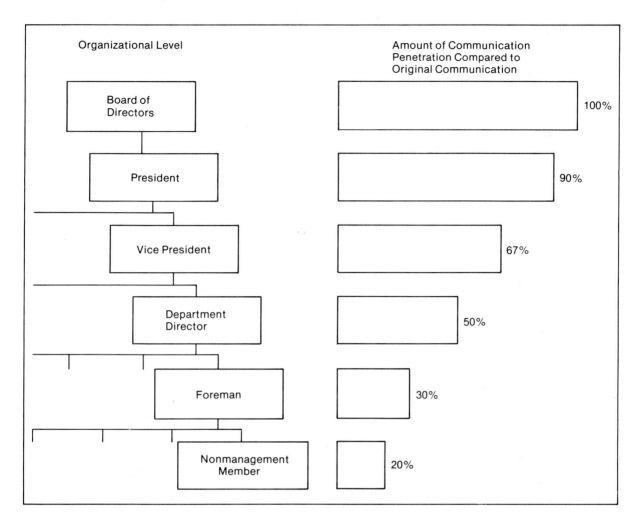

Organizational Level

Board of Directors

President

Vice President

Department Director

Foreman

Nonmanagement Member

Amount of Communication Penetration Compared to Original Communication

100%

90%

67%

50%

30%

20%

2. Does top management provide adequate funding for the hazard control program? _____

3. Does top management support training and education to further professional development? _____

Figure 39. (With permission of Richard D. Irwin, Inc., and George R. Terry, "Principles of Management" Six Edition, 1972.)

The Role of Purchasing

1. Does the purchasing department consider hazard control necessary for equipment and other product acquisitions? _____

2. Are department heads held responsible for assuring that the items they order meet with established safety and health and product safety standards and/or are otherwise ordered with available hazard controls? ____

3. Does purchasing coordinate its efforts with department directors before soliciting bids for products? _____

4. Is the hazard control department conferred with on issues involving the acquisition of products? When? _____

Analysis of Operational and Management Systems for Loss Potential   137

Procedures

1. Have procedures for hazard reduction been written and made available to those in the line organization? _____

2. Are hazard reduction procedures presented in a form that the worker understands and can use? _____

0. Does not apply
1. To a very small extent
2. To a limited extent

3. Are policy manuals maintained? _____

4. Does an employee suggestion program exist? _____
   How does it work? _____ Is the attitude of the employees toward the suggestion program favorable or unfavorable? _____

5. Have procedures been established for the enforcement of hazard control regulations? _____

3. To a moderate extent
4. To a considerable extent
5. To a great extent

6. Do new workers receive indoctrination in hazard control practices and risk assessment? _____

7. Does the indoctrination follow an established format? _____

8. Are organizational rules and procedures explained to new workers? ____
   a. How does the organization convey hazard recognition information to new workers—what techniques do they use?
      Explain _____
      1. Indoctrination speeches _____
      2. Handbooks _____
      3. On-the-job walkthroughs _____
      4. One-to-one supervisor instruction and follow-up.

9. Is special training and education provided to new employees in hazard recognition, evaluation, and control? If yes, what techniques are used?
   a. Stand-up safety meetings _____
   b. OSHA slide programs _____
   c. Other (Explain) _____

9a. Have department heads and supervisors been adequately educated in the purpose and benefits behind the organizations hazard control efforts?
   _____

10. Has the organization assessed each of its operations to determine safety and health hazards? _____
    a. Have hazard analyses been made? _____
    b. Who conducts the analyses? _____
    c. How are analysis data used? _____

11. Is a prompt investigation made of all accidents, regardless of severity in order to determine the causal factors involved? _____

12. Do line managers participate in the accident investigative effort? _____

13. Are no-injury accidents investigated? _____

14. Of the accident reports analyzed, is it evident that the direct and contributing causes of the accident are listed? _____

15. Does a standard accident data reporting and recording system exist?
    _____

16. Does the system produce adequate and reliable data for informed decisions? _____

(See pages 113–116 for additional areas of inquiry to be used in the assessment of accident and injury data systems.)

17. Where potential human error is evident, what means are employed to rectify the problems? _____

18. Are supervisors given authority to enforce company rules and procedures? _____

19. Are pre-employment physical examinations given to all new employees? _____
    a. Is consideration given to hearing impairment? _____
    b. Condition of the cardiovascular system? _____
    c. Condition of respiratory system? _____

20. Does the organization maintain records which indicated a worker's medical history—including number of lost-time injuries and illnesses, medical and first-aid cases, costs of medical treatment, department assigned and/or working at time of injury? _____

21. Are physical and physiological limitations considered in the assignment of workers to particular jobs? _____

22. Does the organization provide periodic medical exams for its employees? _____

23. Has the organization made provisions for dealing with worker injuries and illnesses contacted while at work? _____

24. Does the organization provide a system for medical follow-up for employees with a chronic occupational illness? _____

25. Does the organization maintain programs in alcohol and drug abuse?
    _____

26. Inspections—
    a. Are routine inspections conducted? _____
    b. Who makes the inspections? _____
    c. What items are covered at what intervals? _____
    d. Are committees formed to conduct inspections? _____
    e. What procedures exist to assure that inspection results reach appropriate decision-makers? _____
    f. What system of follow-up exists? _____
    g. How are inspection data used? _____

Performance Measurement
1. What criteria exist to measure hazard control performance? (Specify) _____
2. Are the criteria quantifiable? _____
3. Are the criteria only qualifiable? _____
4. Do the criteria accurately reflect the degree of change? _____
5. Does the organization utilize insurance experience modification indices

Extent Scale
0. Does not apply
1. To a very small extent
2. To a limited extent
3. To a moderate extent
4. To a considerable extent
5. To a great extent

to measure hazard control performance and to assess lower management's contribution to hazard reduction? _____

A discussion of experience modification is found in Note 4.

6. How do the experience modification rates last year compare with those of the past two years? _____

7. What are the experience modification estimates for this year? Are they higher or lower than last year? Explain _____

8. How does the cost of operating the hazard control department compare to total organizational costs? _____

9. Is the organization getting its money's worth on the basis of cost/effectiveness. _____

10. Does the organization utilize control charts to plot hazard control program effectiveness? _____

Extent Scale
0. Does not apply
1. To a very small extent
2. To a limited extent
3. To a moderate extent
4. To a considerable extent
5. To a great extent

Records and Files

1. Are accident, injury, and loss data acquired on a continuous basis? ____

2. Are accident cost trends produced? _____

3. How frequently are they reported? _____

4. How often are the data analyzed? _____

5. Where are the data kept? _____

6. Do all managers and supervisors see the data? _____

7. Is special attention given to those departments that are experiencing higher accident and loss rates? _____

8. Is access to the data possible by anyone in the organization who wants them? _____

9. What provisions exist to guarantee confidentiality of information? ____
_____

Records of Hazard Control Program Performance

1. To what extent are hazard control records (charts, listings on bulletin boards, graphs, etc.) displayed? _____

2. Using the extent scale, indicate how frequently "safety" records are updated for each of the following:

    the company _____
    the department _____
    the division _____
    the work group _____
    the individual _____

3. Using the extent scale, indicate the *extent* to which the record of "safe" work performance

    of each individual is made public to other employees _____
    of groups or division is made public to other groups or divisions ____
    of each individual is made known to that individual _____
    of each group or division is made known to that group or division __

Supervisory Activities

1. Using the extent scale, indicate to what extent supervisors do the following:

   a. set an example by demonstrating hazard control in work practices _____

   b. give workers credit for work well done _____

   c. show respect for workers _____

   d. show concern for each individual _____

   e. make work assignments clear _____

   f. offer constructive criticism of worker's performance _____

   g. give workers increased control over work activities _____

   h. show a concern for employees' safety habits _____

   i. encourage workers to try their best _____

   j. encourage workers to set safety goals _____

   k. evaluate worker's safety performance _____

   l. organize the work well _____

   m. ask workers their opinions on work procedures _____

   n. accept suggestions for improving work procedures _____

   o. give prompt answers to worker's technical questions _____

   p. give accurate answers to worker's technical questions _____

   q. satisfactorily resolve problems between workers _____

2. To what extent are the following used in supervisory training for individuals who supervise workers on this job?

   a. Formal classroom training _____

   b. Supervised on-the-job training _____

3. To what extent is the need for hazard control stressed in supervisory training programs? _____

Extent Scale

0. Does not apply
1. To a very small extent
2. To a limited extent
3. To a moderate extent
4. To a considerable extent
5. To a great extent

Work Group Characteristics

1. To what extent are the following used to encourage safe performance by work groups on the job?

   a. Team training _____

   b. Competition within work groups (among members of work groups) _____

   c. Competition between work groups _____

   d. Cooperation within work groups (Among members of work groups) _____

   e. Cooperation between work groups _____

2. To what extent do group attitudes encourage workers to engage in unsafe activities? _____

3. To what extent are work groups allowed to participate in the formulation of job and hazard control rules and practices? _____

Training Activities

Extent Scale

0. Does not apply
1. To a very small extent
2. To a limited extent
3. To a moderate extent
4. To a considerable extent
5. To a great extent

1. To what extent do entry level workers need special work-related knowledge and skills to perform the job safely? _____

2. To what extent is there a need for continued updating of job knowledge? _____

3. To what extent are each of the following types of training used to train workers for the job?
   a. Classroom training _____
   b. Continuously supervised on-the-job training _____
   c. Occasionally supervised on-the-job training _____
   d. Unsupervised on-the-job training _____
   e. Other (specify) _____

4. During training, are trainees normally required to practice various tasks? To what extent are the tasks practiced during training similar to the actual tasks that make up the job in terms of:
   a. end products (what the trainee is required to produce) _____
   b. the conditions under which tasks are performed (speed requirements, accuracy requirements, emergency conditions, etc.) _____
   c. problem identification activities (e.g., maintenance technician looking for frayed or loose wires, burnt terminals, worn parts; vehicle operator scanning instrument panel; etc.) _____

5. To what extent are the tasks practiced during training similar to the actual tasks that make up the job, in terms of:
   a. distractions (e.g., background noise from other machines or equipment, static on an electronic device, voices of others in the vicinity not related to the task, etc.) _____
   b. problem-solving activities (e.g., deciding how to place cargo in the hold of a ship, a carpenter deciding how much lumber is needed for a project) _____
   c. setting up or controlling machines (setting up a drill press, operating a duplicating machine, operating a meat slicer, etc.) _____
   d. assembling or disassembling parts and equipment (e.g., putting a telephone together, taking an engine apart, etc.) _____
   e. coordinating feet and/or hands to operate vehicles or equipment (e.g., operating a bulldozer, operating a sewing machine, operating a forklift, etc.) _____
   f. general body movements (e.g., climbing, balancing, stooping, etc.) _____
   g. use of tools (e.g., hand tools, power tools, etc.) _____
   h. use of hands and fingers to do precise work (e.g., using a soldering iron or welding equipment, use of saws or other hand held cutting tools, etc.) _____
   i. communication activities (e.g., giving instructions, writing memos, signaling others, etc.) _____

j. amount of teamwork required (e.g., working as part or a work team, etc.) _____

k. characteristics of the physical environment (e.g., noise, illumination, vibration, temperature, etc.) _____

Extent Scale
0. Does not apply
1. To a very small extent
2. To a limited extent
3. To a moderate extent
4. To a considerable extent
5. To a great extent

6. Training programs make use of a number of different incentives to motivate trainee performance. Some incentives may be more effective than others, depending on the trainee involved. In general, when each of the following is used, to what extent is it effective?

a. Verbal approval from supervisor or instructor _____

b. Verbal approval from fellow trainees _____

c. Tangible rewards (money, prizes, etc.) _____

d. Symbolic rewards (position on chart, token, certificate, etc.) ____

e. Competition _____

f. Setting performance goals _____

g. Performance feedback (quantity or quality of product) _____

h. Other (specify) _____

7. Training programs make use of a number of different incentives to motivate trainee performance. Some incentives may be more effective than others, depending on the incentive and the trainee involved. In general, when each of the following is used, to what extent is it effective?

a. Verbal approval from supervisor or instructor _____

b. Verbal approval from fellow trainees _____

c. Tangible rewards (money, prizes, etc.) _____

d. Symbolic rewards (position on chart, tokens, certificate, etc.) ____

e. Competition _____

f. Setting performance goals _____

g. Performance feedback (quantity or quality of product) _____

h. Other (specify) _____

Budget and Cost

1. Does top management envision its hazard control effort merely as a vehicle which will enable the organization to conform with federally promulgated health and safety regulations, or as an effort which can also yield financial gain through loss-reduction and money savings.

2. Are accident cost data readily available? How complete are they?

3. What are the criteria used to arrive at cost estimates?

4. Are costs broken down into direct and indirect cost categories?

5. What formula is used to estimate the direct cost/indirect cost ratio? How was this formula arrived at? Does it seem to accurately portray the organization's total accident loss experience?

6. Does the organization record other liability losses?

7. Are cost estimates considered as factors in preparing budgets?

Extent Scale
0. Does not apply
1. To a very small extent
2. To a limited extent
3. To a moderate extent
4. To a considerable extent
5. To a great extent

8. How does current year's accident costs compare with those of previous three years?
9. What is the cost of the organizations maintenance program?
   a. What extent of the total maintenance costs can be attributed directly and indirectly to ''safety'' and health.

Workplace, Facilities, Equipment

1. Does the plant layout lend itself to work flow?
2. Have adequate environmental controls been provided?
3. Is adequate maintenance provided?
4. Has the maintenance organization been tasked with certain aspects of hazard reduction? What specific tasks?

The Hazard Control Organization

1. What are the stated purposes of the hazard control program? _____
2. Are the hazard control department's objectives compatible with those set by top management? _____
3. Is the hazard control department adequately staffed—by numbers of people and required expertise—to effectively carry out the hazard control mission? _____
4. Does the hazard control department have access to medical and workmen's compensation cost-figures? _____
5. Are written functional responsibilities established for the hazard control department? _____
   a. Have these responsibilities been linked to responsibilities of other members of the management system? _____
6. Is the hazard control department structured well enough to handle ''crash demands'' while maintaining its overall program integrity and fulfilling on-going developmental activities? _____
7. Does a cooperative effort exist between line organization and the hazard control department? _____
   What indicators exist to the contrary? _____
8. What authority has the organization given to the hazard control specialist? _____
9. How much authority does the hazard control specialist actually use?

   _____
10. Does the hazard control department keep top management in the other departments informed of accident, injury, illness, and cost trends? _____
11. To what activities does the hazard control department devote the majority of its time? _____
    How many of these activities are of a maintenance nature (day-to-day) administrative work? _____
    How many of these activities are of a creative (program development) nature? _____
12. Is the hazard control department conferred with on matters of new systems design; facilities or methods modification? _____

13. Is the hazard control department involved in the organization's overall product safety effort? _____
Which specific hazard control department tasks relate to product safety? _____
14. How does the hazard control department fit into the organization's training and education programs? Does the hazard control insure that hazard recognition and control training meet organizational needs? _____
15. Does the hazard control department review all design specifications for equipment, materials, etc? _____
16. Does the hazard control department work closely with the medical department? _____
17. Does the hazard control department involve line departments in safety and health inspections, hazard assessments, and in recommending controls? _____
18. Does the hazard control department provide advice to other departments in the development of their hazard control programs? _____

II. Physical Work Environment

1. There are many possible hazards in the physical work environment. Often these hazards can be identified by reviewing past accident reports. However, hazards can exist for which no accident has occurred or been reported. Thus, observation and interview should also be a means of identifying these hazards. Using the extent scale, indicate the extent to which errors, accidents, illness or injury result from the following.

   Extent Scale
   0. Does not apply
   1. To a very small extent
   2. To a limited extent
   3. To a moderate extent
   4. To a considerable extent
   5. To a great extent

   a. Being struck by:
      (1) falling objects _____
      (2) vehicles _____
      (3) flying objects hurled by machinery _____
      (4) Other (specify) _____
   b. Being contacted by:
      (1) hot substances _____
      (2) extremely cold substances _____
      (3) toxic substances _____
      (4) radioactive materials _____
      (5) other (specify) _____
   c. Striking against:
      (1) protruding objects _____
      (2) other workers _____
      (3) other (specify) _____
   d. Being cut by:
      (1) machinery _____
      (2) tools _____

Extent Scale
0. Does not apply
1. To a very small extent
2. To a limited extent
3. To a moderate extent
4. To a considerable extent
5. To a great extent

    (3) sharp objects _____

    (4) other (specify) _____

  e. Coming in contact with:

    (1) hot surfaces _____

    (2) energized electrical conductors _____

    (3) corrosive chemicals _____

    (4) other (specify) _____

  f. Getting caught in:

    (1) confined spaces _____

    (2) other (specify) _____

2. Using the extent scale, indicate the extent to which errors, accidents, illness, or injury result from the following.

  a. Getting caught on:

    (1) projecting objects _____

    (2) moving machine parts _____

    (3) other (specify) _____

  b. Being caught between:

    (1) points of operations on machines _____

    (2) inrunning rolls, gears, etc. _____

    (3) drive belts _____

    (4) vehicles and stationary objects _____

    (5) other (specify) _____

  c. Falls to below:

    (1) from ladders _____

    (2) from work platforms _____

    (3) on stairs _____

    (4) other (specify) _____

  d. Falls at one level due to:

    (1) tripping over an object _____

    (2) slipping on oil, grease, water, etc. _____

    (3) poor illumination _____

    (4) other (specify) _____

  e. Exposure to:

    (1) toxic gases, fumes or vapors _____

    (2) extreme heat or cold _____

    (3) an oxygen deficient atmosphere _____

    (4) radioactive radiation _____

    (5) U.V. microwave, etc., radiation _____

    (6) other (specify) _____

  f. Overexertion due to:

    (1) improper lifting _____

    (2) pushing or pulling _____

      (3) twisting or turning _____

      (4) other (specify) _____

3. Various hazard control methods are available to respond to hazards in a job. A company may utilize each as needed, or rely solely on one approach (e.g., training). In general, to what extent have each of the following methods been implemented in response to the hazards in *this* job?

    a. Removal of the worker—assigning the function to a machine (automation) _____

    b. Removal of the hazard—eliminating toxic materials or hazardous work procedures _____

    c. Elimination of worker contact with the hazard—using machine guards, barriers, ventilation, etc. _____

    d. Use of personal protective equipment—helmets, gloves, safety shoes, etc. _____

    e. Increased job training—work procedures training, safety training, etc. _____

4. Indicate the extent to which you believe the following *conditions in the work area* contribute to errors, accidents, illness, and injury.

    a. Confined or congested work areas _____

    b. Worker maintaining cramped or uncomfortable positions (e.g., stooping, bending) _____

    c. Requirements for stressful body movements (e.g., turning, twisting, reaching) _____

    d. Obstructed view of warning indicators _____

    e. Noise interference with instructions, commands, warnings, etc. __

    f. Vibration _____

    g. Dust _____

    h. Noise _____

Extent Scale
0. Does not apply
1. To a very small extent
2. To a limited extent
3. To a moderate extent
4. To a considerable extent
5. To a great extent

III. Tools, Machinery & Equipment

1. To what extent have the following been factors in errors, accidents, illness, or injury?

    a. Machine failure _____

    b. Inadequate maintenance of equipment _____

    c. Removal or bypassing of machine or equipment guarding device

       _____

    d. Failure to use personal protective equipment _____

    e. working without the proper tools _____

2. To what extent have each of the following been a factor in job-related errors or accidents?

    a. Non-powered hand tools _____

Extent Scale
0. Does not apply
1. To a very small extent
2. To a limited extent
3. To a moderate extent
4. To a considerable extent
5. To a great extent

b. Portable powered tools/equipment _____

c. Portable non-powered equipment _____

d. Stationary machines/equipment _____

e. Materials transport vehicles—normally used to and from the work site (e.g., trucks, vans, trains, etc.) _____

f. Materials moving or lifting devices—normally used at the work site, (e.g., hoists, cranes, forklift, etc.) _____

3. To what extent do *guarding devices* for the tools, machinery, and equipment used in the workplace:

a. interfere with job performance _____

b. provide the protection intended _____

c. receive adequate maintenance _____

d. to what extent are equipment maintenance inspections performed frequently enough to insure safe operations? _____

e. To what extent are problems spotted during maintenance inspections promptly corrected? _____

4. If a worker does not perform the required maintenance on a piece of equipment, indicate the extent to which each of the following actions would result under normal circumstances.

a. No action would be taken by supervisors _____

b. No action would be taken by co-workers _____

c. The worker would be reminded of the requirements by co-workers _____

d. The worker would be reprimanded—given a written or verbal expression of dissatisfaction with his performance. _____

e. Punitive action would be taken against the worker, such as loss of a merit increase, or in extreme instances, suspension. _____

5. To what extent do workers follow standard operating procedures for:

a. The use of machinery and equipment _____

b. The use of power tools _____

6. If a worker fails to operate equipment in the proper, safe manner, indicate the extent to which each of the following actions would result under normal circumstances.

a. No action would be taken by supervisors _____

b. No action would be taken by co-workers _____

c. The worker would be reminded of the requirements by co-workers _____

d. The worker would be reprimanded—given a written or verbal expression of dissatisfaction with his performance _____

e. Punitive action would be taken against the worker, such as loss of privileges, loss of a merit increase, or in extreme instances, suspension _____

7. Faulty design of equipment is a frequent contributor to accidents. Two important features on equipment are the indicators displays (e.g., gauges, dials, meters, lights, sounds, etc.) and controls (levers, knobs, pedals, cranks, buttons, etc.). In general, to what extent have each of the following difficulties contributed to errors or accidents in the workplace?

a. Failing to use the right control _____

b. Operating a control at the wrong speed _____

c. Moving a control to the wrong setting or position _____

d. Failing to follow the steps in using controls in the proper order __

e. Failing to check, unlock or use a control at the proper time _____

f. Moving a control in the wrong direction _____

g. Accidentally activating a control _____

h. Controls being beyond reach of the worker _____

i. Failing to notice an important change in an indicator (gauge, dial, meter, etc.) _____

j. Failing to notice the right indicator because of its similarity and closeness to other indicators _____

k. Incorrectly interpreting an indicator _____

l. Difficulty in seeing the numbers, letters, or scale on an indicator

_____

m. Failing to check or refer to an indicator at the proper time _____

n. Confusing the controls or indicators on one piece of equipment with the control or indicators on a similar piece of equipment. For example, one model of a power saw is turned off by pushing a button in, while a later model of the same saw is turned off by sliding the button to another position. Another example would be confusing the controls (i.e., accelerator, brake, gears) on one type of bulldozer, with those of another model _____

Extent Scale

0. Does not apply
1. To a very small extent
2. To a limited extent
3. To a moderate extent
4. To a considerable extent
5. To a great extent

8. Indicate the extent to which each of the following pieces of personal protective equipment are used or worn by workers when they are required. If the equipment is not required for this job, assign a value of "0" to the item, and so forth,

a. respirator _____

b. ear plugs or ear muffs _____

c. safety glasses _____

d. safety goggles _____

e. face shields _____

f. hoods _____

g. safety helmet (hard hats) _____

h. safety caps (cotton, plastic, rubber, etc.) _____

i. gloves, mittens _____

j. hand leathers _____

Extent Scale
0. Does not apply
1. To a very small extent
2. To a limited extent
3. To a moderate extent
4. To a considerable extent
5. To a great extent

k. barrier creams _____

l. sleeves _____

m. leggings _____

n. spats _____

o. aprons _____

p. protective suits _____

q. safety shoes (wooden soles, nonskid, steel toes, etc.) _____

r. foot guards _____

s. safety belts for climbing _____

t. other (specify) _____

9. Often personal protective equipment is available, but workers decline to wear it. In general, to what extent are each of the following reasons given? The equipment is:

a. uncomfortable _____

b. ineffective _____

c. dirty or unsanitary _____

d. in need of repair _____

e. difficult to obtain _____

f. of poor design, such that it interferes with performance _____

10. If a worker does not use the proper personal protective equipment, indicate the extent to which each of the following actions would result under normal circumstances.

a. No action would be taken by supervisors _____

b. The worker would be reminded to wear the equipment by supervisors _____

c. The worker would be reprimanded—given a written or verbal expression of dissatisfaction with his performance _____

d. Punitive action would be taken against the worker, such as loss of a merit increase, or in extreme instances, suspension _____

IV. Individual/Job Compatibility

1. To what extent do workers performing at or below minimum acceptable levels have difficulty:

a. making decision (planning, making work assignments, etc.) _____

b. Processing information (trouble-shooting, making calculations, etc.) _____

c. Using and controlling machinery (setting the blade height on a table saw, setting mixture valves on an oxy-acetylene torch, setting up a drill press, etc.) _____

d. performing activities requiring the use of the arms and hands (e.g., assembling, painting, etc.) _____

e. operating vehicles or equipment requiring the coordination of feet and hands (e.g., driving a bulldozer, operating a forklift, operating a sewing machine, operating a steam pressing machine in a laundry, etc.) _____

f. performing activities requiring general body movement (e.g., climbing, balancing, lifting, etc.) _____

g. performing activities requiring the use of the fingers (e.g., typing, drawing, etc.) _____

h. using devices of a technical or precision nature (soldering electronic components, welding metal plates or pipes, cutting with a diamond or carbide wheel, etc.) _____

i. explaining decisions or relaying information (restating a given idea in a number of different ways, rapidly and fluently putting ideas into words, etc.) _____

j. getting along with supervisors or subordinates (maintaining friendly relations, helping out during rush situations, etc.) _____

Extent Scale
0. Does not apply
1. To a very small extent
2. To a limited extent
3. To a moderate extent
4. To a considerable extent
5. To a great extent

2. To what extent do workers performing at or below minimum acceptable levels have difficulty:

a. adjusting to working under unpleasant condition (working in a hot or noisy areas, etc.) _____

b. Adjusting to the demands of the job (keeping up with production schedules, overtime, etc.) _____

c. maintaining good work habits (keeping work hours, dressing appropriately, etc.) _____

d. staying alert for changes or paying attention to detail (repairing micro-electronic circuits, monitoring an automatic production process, inspecting for defects or quality, etc.) _____

e. planning and carrying out own work activities (exercising one's own ideas, etc.) _____

f. adjusting to an irregular work schedule (variable hours, changing shift work, etc.) _____

3. Indicate the extent to which workers are required to perform activities requiring:

a. finger/hand/arm strength (using hand shears to cut sheet metal, using a crow bar to open crates, cutting metal rods with bolt cutters, loosening tire lugs with a lug wrench, etc.)

b. dynamic strength—exerting force repeatedly or continuously over time (riveting sheet metal to an airplane wing, one rivet after another, for eight hours; breaking up concrete with a jackhammer, etc.) _____

c. general body strength (moving bricks from truck to construction site, stacking 100 pound sacks of grain, moving furniture, etc.)

_____

d. endurance/stamina—exerting the body through continuous effort over a long period of time (e.g., long-shoremen unloading cargo, etc.) _____

e. speed in performance (sorting products as to quality, performing specific step in an assembly line, etc.) _____

0. Does not apply
1. To a very small extent
2. To a limited extent
3. To a moderate extent
4. To a considerable extent
5. To a great extent

4. To what extent does this job involve:
   a. repetitive actions which can be done "automatically" (without thinking) _____
   b. performing several different activities at once _____
   c. observing indicators (gauges, meters, dials, etc.) or equipment for continually changing information _____
   d. observing indicators (gauges, meters, dials, etc.) or equipment for infrequently changing information _____
   e. working with a variety of systems or types of equipment _____

5. To what extent does this job involve:
   a. making decisions under time pressure _____
   b. solving problems under time pressure _____
   c. recognition of hazardous conditions (e.g., recognizing when equipment is operating at or beyond safety limits, etc.) _____
   d. problem identification _____
   e. need to remember facts, work procedures, machine settings, etc.
   _____
   f. maintaining high levels of attention and concentration over an extended time span (e.g., several hours) _____
   g. unexpected events can occur in jobs bringing about potentially hazardous conditions requiring immediate attention. To what extent are workers in this job exposed to these emergency situations? _____

6. To what extent have emergency conditions resulted from:
   a. the failure to recognize the seriousness of hazards _____
   b. the failure to detect and report the need for warning signals _____
   c. the failure to take corrective actions _____

7. To what extent have accidents, errors, injuries, or illnesses resulted from:
   a. the failure to perform required job functions during emergencies
   _____
   b. the failure to follow established emergency procedures _____

8. To what extent does this job involve:
   a. repeating the same activities on a moment-to-moment basis _____
   b. repeating the same activites on an hourly or daily basis _____
   c. performing work activities in a prescribed sequence (e.g., following a checklist or manual, following start-up and shut down procedures, etc.) _____
   d. performing tasks that frequently approach the limits of human capabilities or tolerance (e.g., performing many different activities at one time; lifting over 100 pounds; following rigidly structured procedures; monitoring a process for extended time periods, etc.) _____

e. working at a pace set by machinery rather than at one's own speed _____

f. working as part of a team, when the work could be done better by an individual (e.g., a worker having to coordinate activities with a number of people vs. establishing his own work schedule; responsibility spread over a number of workers vs. one worker responsible for the project; a worker has to wait on others to finish their job before he can work on his, etc.) _____

g. individuals performing tasks that could better be performed by teams (e.g., tasks requiring knowledge of many different subject fields; requirements for two tasks requiring use of the left hand to be performed simultaneously, etc.) _____

h. working under pressure or against deadlines _____

i. frequent interruptions by others _____

For many years, the issue of whether the hazard control function should be a staff or line position has met with widely differing views. Generally speaking, the hazard control function is most often found to be part of the staff organization. However, in certain cases, military organizations for instance, the position is often set up in the line organization and functions reasonably well. Since the hazard control function is more often than not set-up as a staff function, it is worth a few minutes to examine the relationship between the hazard control staff officer and those in line managerial positions.

Note: 1 Staff and Line Managerial Officers

To begin with, the concept of "staff" connotes an advisory position. Thus, the role of staff people in an organization is to provide information to the decision makers in an area of expertise which the decision makers are not sufficiently knowledgeable. Thus, the staff officer does not exercise direct command over anybody in the organization—save those within his own department.

Essentially, staff people, for the most part, are to increase and apply their specialized knowledge in problem areas, and to advise those officers who make up the "line" organization and have authority over production processes. Many of the major functions of the hazard control department as a staff entity are summarized in Chapter 3, under the discussion of the roles of management systems in the hazard control process. Tarrants[3] visualizes the function of the safety staff organization as encompassing part or all of the following duties: (1) assembling facts; (2) summarizing and interpreting data: (3) recommending courses of action; (4) discussing proposed plans with various executives and obtaining their concurrence or reasons for objection; (5) preparing written orders and other documents necessary to put a plan into action for submission to line authority; (6) explaining and interpreting the technical aspects of orders that have been issued; (7) appraising actual operations to ascertain if the orders issued are achieving desired results; (8) developing new plans on the basis of operating experience and anticipated conditions; (9) promoting an exchange of information among operating officials to increase voluntary coordination; (10) developing enthusiasm among operating people for established policies and programs.

An important point to keep in mind is that staff and line must not exist as two separate entities within the organization—each establishing its own path of direction and operating at exclusion of the other. Instead, and critically important, is that both entities blend their contribution in the true spirit of a cooperative effort. Many in the past have failed to realize that staff exists because of the line, not in spite of it. For without the line organization, tending to and accomplishing the organizations objectives, there would be no need for staff as there would be no organization left for them in which to operate.

Rights of Staff

Pope[4] envisions the staff officer as being in a position where no other manager owes any allegiance to him. The way that staff people are able to get things done is by using three inherent rights of their position:

1. The right to ask questions (The line manager has an obligation to provide answers).
2. The right to give advice (The line manager has an obligation to listen).
3. The right to warn (The line manager has an obligation to heed or ignore that warning at his own peril).

Limitations of Staff

Among the many limitations associated with staff positions, one of the worst is the danger that the staff officer, by virtue of what he is trying to do, will portray the illusion that he is taking authority away from the line. A second major limitation is that staff, by the very nature of their work, are constantly proposing plans and programs which line is responsible for implementing. Implicit in this arrangement is the fact that line is held accountable for the successful implementation of the plan or program, and is rated accordingly. Thirdly, is the limitation that occurs when staff engineers an idea for implementation by line without a thorough working knowledge of the system in which the idea must function. This problem has been a significant deterrent in establishing good working relationships between the staff and line organizations. In a situation like this, the line officer verbalizes that those guys up there in staff ought to come down here and find out what's happening, before they go off half-cocked and end up creating more problems than they are helping to eliminate. Actually, if staff people everywhere would take the time to get to thoroughly understand the systems with which they are working and the line officers in charge of the operation of these systems, greater productivity could be realized and many internal conflicts could be eliminated. Lastly, unless the staff officer is shrewd enough to perceive and handle the problem, it is likely that line may often perceive what he is doing as a blatant smear on their abilities to offer creative solutions to problems.

From the standpoint of the hazard control specialist's overall contributions to the organization, it is perhaps best if he handles his job in such a way that the line is involved in the solutions and, once the solution is implemented, line takes full ownership of the idea and its subsequent improvements. In effect, the hazard control specialist loses ownership of his idea, and that is the way it ought to be. The hazard control specialist's rewards shouldn't have to come from his association with all the things he made happen, but instead from the hazard reduction benefits accrued from the ideas, plans, and programs he was able to get the line organization to implement, and enjoy the benefits of.

The organization chart in Figure 40 shows that the Hazard Control department is set up as a staff unit that reports directly to the Vice President of Operations. The two-way communication that exists between the hazard control unit and the other key members of the organization can be summarized as follows:

Note: 2 Linkages Between the Hazard Control Department and Organizational Subsystems

Corporate Chart

1. Hazard Control Department to Chairman of the Board (through the V.P. of Operations)
   a. formulates for approval corporate safety policy.
   b. keeps appraised of hazard issues, major changes in policy, etc.
1a. Chairman of Board to Hazard Control
   a. provides support for program.
   b. listens to recommendations to Vice President of Divisions.
2. Hazard Control to Vice President of Divisions
   a. keeps informed of accident and loss trends.
   b. works out problems unique to specific division.
   c. keeps appraised of any problems located during hazard control audits.
2a. Vice President to Hazard Control
   a. present safety awards within their divisions.
   b. provide support within their division through their managers.
   c. assist on accident investigations and safety and health inspections.
3. Hazard Control to Process Engineer—keeps Process Engineering aware of hazard data that pertain to their operations.
3a. Process Engineering to Hazard Control
   a. Confers with Hazard control when new or modified processes are in the conceptual and design phases.

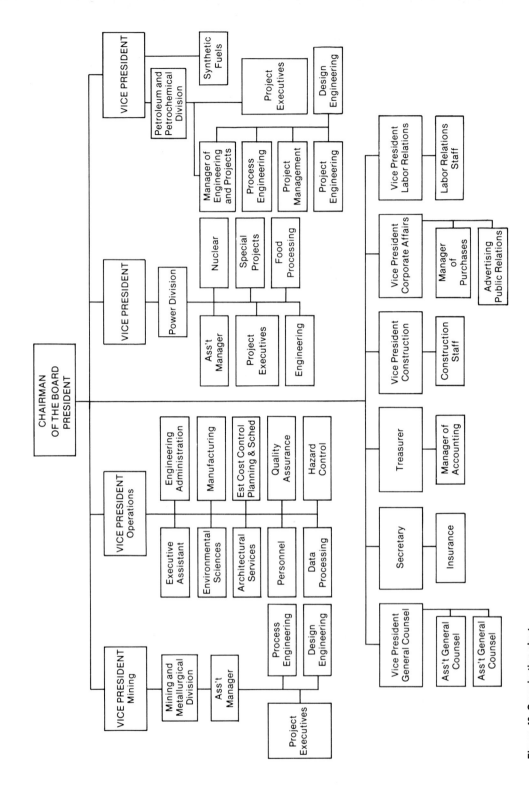

Figure 40. Organization chart.

4. Hazard Control to Design Engineering
   a. Hazard control provides council on CFR Part 1910, and 1926 Standards, and safety and building codes to assure that company will design a facility which is safe for customer to operate.

4a. Design Engineering to Hazard Control Department
   a. Collaborates with Hazard Control on matters of standards interpretation and use.

5. Hazard Control to Estimating Cost Control and Planning and Scheduling
   a. Provide cost figures for hazard control and first-aid programs during operations, i.e., personnel, facilities, equipment, etc.

6. Hazard Control to Environmental Sciences
   a. Assists with environmental surveys.
   b. provides suggestions on control alternatives.

6a. Environmental sciences to Hazard Control
   a. provides hazard control with industrial hygiene services.
   b. loans hazard control department sampling equipment for preliminary surveys.

7. Hazard Control to Architectural Services
   a. provides hazard control inputs to new designs.
   b. provides feed-back of hazard problems located during inspection.

8. Hazard control to Personnel Department
   a. provide hazard recognition information for personnel training and education.
   b. provides loss time, accident and workmen's compensation information.
   c. collaborates with personnel assignment.

8a. Personnel Department to Hazard Control
   a. Collaborates on matters of motivational and incentives aspects of hazard control program.
   b. Utilizes hazard control department to assist in the preparation of hazard recognition and assessment training and educational information.

9. Data Processing to Hazard Control
   a. provides hazard control with reports on monthly workmen's compensation premium runs broken down by job, supervisor, craft.
   b. provides absenteeism reports.
   c. provides cost gudget reports for hazard control.

10. Hazard Control Department to Purchasing
   a. Consults on hazard control requirements for new purchases.
   b. Assist evaluating or purchasing alternatives where hazard control is a factor.

10a. Purchasing to Hazard Control—collaborates on needs for hazard controls in items to be purchased.

11. Hazard Control Department to General Counsel
   a. keeps informed of any changes in product, environmental and health and safety laws and regulations.

11a. General Counsel to Hazard Control Department
   a. General Counsel handles all OSHA violation cases.
   b. Informs hazard control of all loss cases, e.g., liability, W.C., etc.

12. Hazard Control to Accounting
   a. Hazard Control provides budget reports—semi—and annual.
   b. quarterly estimates of savings on insurance.
   c. Cost estimates of losses.

12a. Accounting to Hazard Control
   a. provides current liability and workmen's compensation Insurance data.
   b. provides overall cost figures.

13. Hazard Control to Construction
   a. provide field monitoring of projects
   b. specifies Safety and Health standards for material and equipment.
   c. supplies hazard control specialists and nurses to field jobs.

14. Hazard Control Department to Corporate Affairs
   a. Assist in matter of Public Relations.

14a. Corporate Affairs to Hazard Control Department—coordinates with the Hazard Control Department in matters of programs.

15. Hazard Control to Labor Relations
   a. coordinate all matters of disputes through Labor Relations.
   b. assist Labor Relations on union problems involving issues of safety and health—especially NLRB cases.

15a. Labor Relations to Hazard Control
   a. Keeps hazard control aware of any worker problems involving physical, environmental and human factor problems in the workplace.

Note: 3 Policy Statements

A well designed policy statement will provide the needed direction for an organization's hazard control mission. The policy statement should reflect the attitude of management, with regard to hazard reduction; indicate the importance that is placed on accident and injury reduction; specify that hazard control will be integrated into all organizational operations; state the requirement for active leadership and direct participation among the staff and line organizations; specifically who is held accountable, and how accountability will be measured.

The sample policy statement which follows reflects a good attempt by the company's top management to develop a blueprint upon which its total hazard control program may be built. However, there is one weak area. No mention is made of accountability, and how it will be measured. Among the ways of setting accountability may be to state that accountability would be established by: charging accidents and losses to the department where they occur (the experience modification index is valuable in demonstrating these losses), or including accident and loss costs into the criteria for manager's and supervisor's performance ratings.

SAMPLE POLICY STATEMENT*

It is the policy of the Company to establish throughout the entire organization the firm and fully-accepted concept that people and property are our most important corporate assets and the conservation thereof has management's highest priority support and participation.

The corporation considers no phase of operation or administration of greater importance than hazard control. Accidents which result in personal injury and/or damage to property and equipment represent needless waste and loss. To mitigate the effects of accidents on corporate resources, both human and material, all operations shall be conducted in a safe and efficient manner.

Planning for safety shall start with design and continue through purchasing, fabrication, construction, operations, and maintenance. All practical steps shall be taken to maintain safe, healthful places of work by building in safe and healthful condition. To minimize existing accident and health hazards, adequate protective equipment shall be provided and shall be used by all persons, including subcontractors at work locations in accordance with Company Hazard Control Standards.

Responsibility

Operating management shall leave the prime responsibility for the implementation of this policy and the integration of accident prevention and property conservation within their operating functions.

All supervisory employees shall accept responsibility for the implementation of this policy and the integration of accident prevention and property conservation within their operating functions.

The Hazard Control Department functions as a staff service and is responsible for assisting management in the formulation of sound policy designed to meet stated objectives. It is accountable for effecting plans and programs for safe work procedures, fostering an attitude of safety-mindedness, and initiating recommendations associated therewith. It will actively work with operating management in achieving the goals set forth in this policy. Hazard Control has the additional responsibility of monitoring and auditing all aspects of corporate loss prevention and reporting results thereof to appropriate management.

The purchase of insurance by the Hazard Control Department to cover the occurrence of any loss which significantily affects the company's operations or

*Courtesy: The Dravo Corporation, Pittsburgh, Pennsylvania.

financial position is not a substitute for an affective hazard control program. By reducing, eliminating or controlling losses, the Company will reduce both the immediate and future cost of insurance and will also minimize the many indirect and unrecoverable costs associated with losses.

Communications

It is the responsibility of corporate officers, general managers, and officers of subsidiary companies to communicate this policy to all members of management and others who are in a position to help execute the general policy.

(1) Purpose and Scope

    1.1 To channel all management hazard control activities toward a single goal. This goal is the elimination of injuries to people and damages to property, and where this is not achieved, the minimization of their effects on the earning potential of the individual and the Company.

    1.2 This standard designates the basic components of a sound hazard control program and specifies minimum activities expected within each. Less than these minimums will be considered sub-standard. Limitation or restriction of hazard control activities is in no way intended. Desire, initiative and imagination are the only limits.

    1.3 This standard has been approved by the General Management Committee and will apply throughout the Corporation and its subsidiaries.

(2) Responsibility

    2.1 The President will assure continuing support of the program and insist upon its progress.

    2.2 General Managers and other officers are responsible to the President for implementing hazard control and for integrating it, by example and dedicated interest, with all operations within their respective divisions, departments and subsidiaries.

    2.3 Managers, superintendents, and others in operating management are responsible to their general managers for the achievement of not less than the minimum activities set forth in this standard, and for setting a consistent personal example of performance.

    2.4 Foremen, and others in supervisory management shall be responsible to operating management for satisfactory performance in all hazard control activities having application to operations and personnel under their direction.

    2.5 The Hazard Control Department is responsible to management for the preparation and distribution of program material and is to lend any assistance required to further activities under this standard. The Hazard Control Department is responsible for periodic audit of operating locations, including performance under this standard, program status, statistics, and for reporting results to the General Management Committee.

(3) Organization and Administration

    3.1 All officers shall evidence in contacts with operating personnel their determination to improve our loss record.

3.2 General Managers, managers, and superintendents shall meet regularly with their respective key personnel to discuss hazard control. This may be done in special meetings or in operating meetings. In the latter case, hazard control shall be placed on the agenda and thoroughly discussed.

3.3 Where distance or other difficulties prevent regular meetings between operating managers and their supervisors, personal safety discussion in their field contacts may be substituted.

3.4 General Managers and their operating managers will employ every reasonable and practical means to impress upon their managers, superintendents, and captains the necessity of making hazard control an inseparable part of operation functions. Managers, superintendents and captains will similarly impress this necessity upon all supervisors under them.

3.5 Subcontractors, at the time of negotiating the contract, shall be fully informed by the Purchasing Department of Hazard Control Standards applicable to them. Upon the arrival of a subcontractor at the job site, the company manager or superintendent shall see to it that the employees of the subcontractor have been fully informed as to their hazard control responsibilities.

(4) Training

4.1 Newly employed, promoted, and transferred personnel shall be fully instructed in safety practices for their areas of responsibility. Instruction will include discussion of applicable instruction materials with foremen and employees.

4.2 Operating instructions will include specific attention to safety in all instances where experience indicates the possibility of personal injury or property damage.

4.3 Supervisors shall hold regularly scheduled safety or "huddle" meetings with men under their direction. Operating management shall attend these meetings periodically. If meetings are not practical, regular recorded personal contacts similar to Paragraph 4.4 may be substituted for "huddle" meetings.

4.4 Supervising management shall make a specific effort to periodically call to the attention of those under their direction pertinent safety-efficiency items.

4.5 Program materials such as posters, monthly reports, booklets, courses, etc. will be furnished by the Hazard Control Department and their use discussed by members of this department.

(5) Work Practice Control

5.1 Each manager and superintendent is responsible for:
   a. A continuous survey of his operations, so that he is aware of the principal sources and causes of possible injury or losses due to unsafe work practices or procedures.
   b. Initiating corrective action.

5.2 Periodic supplemental surveys will be made by the Hazard Control Department to assist and advise operating personnel in complying with Paragraph 5.1.

5.3 Control under this section will be achieved through:
  a. The practical experiences of our operating supervision in safely directing the actions of those under their guidance.
  b. Effective application of Section 3, "Organization and Administration," and Section 4, "Training—Instruction."
  c. Compliance with other applicable Hazard Control Standards.

(6) Physical Conditions Control

6.1 Each manager and superintendent is responsible for:
  a. A continuous survey of his operations so that he is aware of the principal sources and causes of possible injury or losses due to unsafe physical conditions.
  b. Initiating corrective action.
  c. Maintaining orderly housekeeping conditions to assure maximum safety and efficiency in work areas and fire prevention.
6.2 Periodic supplemental surveys will be made by the Hazard Control Department to assist and advise operating personnel in complying with Paragraph 6.1 above.
6.3 Control under this section will be achieved through the use of all practical steps to maintain safe and healthful places of work. This can be done only if accepted principles of hazard control are applied, beginning with planning and continuing through design, purchasing, fabrication, construction, operation, and maintenance.
6.4 Based on mutual respect for the problems peculiar to each, the various departments concerned with planning, design, purchasing, fabrication, construction, operation, maintenance, and hazard control shall freely exchange any information that may contribute to safe and casualty-free operations. Especially, this course is to be followed in the acquisition or alteration of plant, equipment, process, procedure and in pre-planning conferences for field contract.8

Where the Hazard Control Department normally has no access to information on contemplated acquisitions or alterations, it shall be the responsibility of the General Manager involved to notify the Hazard Control Department of such plans.

*****

**Note: 4
Experience
Modification**

An index of hazard control program effectiveness comes from the workmen's compensation insurance carrier in the form of a computation referred to as experience modification.

What Is Experience Rating?

Experience rating is a comparison of the actual losses of an individual risk (company) with the losses expected from a risk of such size and classification, and a modification of the applicable premium to reflect the variation of actual losses from expected losses. The extent to which such deviation is recognized in the experience modification is determined by two values in the rating plan, the

"B" or ballast value and the "W" value. The latter value is used only in connection with the rating of the larger risks. Thus, experience rating determines whether the individual risk is better or worse than the average, and also how much the premium should be modified to recognize this variation. When the losses are less than those expected from an average risk of the same size and type, a credit is produced and the premium is reduced; when they are greater, a charge results and the premium is increased. The information contained in the experience rating plan constitutes a summary of the organization's injury loss experience along with an index against which the organization is able to get a fix on its success or failure in preventing lost-time injuries. In addition, the index lets the organization know where it stands in relation to organizations like it from the standpoint of whether its costs for workmen's compensation coverage is average, above average, or below average.

How It Works

Each state calculates manual rates, average rates for all insured within a given classification representing their types of business. These rates are applied to each $100 of employee payroll to develop the annual premium. At a $750 non-modified premium level, the employer automatically qualifies for an Experience rating which is used to recognize the extent to which his experience is better or worse than other insureds with similar types of operations.

Using loss experience, the rating bureau within the state, is able to predict expected or potentially predicted losses. The insurance company, although it is prepared to pay on those losses, is not in business to lose money. Therefore, the state rating bureau, includes the insurance company's cost of providing services to their risks, into the computation of the manual rate. A rule of thumb indicates that the higher the risk of loss associated with a given classification, the higher the rate. The experience modification is expressed as a factor, as for example 1.10 (or a 10 percent surcharge), and is applied to the annual premium prior to premium discount. The following example may clarify this point. Assume that a company has an experience modification of 1.00 indicating that it will pay $1.00 for every dollar's worth of insurance coverage. On the other hand, if it had a rate of .85, it would indicate that the organization's accident experience is below average as compared to organizations in the same industry, and thus the organization will pay 15 percent less for the same coverage. Of course, the same rule applies in reverse. If the modifier is above 1.00, let's say 1.09, the organization will pay 9 percent more for the same coverage.

Experience modification is determined in accordance with the Experience Rating Plan (ERP) Formula which has been approved by the Insurance Commissioner and is the same plan used in all National Council States. Those States not included are: New Jersey, Delaware, Pennsylvania, and California, which use their own experience modifications based on premiums developed in those states. The ERP compares actual losses with expected losses for three years prior, excluding the current year. Loss frequency is penalized more heavily than loss severity, by limiting losses over $2,000 to a specified amount. Losses under $2,000 are included at full values. Loss frequency is penalized more heavily, since it is felt that the insured can more easily control the small losses than the less frequent severe loss. Simply stated, the ERP formula assigns more weight to loss frequency than to loss severity, because loss severity is assumed to be more influenced by chance.

In summary, the experience rating plan develops expected losses for the three years covered by the plan by applying the pure loss rate, which is that part of the current manual rate required to pay losses (excluding any expenses), to the insured's audited payrolls by classification for the same period of time. The insured's actual losses are then compared with the expected losses, giving greater weight to losses under $2,000 for both actual and expected losses. If the formula actual losses are greater than formula expected losses, the experience modification will be a debit. If the reverse is true, the experience modification will be a credit.

The Rating Procedure

Figure 41 illustrates an actual experience rating calculation showing information on payrolls and losses as reported by the insurance carrier, and expected losses and the modification calculation using the experience rating factors from Tables I, II, and III of the ERP. The experience rating plan form in Figure 41, is divided into three parts: Part I shows the company's actual losses; Part II is an exhibit of the Company's expected losses; Part III is the rating procedure where the data from Part I and II are completed.

Following is a description of the categories in each part of the plan.

Part I—Actual Losses

COL (8) policy year.

COL (a) claim number as reported by carrier, reduced to last five digits.

COL (10) Actual incurred losses as reported by carrier.

COL (11) Primary Actual Losses is determined from Table I of the ERP, and, in effect, discounts the actual losses so that frequency is more heavily penalized. The formula assigns more weight to accident frequency than to accident severity.

Part II—Expected Losses

COL (1) Code numbers.

COL (2) Policy years.

Figure 41.

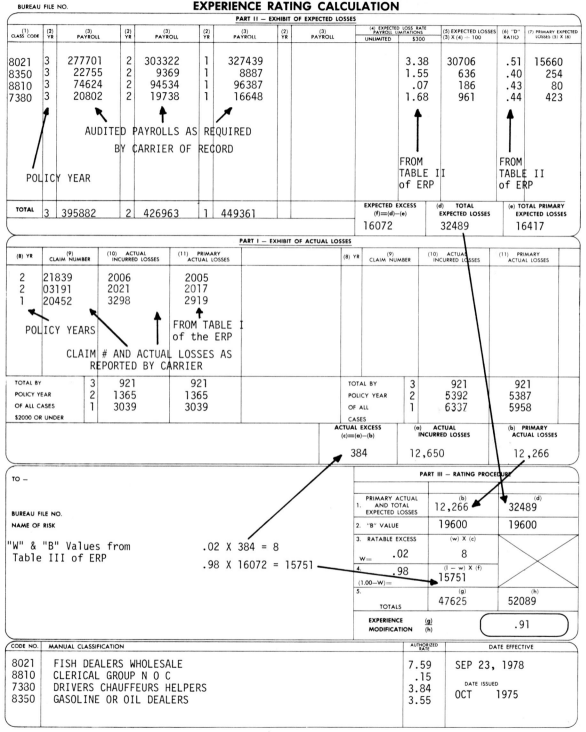

THE WORKERS' COMPENSATION RATING AND INSPECTION BUREAU OF MASSACHUSETTS
EXPERIENCE RATING CALCULATION

BUREAU FILE NO.

PART II — EXHIBIT OF EXPECTED LOSSES

(1) CLASS CODE	(2) YR	(3) PAYROLL	(2) YR	(3) PAYROLL	(2) YR	(3) PAYROLL	(2) YR	(3) PAYROLL	(4) EXPECTED LOSS RATE PAYROLL LIMITATIONS UNLIMITED	$300	(5) EXPECTED LOSSES (3) X (4) ÷ 100	(6) "D" RATIO	(7) PRIMARY EXPECTED LOSSES (5) X (6)
8021	3	277701	2	303322	1	327439				3.38	30706	.51	15660
8350	3	22755	2	9369	1	8887				1.55	636	.40	254
8810	3	74624	2	94534	1	96387				.07	186	.43	80
7380	3	20802	2	19738	1	16648				1.68	961	.44	423

AUDITED PAYROLLS AS REQUIRED
BY CARRIER OF RECORD

POLICY YEAR

FROM TABLE II of ERP (for column 4)

FROM TABLE II of ERP (for column 6)

| TOTAL | 3 | 395882 | 2 | 426963 | 1 | 449361 | | | EXPECTED EXCESS (f)=(d)—(e) 16072 | (d) TOTAL EXPECTED LOSSES 32489 | (e) TOTAL PRIMARY EXPECTED LOSSES 16417 |

PART I — EXHIBIT OF ACTUAL LOSSES

(8) YR	(9) CLAIM NUMBER	(10) ACTUAL INCURRED LOSSES	(11) PRIMARY ACTUAL LOSSES		(8) YR	(9) CLAIM NUMBER	(10) ACTUAL INCURRED LOSSES	(11) PRIMARY ACTUAL LOSSES
2	21839	2006	2005					
2	03191	2021	2017					
1	20452	3298	2919					

POLICY YEARS

FROM TABLE I of the ERP

CLAIM # AND ACTUAL LOSSES AS REPORTED BY CARRIER

TOTAL BY POLICY YEAR OF ALL CASES $2000 OR UNDER	3	921	921		TOTAL BY POLICY YEAR OF ALL CASES	3	921	921
	2	1365	1365			2	5392	5387
	1	3039	3039			1	6337	5958

| ACTUAL EXCESS (c)=(a)—(b) 384 | (a) ACTUAL INCURRED LOSSES 12,650 | (b) PRIMARY ACTUAL LOSSES 12,266 |

TO —

BUREAU FILE NO.

NAME OF RISK

"W" & "B" Values from
Table III of ERP

.02 X 384 = 8

.98 X 16072 = 15751

PART III — RATING PROCEDURE

		(b)	(d)
1.	PRIMARY ACTUAL AND TOTAL EXPECTED LOSSES	12,266	32489
2.	"B" VALUE	19600	19600
3.	RATABLE EXCESS w= .02	(w) X (c) 8	
4.	(1.00—W)= .98	(1 — w) X (f) 15751	
5.	TOTALS	(g) 47625	(h) 52089

| EXPERIENCE MODIFICATION (g)/(h) | .91 |

CODE NO.	MANUAL CLASSIFICATION	AUTHORIZED RATE	DATE EFFECTIVE
8021	FISH DEALERS WHOLESALE	7.59	SEP 23, 1978
8810	CLERICAL GROUP N O C	.15	
7330	DRIVERS CHAUFFEURS HELPERS	3.84	DATE ISSUED
8350	GASOLINE OR OIL DEALERS	3.55	OCT 1975

Analysis of Operational and Management Systems for Loss Potential

TABLE 1
Primary Rating Values of Actual Losses

EXPERIENCE RATING PLAN MANUAL

Effective January 1, 1977

Actual Loss	Primary Value	Actual Loss	Primary Value	Actual Loss	Primary Value	Actual Loss	Primary Value	Actual Loss	Primary Value
0-2000	Actual	2025	2020	2050	2040	2075	2060	2101	2080
2001	2001	2026	2021	2051	2041	2077	2061	2102	2081
2002	2002	2027	2022	2053	2042	2078	2062	2103	2082
2004	2003	2029	2023	2054	2043	2079	2063	2105	2083
2005	2004	2030	2024	2055	2044	2081	2064	2106	2084
2006	2005	2031	2025	2056	2045	2082	2065	2107	2085
2007	2006	2032	2026	2058	2046	2083	2066	2109	2086
2009	2007	2034	2027	2059	2047	2084	2067	2110	2087
2010	2008	2035	2028	2060	2048	2086	2068	2111	2088
2011	2009	2036	2029	2061	2049	2087	2069	2112	2089
2012	2010	2038	2030	2063	2050	2088	2070	2114	2090
2014	2011	2039	2031	2064	2051	2089	2071	2115	2091
2015	2012	2040	2032	2065	2052	2091	2072	2116	2092
2016	2013	2041	2033	2067	2053	2092	2073	2117	2093
2017	2014	2043	2034	2068	2054	2093	2074	2119	2094
2019	2015	2044	2035	2069	2055	2095	2075	2120	2095
2020	2016	2045	2036	2070	2056	2096	2076	2121	2096
2021	2017	2046	2037	2072	2057	2097	2077	2123	2097
2022	2018	2048	2038	2073	2058	2098	2078	2124	2098
2024	2019	2049	2039	2074	2059	2100	2079	2125	2099

NOTE: If an actual loss lies between any two adjacent figures in the "Actual Loss" column, the primary value shall be the primary value for the lower of the two figures.

TABLE 2
Manual Rates, Expected Loss Rates and D Ratios

MASSACHUSETTS—Experience Rating Plan Manual

State No. 20

Effective July 11, 1977

Code No.	Rate	Loss Rate	Ratio Std.	Code No.	Rate	Loss Rate	Ratio Std.	Code No.	Rate	Loss Rate	Ratio Std.	Code No.	Rate	Loss Rate	Ratio Std.
4024D	6.12	2.51	.59	4250	4.29	1.84	.51	4439	4.24	1.79	.49	4653	5.57	2.39	.47
4034	7.51	3.18	.57	4251	3.36	1.44	.53	†				4665	8.14	3.46	.53
4036	5.69	2.39	.49	4263	7.46	3.18	.52	4452	5.50	2.34	.57	4692	1.26	.55	.51
4038	2.91	1.23	.50	4273	4.92	2.10	.55	4459	4.52	1.90	.52	4693	2.31	.99	.54
4053	1.14	.50	.60	4279	3.54	1.51	.52	4470	4.04	1.73	.47	4710	3.85	1.65	.50
4061	3.43	1.46	.51	4283	6.41	2.72	.52	4479	2.14	.91	.71	4712	3.22	1.39	.48
4062	3.43	1.46	.51	4299	2.01	.86	.56	4484	4.76	2.03	.51	4720	3.55	1.50	.64
4111	3.54	1.53	.45	4301	3.66	1.56	.55	†				4730	3.54	1.49	.52
4112	.98	.42	.52	4304	1.82	.79	.53	4493	6.90	2.94	.52	4740	9.77	4.10	.49
4113	1.14	.50	.60	4307	2.92	1.23	.63	4511	.95	.41	.45	4741	13.50	5.73	.51
4130	3.89	1.65	.56	4308	.75	.33	.56	4557	2.91	1.24	.49	4761*	31.79	12.87	.42
4131	3.54	1.53	.45	4350	.98	.42	.63	4558	4.69	2.00	.52	4766*	9.07	3.67	.42
4133	1.93	.83	.56	4351	.84	.37	.50	4561	3.61	1.54	.53	4767*	7.69	3.21	.42
4150	1.23	.53	.56	4352	1.28	.55	.50	4581	8.42	3.54	.48	4770*	13.60	5.52	.42
4206	7.06	3.01	.46	4360	.63	.28	.55	4583	10.45	4.37	.50	4773*	31.79	12.87	.42
4207	7.06	3.01	.46	4361	.85	.37	.55	4597	3.85	1.65	.50	4774*	22.71	9.19	.42
4239	4.64	1.98	.53	4362	.49	.21	.52	4611	1.58	.67	.57	4775*	18.16	7.35	.42
4240	4.59	1.96	.54	4410	4.25	1.80	.63	4627	5.39	2.26	.65	4776*	27.26	11.04	.42
4243	4.67	1.99	.53	4417	6.13	2.62	.52	4628	1.58	.67	.57	4779*	22.71	9.19	.42
4244	7.46	3.18	.52	4432	1.51	.64	.63	4635	3.64	1.49	.45	4799*	49.99	20.23	.42

†Effective July 1, 1977

TABLE 3

W & B Values

MASSACHUSETTS—Experience Rating Plan Manual

State No. 20 **Issued July 11, 1977**

Expected Losses	W	B	Expected Losses	W	B	Expected Losses	W	B
25000 & Below	.00	20000	97100-101219	.18	16400	171260-175379	.36	12800
25001- 31179	.01	19800	101220-105339	.19	16200	175380-179499	.37	12600
31180- 35299	.02	19600	105340-109459	.20	16000	179500-183619	.38	12400
35300- 39419	.03	19400	109460-113579	.21	15800	183260-187739	.39	12200
39420- 43539	.04	19200	113580-117699	.22	15600	187740-191859	.40	12000
43540- 47659	.05	19000	117700-121819	.23	15400	191860-195979	.41	11800
47660- 51779	.06	18800	121820-125939	.24	15200	195980-200099	.42	11600
51780- 55899	.07	18600	125940-130059	.25	15000	200100-204219	.43	11400
55900- 60019	.08	18400	130060-134179	.26	14800	204220-208339	.44	11200
60020- 64139	.09	18200	134180-138299	.27	14600	208340-212459	.45	11000
64140- 68259	.10	18000	138300-142419	.28	14400	212460-216579	.46	10800
68260- 72379	.11	17800	142420-146539	.29	14200	216580-220699	.47	10600
72380- 76499	.12	17600	146540-150659	.30	14000	220700-224819	.48	10400
76500- 80619	.13	17400	150660-154779	.31	13800	224820-228939	.49	10200
80620- 84739	.14	17200	154780-158899	.32	13600	228940-233059	.50	10000
84740- 88859	.15	17000	158900-163019	.33	13400	233060-237179	.51	9800
88860- 92979	.16	16800	163020-167139	.34	13200	237180-241299	.52	9600
92980- 97099	.17	16600	167140-171259	.35	13000	241300-245419	.53	9400

(a) State Per Claim Accident Limitation $43,700
(b) State Multiple Claim Accident Limitation $87,400
(c) U.S. Longshoremen's and Harbor Workers' Act Per Claim Accident Limitation $46,000
(d) U.S. Longshoremen's and Harbor Workers' Act Multiple Claim Accident Limitation $92,000
(e) Employers' Liability Accident Limitation $55,000
   U. S. L. & H. W. Act—Expected Loss Factor—Non-F Classes 61.3% ★

COL (3). Audited Payrolls from statistical unit reportings.

COL (4) Expected Loss Rate (from Table II of the Experience Rating Plan) is defined as that part of the current manual rate necessary to pay losses. The rate is multiplied by the payrolls for the three year period to produce expected losses (Col 5) for the three year period.

COL (5) Expected losses—Payrolls × Expected Loss Rate = 100.

COL (6) D ratio (from Table II of the Experience Rating Plan) separates the expected losses into excess and primary losses, just as is done for actual losses.

Part III—Rating Procedure

1. Primary actual losses derived from exhibit of Actual Losses and Total Expected Losses.

2. B value (from Table III of the ERP) is a stabilizing factor which limits the swing of the modification from neutral.

3. W value (from Table III or the ERP) is a weighing factor which increases as the size of the risk increases. In the rating attached, the value of .02 is applied to actual excess losses of 747 and .98 of 16,072. Eventually, a point is reached where the large employer is experience-rated on his own experience.

Experience Modification Comparisons

The charts in Table 4 show the effect of the experience modification at different standard premium levels. The charts show the experience modifications, net premiums after stock company premium discount and the total range between premiums at the lowest and highest experience modifications indicated. In actual practice, experience modifications can be lower as well as higher than the illustrations.

It is clear that the experience modification is the most important single factor affecting the insured's workers' compensation premium.

Revising Experience Rating Calculations

Among the three reasons by which an experience rating calculation may be revised are: (1) in cases where loss values are included or excluded through mistake other than error in judgement; in other words, a clerical error; (2) where the claim is noncompensable; (3) where the employee collects workers compensation benefits but the insurance company subsequently recovers the benefits paid from a negligent third party.

TABLE 4

Experience Modification	Non-modified Premiums				
	5,000	10,000	15,000	20,000	
.80	3,716	7,184	10,596	14,000	Modified Premiums
.85	3,944	7,607	11,233	14,858	
.90	4,171	8,037	11,880	15,714	
.95	4,398	8,463	12,511	16,568	
1.00	4,625	8,890	13,155	17,420	
1.10	5,049	9,746	14,437	19,118	
1.20	5,478	10,956	15,714	20,832	
1.30	5,902	11,453	16,984	22,542	
1.40	6,328	12,306	18,270	24,248	
1.50	6,757	13,155	19,552	29,950	
RANGE	3,041	5,971	8,956	11,950	

Experience Modification	Non-modified Premiums				
	25,000	50,000	100,000	150,000	
.80	17,420	34,480	68,560	102,360	Modified Premiums
.85	18,487	36,592	72,845	108,630	
.90	19,552	38,745	77,130	115,020	
.95	20,615	40,897	81,415	121,267	
1.00	21,675	43,000	85,700	127,500	
1.10	23,815	47,300	94,050	140,085	
1.20	25,950	51,540	102,360	152,640	
1.30	28,080	55,835	110,760	165,165	
1.40	30,205	60,060	119,140	177,660	
1.50	32,362	64,350	127,500	190,350	
RANGE	14,942	29,870	58,940	87,990	

Factors Which Affect Experience Rating Modifications

The single most positive factor which affects experience rating modifications is an effective hazard control program. Quite simply, by keeping accident frequency to a minimum, the company will enjoy the benefits of lower workman's compensation rates. A second factor involves the willingness of the company to absorb certain costs, for example in-plant first aid or medical services. Thirdly is the company's cooperation in rehabilitating the injured worker. Fourth, the company's ability to demonstrate comprehensive preemployment medical services. Fifth, but certainly very important, is sensitivity to and concentrated effort to reduce loss by all members of the management team. In this regard, the experience modification may serve as a powerful tool for measuring the responsibility of those tasked with hazard control.

Conclusion

The experience rating plan is designed to stimulate an organization to take positive action to reduce losses and their associated costs. From the standpoint of dollars and cents, it can readily be seen that experience rating pays the employer a return for hazard controlled work practices. On the other hand, a financial penalty is imposed upon the policy holder who has an undue number of accidents. There is also a humanitarian factor which should not be overlooked. The effect of the rating plan is to secure a reduction in accidents, which means reduction in loss of life and limb, and of suffering on the part of the injured employee and his dependents. This is a very worthwhile result.

Note: Experience rating plan and tables may be obtained from: (1) your insurance company or (2) for a price from the National Council on Worker's Compensation Insurance, One Penn Plaza, New York, 10001. Acturarial technical type explanation of the experience rating plan can be found in Volume II pages 32–36 of the Supplemental Studies for the National Commission on State Workmen's Compensation Laws available through the Government printing office.

Special appreciation to the Workers' Compensation Rating and Inspection Bureau of Massachusetts for its contributions to this section.

Browning, R. L., "Estimating Loss Probabilities," Chemical Engineering, December, 1969.
Koontz, H., and O'Donnell, C., "Principles of Management," McGraw-Hill, 1968.
Martin, J. A., "Large Plant Safety Program Management," American Society of Safety Engineers Journal.

Bibliography

Mills, R., "Setting Up and Auditing a Corporate Safety Program," ASSE Journal, October, 1973.

Optner, S. L., "Systems Analysis for Business Management," Prentice-Hall, Inc., Englewood Cliffs, New Jersey, 1960.

Tarrants, W., "Management for Accident Control," Society of Safety Engineers Journal, February, 1972.

Terry, G. R., "Principles of Management," Fourth Edition, Richard D. Irwin, Inc., Homewood, Illinois, 1964.

Walton, E., "Communicating Down the Line: How They Really Got the Word," Personnel, July-August, 1959.

Weaver, D. A., "A Management Index of Safety Performance," American Society of Safety Engineers Journal, May, 1971.

Notes
1. Eugene Walton, "Communicating Down the Line: How They Really Get the Word," Personnel, July-August, 1959, pp. 78–82.
2. George R. Terry, "Principles of Management," Fourth Edition, 1964, Richard D. Irwin, Inc., Homewood, Illinois.
3. W. Tarrants, "Management for Accident Control," Society of Safety Engineers Journal, Feb. 1972.
4. W. Pope, "Authority and How to Make Use of It," SSM National Safety Management Society, 1973.

Special Note: Appreciation to Thomas Tuttle, Psycon, Inc. for his contribution to the checklists—Areas for Inquiry.

Hazard Identification and Evaluation 6

Introduction

Over the past decade we have witnessed the development of increasingly complex transportation, weapons, construction, production and numerous other systems which have been designed to better life in our society. Accompanying such progress are hazards having the capacity to induce situations with accident potential. In an effort to examine these systems in an orderly manner, to identify, evaluate, and reduce accident potential situations, several analytical techniques have been quite successfully developed and utilized. This chapter will discuss these analytical techniques in order to acquaint the reader with the purpose and utility of the methods, while at the same time demonstrating the use of these techniques in the actual problem solving process.

The systems engineering methods described in this chapter reflect those which have been accepted as most practical aids to analyze and improve the "safety" performance of a total system, while at the same time improving the acceptability of each of the systems' individual components. The systems engineering methods described represent an attempt to recognize events or conditions that have potential for negatively affecting system performance and which can lead to damage, injury, or other undesired outcomes such as facility loss, schedule interruption, and increased operational costs. The assumption underlying these methods is that once hazards are identified, resources can be mobilized to set forth the necessary corrective or preventive actions. The effectiveness of the methods is best judged in terms of their potential impact on management decision-making to improve the state of their systems. Simply stated, hazard analytical techniques are, in themselves, only tools used to assist management in making decisions for the right reasons, while understanding as much as possible the potentials for and impact of risk and loss situations.

These techniques are not cure-alls. They are not designed to produce miracles. They cannot think for the analyst. Their primary utility is: to force people to examine their systems in as thorough manner as is possible; ask the right questions—those which are important to locating problems which adversely effect the success of that systems operation; uncover problems of importance; evaluate a hazard's importance by virtue of an established hierarchy and recommend alternatives to rectify hazardous situations of high consequence.

A Shift in Tradition

Traditionally, work operations have been analyzed during the operational phase of their life cycles for potential failures capable of detracting from overall system effectiveness. Hazard analytical techniques applied during this phase of a systems' life cycle have returned substantial dividends in the form of reductions in both accidents and overall system losses. During the past decade, a shift has taken place. No longer are hazard control specialists concentrating their efforts solely on operations but instead are taking a hard look at the systems for which they are accountable back at their conceptual and design stages. They are using analytical methods and techniques before accidents happen to identify and judge the evident nature and ramifications of hazards associated with their systems. The results of this widening of the assessment effort has, in many instances, significantly altered the direction of some hazard control efforts, due to the realization that finding potential failures in a system prior to the production or process stages can be most beneficial on a cost-effectiveness basis to say nothing of the injuries, deaths, and damage which can be avoided.

Hazard Analysis— An Evolutionary Process

Hazard analytical techniques are not in themselves revolutionary. Instead, such techniques have been born out of an ever-increasing demand for more precise methods for uncovering and assessing hazards over a long period of time. Among the supportive factors behind this evolutionary process is the fact that (1) the high costs associated with accidents necessitate a hard look at operations to do whatever is possible to reduce such economic losses; (2) the ever-increasing complexity of today's production, construction, and other processes have created situations which cannot any longer be informally "eyeballed" to locate key systems failures. The sophistication of system components, the interaction among these components, and the potentials for excessive loss have necessitated a more precise approach; (3) the increasingly intolerance of failures and accidents voiced by society. We can see examples of this demonstrated by recent citizens committees who scrutinize the potential risk of the use of nuclear energy, as well as the risk associated with the products they use at home, work, and recreation. Product liability, as a current issue, will be discussed in chapter 10. It will suffice here to say that today's consumer is no longer willing to accept products which contain hazards capable of causing harm, when such hazards can be recognized and eliminated, or at least reduced to acceptable levels.

The hazard control specialist must keep abreast of current hazard assessment techniques in order to maximize the service for which he or she was hired. While it is not always necessary for hazard control personnel be thoroughly familiar with all the intricate mathematics and engineering methods which usually accompany analytical processes, they nevertheless must be knowledgeable of the basic methods and objectives of these methods, as well as how they can be used to assist in fulfilling the organization's hazard control mission.

The Role of the Hazard Control Specialist in Risk Assessment

The idea of analyzing a problem or situation to extract data for decision-making is not new and, in reality, most data from an analysis never is recorded on paper. The fact of the matter is that good production, construction, and other workers are always, sometimes unconsciously, making assessments. The results of these guide their actions on a day-to-day basis. While such informal analysis and the resultant actions based on such inquiry are critical to progress, at times it is beneficial to record the results of such mental activity on paper. Written analysis, prepared when necessary, will serve as the basis for communicating hazard and risk potential data to those in command positions. Furthermore, written hazard analyses serve as the basis of more thorough inspection activity, as well as education of people in the line and staff organization to the ramifications of hazards existing within their operations, and the purpose and logic behind established control measures. Organizational leaders may wish to require that formal written analyses be prepared for each of their critical operations. In so doing, not only can they benefit from the information immediately but can, in addition, reap benefits over the long run. Once important hazard data are committed to paper, they become part of the organization's formal documentation. Regardless of whether line personnel or perhaps even the hazard control specialist leave the organization, sufficient data is left behind for those who will succeed them.

The Essence of Systems Analysis

Systems analysis had its antecedence in the military operations analysis of 1939–45. However, operations analysis differed from the longer-range problem solving of "systems analysis" and concerned itself mainly with "tactical" problems that involved the immediate use of equipment in operations, primarily a function of effective utilization.[1] Systems methods came into their own in the aerospace industry, when it was realized that time-honored production evaluation was no longer practical. As a result of this shift in thinking, various systems methods were employed to increase reliability and safety of the developing man-machine systems. Soon after, the Department of Defense promulgated military specifications which require the application of systems

Systems Analysis In Retrospect

safety as an integral part of contract terms. Military Standard 882—"Requirements for System Safety Program for Systems and Associated Subsystems and Equipment"—July 15, 1969, is an example of such a specification. It was put forth mainly to conserve resources, force the contractor to produce failure data prior to system development, and prevent injury to the public and government personnel. Systems engineering initially was concerned with activities that were effectiveness-oriented rather than profit-oriented. However, if properly applied, it can define profitable solutions to many of top management's most concerning operational problems.

Understanding the Terminology

System

Before we launch into a discussion of various systems methods, an examination of several terms will be useful. To begin with, let us examine the phenomenon of *"system"* from the standpoint of what it is, what it does, and where it does it. A "system" is defined in different ways. For example, Fitts (1969) defines *a system as "an assemblage of elements that are engaged in the accomplishment of some common purpose(s), and are tied together by a common information flow network, the output of the system being a function not only of the characteristics of the elements but of their interaction or interrelationships."*[2] *"Interaction,"* as considered in the pages to follow, *is the effect of one variable acting on another. It can also be defined as the effect produced by either variable acting alone."* Once we speak of interaction we admit nonindependent systems failure—that is, failure which occurs from the combined effects of one or more system variables. Hall (1962) considers a system to be a set of objects with relationships between the objects and their attributes.[3] Miller (1954), in a more behavioral vein, describes a system of consisting of machines and men plus the process by which they interact within an environment.[4] Shapero and Bates (1956) describe their system concept in terms of what they call systems components consisting of mechanisms (equipment), human operational components (personnel), facilities (installations), and integrators.[5]

The Department of Defense, in its Military Systems Safety Standard 882 defines "system" as *"a composite of operational and support equipment, personnel, and facilities, that forms an entity capable of supporting an operational role within a given environment."* Implied in this definition is worker-machine interaction which refines our broad system definition to a specific man-machine system. While these definitions seem somewhat less than uniform, they do share certain commonalities. Among these:

1. Systems are deterministic entities having a purpose. They consist of an interacting set of discrete elements (parts and subsystems) that influence each other. Interaction in this sense, implies nonindependent failure of elements.

2. Machines are required to achieve system goals.
3. Both people and equipment are required for system operation.
4. The worker-machine relationship is directed toward an object or a purpose.
5. The system has both an internal and an external environment.

In summary, a system is characterized by some purpose, it is directional; second, it exists for a reason; third, it consists of an interacting set of discrete variables (human, physical, environmental).

With reliable hazard data, the hazard control specialist is able to generate necessary control required to keep the system on course, consequently enabling it to reach its designed objectives.

In order to assist the reader in conceiving the relationship of a system to its components, the following example is listed. Think of the family automobile as the parent system. With this as a given, then, the steering mechanism can be considered as a major subsystem of the entire automobile; the tie rods would qualify as components of the system; and the tie rods ends would be referred to as parts—the smallest unit of a system.

A question which constantly arises deals with the issue of what a "safe" system is—indeed, if such a phenomenon can ever really exist. Although there are many views on this subject, one definition, one which the work in this chapter will address itself, is offered for consideration. *A safe system may be conceived as one in which the likelihood of occurrance of all identifiable hazards are maintained at an acceptable level.* This definition offers some key points for discussion. To begin with, "all identifiable hazards" connotes, perhaps, some limitations of man. Limitations of knowledge, experience, or perhaps limitations in comprehending the ramifications of hazard control advancements. Secondly, the definition speaks of "acceptable level." In such wording, this definition admits to less than totally successful—one hundred percent efficient and effective—operations. Instead, the definition concedes the probability of accidents occurring in a system despite all efforts to counter them. On behalf of the hazard control specialist and his or her management, agreement with this definition expresses a sign of maturity—the ability to accept uncertainty—in that, if the full thrust of an organization's hazard control effort is trained on eliminating or at least reducing the destructive potential of the significant hazards in a system, then, perhaps, such an organization can live with problems which are less of a threat to its mission.

Analysis

Having defined "system" our next job is to examine *"analysis."* Once again, we find numerous suggested encapsulations.

A definition, offered by Quade, (1968) is *"a systematic approach to helping a decision-maker choose a course of action by investigating his total problem, searching out objectives and alternatives, and comparing them in the light of their consequences, using an appropriate framework—insofar as possible analytic—to bring expert judgment and intuition to bear on the problem.''*[6]

Haasl, (1969) defines analysis as being a *"directed process for the orderly acquisition of specific information (failure data) pertinent to a given system.''*[7]

Haasl's definition is basic to all analysis insofar as it uncovers two important elements: (1) it is a directed process which portrays a methodical, careful, purposeful process; (2) its purpose is to acquire specific information; in the context of Systems Safety: the information specifically germane to those failures which have adverse affect upon the system under analysis.

The true purpose of analysis is simply to provide data for informed management decisions. We in effect, will attempt to locate hazardous situations occurring in operations intent on identifying the most probable and/or the most severe hazards in order to arrive at a system which, in addition to being safe, will meet such requirements as performance, reliability, and cost. The underlying purpose of hazard analysis, then is to assist the hazard control specialist in maximizing time and effort in locating and correcting the vital few problems of importance, while leaving behind many of the trivial problems to be attended to at a later date.

A thought provided by Eddie Rickenbacker on safety and safe systems will serve to tie together many of the points already made. Rickenbacker stated, that he "never liked to use the word 'safe' in in connection with either Eastern Air Lines or the entire transportation field. Instead, he preferred the word 'reliable.' For as Rickenbacker saw it, whenever motion is involved there can be no condition of absolute safety. The only time man is safe is when he is completely static, in a box underground. With motion comes the inexorable possibility of accidents.[8] The hazard control specialist, due to the nature of the job he or she is hired for, might appreciate Captain Eddie's remarks, if only because the best made-plans and best-executed programs for hazard control will remain subject to unpredictable events. This is the price we pay for progress. But looking at this problem from a positive standpoint, if we can make the fullest use of what we have to work with, perhaps then, we stand a better chance of keeping the systems under our jurisdiction within tolerable levels of safety.

Acquiring Hazard Data

Although the primary emphasis of this chapter is the acquisition of hazard information through the analysis process, a few moments spent on reviewing other ways that the analyst may obtain hazard data may be worthwhile.

As we learned in chapter 4, when attempts are made to acquire information pertaining to any given subject, several alternatives exist. To begin with, we may obtain information directly from those in our own organization or from those in other organizations like ours—relying on their *direct experience* with a specific method, problem, etc. Information acquired as a result of direct past experience is said to be most desirable, providing that the information is reliable. Indeed, to find out exactly how an operation or part of an operation would fail, the most reliable information would come from the people who have worked with that system, who understand all its complexities, and who have either discovered and corrected problems themselves or who were part of group problem-solving and decision-making.

Among the sources of experiential information available to the hazard control specialist are line supervisors and workers, accident report data, inspection information, insurance company audits and studies, manufacturers information and so on.

Although direct past experience is desirable, it is not always available, especially when information is wanted either on a system in design, or one that has not been used long enough to have data on its inherent hazards become known. An example of this situation happened when a chemical company began processing a new substance. During the process, a toxic vapor was produced which affected the workers working with the process very much the same way as if they had consumed a fifth of alcohol within a four hour period. The company became aware of the problem only after one of its most experienced chemists was arrested on his way home from work on a charge of driving while intoxicated. Until this situation occurred, the company was satisfied that they had taken all necessary precautions to assure that the workers would be "safe" during the work process. The company based its hazard control measures on hazard data that they had accumulated from those who had worked on other chemical processes which required the use of similar materials. As it turned out, the control measures which worked successfully on the former projects, were inadequate to meet the hazard demands of the new one. The precise mix of materials in the current process produced, through a synergistic effect, an airborne toxic vapor problem which existing control measures were not designed to control properly.

Because direct experience is not always available, a second alternative is often chosen—acquiring information from those with *related experience.* When people who have worked on projects exactly like your own are not available, then you need to look for those who have had related experience with projects or processes similar to the one of concern. Of course, related experience information has drawbacks. As we noted above, it may not be as sufficiently relevant as one would like. However, even such less than precise information may serve well in helping to frame out a problem area or set directions for continued inquiry.

Thirdly, hazard data may be acquired from *testing.* When neither direct or related experience is available, another alternative is to "test-out" the system to see how it behaves and where the pitfalls lie. Testing can take on one of two objectives. First, testing can be conducted to experiment, that is to learn what happened to the item under test, as it passes through many simulated real-world conditions. In this case we are essentially saying: now that we built it, what possible things can happen, while it is being used, which can cause problems? Secondly, testing can be utilized as a verification method. In this instance, we are reasonably sure of the items' capabilities and limitations and resort to test to "prove" that our ideas are correct. There will be times when the hazard control specialist becomes involved with the test of a particular operation or method. Then, he or she must be familiar with the limitations of testing and test data. To begin with, testing may not be economically, physically, or politically feasible. Secondly, testing is expensive in both time and dollars. Thirdly, and perhaps the most serious limitation of all, it may not be possible to imagine and simulate all the possible failure modes to which the item or system under test will be subjected during actual operation. It will suffice here to say that test data serves a valuable purpose, and when used judicially will provide an extra dimension of knowledge to hazard control decisions. However, one must be certain to use test data with a full knowledge of its capabilities and limitations.

The fourth method of information acquisition relies on the process of *analysis*. An orderly process to acquire specific information (hazard and failure data) pertinent to a given system.

Why Analysis?   Perhaps the primary motive behind any hazard analytical process is the fact that the method, to a great extent, can foster decisions which have a higher probability of having things work out right for the right reasons. In addition, analysis forces us to ask many of the right questions and assists us in attempting to answer them.

When Analysis?   It is not the intent of this chapter to suggest that all operations need to be evaluated via formal written analyses. The fact is that in many instances such sophistication is unnecessary and perhaps not cost-effective. On the other hand, there are instances when consideration should be given to the formal methodology. Among these occasions are:

1. When we don't know any of the hazards associated with a particular job.
2. When we anticipate potential problems which have severe consequences on an operation.
3. When we are finding repeated problems of damage, delay, injuries, fatalities in an operation.
4. When ground rules for safety must be established before a job begins.
5. When hazard information must be communicated accurately and when reliance is placed on others to understand the necessity for and purpose behind specific safety procedures and/or hazard controls.

Consistent with our outline, methods of acquiring information will be divided into two broad categories—*informal* and *formal*. Although the formal analytical methods are the ones which will be explored in some detail in this chapter, it may be worthwhile to briefly discuss two of the popular informat approaches.

Broad Categories of Information Acquisition

Intuition

The Informal Methods

Intuitive decisions, as will be explained later, differ from those made from either the inductive or deductive process. Instead of proceeding logically, a step at a time, intuition provides an instantaneous perceptual insight into a problem. It may be extrasensory in nature—a decision coming in a flash of light—happening so fast that the decision-maker is unaware that the process is taking place. Although intuitive decisions have advantages under certain circumstances, they will not receive attention here. Primarily because few people possess intuitive ability, decisions coming out of the intuitive process cannot be relied on consistently to take evasive actions when it comes to hazard reduction. Furthermore, if an intuitive decision is erroneous, it may have a profound catastrophic effect on the attainment of a mission.

Conjecture

Conjecture is another informal method of acquiring information. With this method, the decision-maker finds himself taking guesses or predicting outcomes of situations from incomplete or uncertain data. If there has ever been a time in the history of hazard control in this country when we cannot be guessing, especially when an incorrect guess could be the very trigger of catastrophic situations, where death, injuries and illnesses may occur, and damage and other losses may be sustained. Now is the time.

Formal Analysis

The Formal Methods

Formal hazard analytical methods may be divided into two broad categories for ease of discussion—those that are of the inductive variety and those classified as deductive.

Inductive Method

The inductive analytical process is based on prediction from observable data. Such a process involves postulating a possible state of existence of the component parts of a system, and then determining the effect of these component parts on the overall success of the system of which they are a part. Simply stated, inductive analysis tells us *what can happen,* not how problems are caused. Inductive analysis forms the basis for what is called the ''single thread

Component	Component Failure Mode	System Operating State	Effect of Component Failure on System
Fuse	Detonates During Assembly	While Being Threaded into Round	Detonation System Destroyed

Figure 42. Single—thread analysis.

analysis'' (Figure 42)—method that considers the effects of failures on a system's operation from the standpoint of its components, their failure in a particular operating state, and finally, the effect of the component failure on the system. Examples of single-thread analyses will be illustrated when Preliminary Hazard Analysis, Failure-Mode Effect Analysis, Systems Hazard Analysis, Construction Hazard Analysis, and Product Hazard Analysis are discussed.

Deductive Method

Deductive analysis involves postulating a possible failure state of the overall system and identifying those component states that may contribute to its occurrence. Unlike inductive analysis the deductive approach tells us how undesired events can occur. The combined events analyses depicted by the ''Fault-Tree'' are illustrative of deductive analysis.

Factors Which Determine the Type of Analysis That Is Best for a Given Situation

Among the most important factors which will determine which analytical approach is best for a given situation, the hazard control specialist must consider the following:

1. How much and what quality information is desired?
2. The information which is already available.
3. The cost of setting-up and conducting the analyses.
4. The amount of time available before decisions must be made and actions must be taken.
5. The availability of people to assist in the hazard analysis process.

Types of Inductive Analyses

Preliminary Hazard Analysis

A preliminary hazard analysis (PHA) Figure 43, is a qualitative study conducted during the conceptual or early development phase of a systems life, which has as its objective: to identify hazardous conditions, and potential failures which are evident or which could develop during operations; to determine their potential effect; and to establish initial design and procedural re-

Part I

Subsystem or Function	Mode	Hazardous Element	Event Causing Hazardous Condition	Hazardous Condition	Potential Accident
Drill press	Drilling holes in casting	Chuck and drill	Operating drill press	Proximity of worker to rotating chuck and drill	1. Catching clothing and hair around rotating parts 2. Drill failure 3. Casting coming loose from clamp
	Inspect and set-up press	Key-jig-drill	Operating drill press	Damaged or broken chuck	Chuck coming apart and striking worker
				Key left in chuck with chuck revolving	Key flying out of chuck and striking worker
				Worker exposed to rotating parts of machine	

Part II

Effect	Hazard Classification	Accident Prevention Measures		
		Hardware	Procedures	Personnel
Injury Delay Damage	III	Point of operation guard Chip breaker	Inspection of drills prior to and after use	Head covering Snug fitting clothing Avoid wearing rings, bracelets, etc. Face protection
Injury Interrupt production Equipment damage	III	Use self-rejecting keys	Tag-out defective equipment	Safety glasses or face shields Stopping machine before making adjustments

Figure 43. Preliminary hazard Analysis.

quirements to eliminate or control these identified hazardous conditions and potential accidents. Figure 44 illustrates a PHA utilized by the Navy Department in their quest for control of hazards in weapon system manufacture.

The PHA is normally used during the initial assessment of the design concept. This analysis identifies the known source of hazards, such as radiation sources, toxic materials, electrical energy, etc., specifying where each will occur in the system, and provides recommendations for control of the hazard. The primary purpose of the PHA is to develop a data bank of safety design requirements specific to a given system. It serves to verify the practicability, from a hazard control aspect, of the design concept, and is useful for follow-up, to ensure that all hazards recognized at earliest stages are eliminated or controlled to an acceptable level. The completed PHA provides baseline information for all future hazard analyses to be conducted on the same process line (or system) and, therefore, must be updated as required to remain current with line development.

PROGRAM **PG/ARM-1**
SYSTEM **ARM-1 Missile**
SUBSYSTEM **ARM-1 Warhead Design**
REVISION _____ REV. DATE _____

PRELIMINARY HAZARD ANALYSIS
(PHA)*

COMPLETED BY _____
DATE STARTED _____
DATE COMPLETED _____
PAGE ____ OF ____ PAGES

ITEM NO.	NOMENCLATURE AND PART NO.	OPERATING MODE 3 **	FAILURE MODE 4 ***	ESTIMATED PROBABILITY 5 ****	FAILURE EFFECTS 6	HAZARD DESCRIPTION 7	HAZARD CAT. 8	RECOMMENDED CONTROL 9	AMPLIFYING REMARKS (INCLUDE VERIFICATION) 10
1	Warhead explosive	All	(1) Shock (2) Friction (3) Heat (4) Incompatible materials	(1) High (2) Low (3) High (4) Unk	(1) Cracking powerizing (2) Localized heating (3) Melting, exudation (4) Chemical reaction	(1), (2), (3), (4) Detonation, deflagration, burning of explosive prior to safe separation from launch vessel	IV	a. Qualify explosive for service application b. Examine all materials for chemical compatibility c. Use only Navy approved explosives for intended application d. Design smooth interfaces between explosive and adjacent parts	Main charge warhead explosives must be compatible with intended weapon application. Use of sensitive primary explosives is forbidden - use of secondary (booster) explosives for main charge applications is highly hazardous. OD-44811 provides qualification procedures and testing for non-service approved explosives.
2	Warhead/fuze booster explosive	All	See: 1-4 (1) 1-4 (2) 1-4 (3) 1-4 (4)	See: 1-5 (1) 1-5 (2) 1-5 (3) 1-5 (4)	See: 1-6 (1) 1-6 (2) 1-6 (3) 1-6 (4)	See: 1-7	IV	See: 1-9a, 1-9d 1-9b 1-9c	Booster explosive must be critically examined for its intended application. If main charge does not require boosting to achieve detonation its shock sensitivity is suspect.
3	Warhead safety and arming device S&A	All uncontainerized handling of "safe" device	Detonator and lead initiation	Low	Damage to and loss of S&A device	Blast, burn and fragment dispersion hazards to personnel	III	Design S&A to: (1) Use small quantity of explosive, (2) Provide for internal dissipation of explosive initiation effects.	A properly designed S&A device will present no explosive hazard to personnel during handling.

*THIS FORM MAY ALSO BE USED TO DOCUMENT THE INITIAL SSHA AND SHA

**INCLUDES LOGISTIC PHASES

***FAILURE MODE INCLUDES EFFECTS OF HUMAN ERROR, NORMAL AND ABNORMAL ENVIRONMENTS, DESIGN DEFICIENCIES, INCOMPATIBILITY

****ENTER ONE OF THE FOLLOWING:

- LOW – LOW OR REMOTE PROBABILITY
- MEDIUM – APPROXIMATELY 0.001 TO 0.0001 PROBABILITY
- HIGH – GREATER THAN 0.001 PROBABILITY
- UNK – UNKNOWN PROBABILITY

Figure 44. Sample PHA worksheet (Sheet 1 of 8)

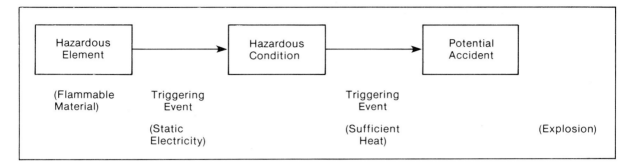

Figure 45.

Using checklists and applicable experience with, or knowledge of, the system hazardous elements, conditions, potential accidents, and their effects can be predicted, and accident prevention or reduction methods can be systematically developed.

In filling out the columnar PHA form the dynamic relationship between the entries should be kept in mind. This relationship between the entries is illustrated in Figure 45. The hazardous element (i.e., flammable material) nust be acted upon or be influenced by some (discrete) event or condition (i.e., static electricity) in order for it to become a hazardous condition. Then when the hazardous condition exists, it must be acted upon by some event or condition in order for it to result in the potential accident (i.e., sufficient heat).

Hazardous Element—That part having natural properties which make it inherently hazardous.

Hazardous Condition—Those circumstances under which the hazardous element is placed in a situation where an accident is much more probable.

Potential Accident—Any undesired event which could possibly result from the previous set of circumstances.

When to Use a Preliminary Hazard Analysis

The following are offered as guides to the selection and use of the PHA:

1. When we have insufficient information concerning the basic elements in a system which have accident potential.
2. Before designs are frozen.
3. Before decisions are made and actions taken to establish hazard controls.

The Results of PHA

In summary, Preliminary Hazard Analyses will assist in the definition of requirements for accident prevention; identification of hazards for which accident prevention methods are inadequate; identification of hazards for which further testing or analysis may be necessary; and finally, personnel requirements for training, etc.

Severity Grading Analyses

This class of analyses includes the Failure-Mode and Effect analysis (FMEA), Failure-Mode, Effect and Criticality Analysis (FMECA), systems hazard analysis (SHA), task analysis, and a host of variations of these analytical methods.

When Severity Grading Analysis?   The many types of hazard analyses which come under the category of severity grading analyses have one basic thing in common—each is chosen for use after preliminary decisions about the systems hazardous elements have been made, when we don't know which failures in a system will cause the most severe damage or injury and when the interrelationships between the elements of the system can be identified.

1. *Failure-Mode and Effect Analysis (FMEA)*—The Failure-Mode and Effect Analysis is both a system safety as well as a reliability analysis used to identify the critical failure modes having a serious effect on the safe and successful life of the system. This analytical technique also permits system changes, in order to reduce the severity of failure effects.

The analysis consists of a critical review of the system, coupled with a systematic examination of all conceivable failures and an evaluation of the effects of these failures on the mission capability of the system. A level of resolution must be specified with the FMEA, as it must with other severity grading and combined events analyses, and must remain consistent throughout the analysis. If time permits, the analysis should be performed at the lowest system element level when failure modes can be identified.

Throughout this analysis the analyst asks how the assumed functional failure can occur, what is the root cause, what are the effects of the failure on adjoining functions and on the system output, what is the failure or hazard category, and how can the failure mode be removed or its effects made less severe. Failure information is listed using the columnar format illustrated in Figure 46, an FMEA conducted on the hot water system is illustrated in Figure 47.

The output of the FMEA will be a listing of failure modes for each critical component, and the corresponding failure causes, along with further designation of the failures which will have unacceptable effects on the overall system performance. Thus the method yields relative hazard severity levels, and other qualitative information useful in management decisions. However, it does not provide absolute probabilistic information or relative hazard frequency levels. Further, as normally used, FMEA concentrates on system components rather than system linkages, which account for a larger number of system failures.[9]

A final limitation of the method is that it concentrates on the hardware components of the system and does not adequately deal with the question of

Component	Failure or Error Mode	Effects on Other Components	Effects on Whole System	Hazard class 1	2	3	4	Failure Frequency	Detection Methods	Compensating Provisions and Remarks
Pressure relief valve	Jammed open	Increased operation of temperature sensing, controller, and gas flow due to hot water loss	Loss of hot water, greater cold water input, and greater gas consumption	x				Reasonably probable	Observe at pressure-relief valve	Shut off water supply, reseat or replace relief valve
	Jammed closed	None	None	x				Probable	Manual testing	Unless combined w/other component failure, this failure has no consequence
Gas valve	Jammed open	Burner continues to operate. Pressure-relief valve opens	Water temperature and pressure increase. Water→steam			x		Reasonably probable	Water at faucet too hot. Pressure-relief valve open (observation)	Open hot water faucet to relieve pressure. Shut off gas supply. Pressure-relief valve compensates
	Jammed closed	Burner ceases to operate	System fails to produce hot water	x				Remote	Observe at output (water temperature too low)	
Temperature measuring and comparing device	Fails to react to temperature rise above preset level	Controller, gas valve, burner continue to function "on." Pressure-relief valve opens	Water temperature too high. Water→steam			x		Remote	Observe at output (faucet)	Pressure-relief valve compensates Open hot water faucet to relieve pressure. Shut off gas supply
	Fails to react to temperature drop below preset level	Controller, gas valve, burner continue to function "off"	Water temperature too low	x				Remote	Observe at output (faucet)	
Flue	Blocked	Incomplete combustion at burner	Inefficiency. Production of toxic gasses			x		Remote	Possibly smell products of incomplete combustion	No compensation built in. Shut down system
Pressure-relief valve and gas valve	Jammed closed Jammed open	Burner continues to operate, pressure increases	Increased pressure cannot bleed at relief valve Water→steam If pressure cannot back up cold water inlet, system may rupture violently			x		Probable + reasonably probable = reasonably probable	Manual testing of relief valve. Observe water output (temperature too high)	Open hot water faucet. Shut off gas supply. Pressure might be able to back up into cold water supply, providing pressure in supply is not greater than failure pressure of system

Figure 46. Sample FMEA Form (National Safety News, 1966).

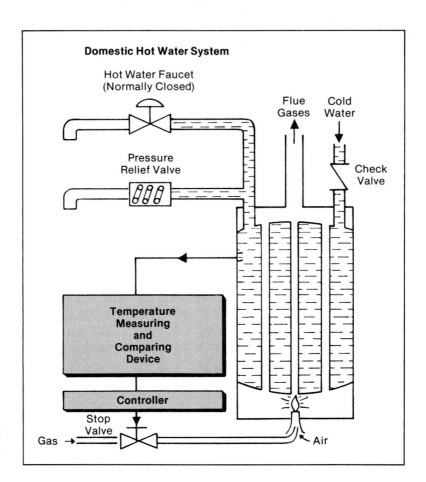

Figure 47. Domestic hot
water system (Courtesy of
J. L. Recht, National Safety Council).

human error. The FMEA is best suited in assessing those failures which have single or a small number of causes rather than failures resulting from a large number of interacting factors, as is the case with human error. The FMEA in Figure 48 illustrates the utilization of the hazard analytical technique to analyze the limitations of a respiratory device in order to make recommendations for system upgrading.

2. *Failure-Mode Effect and Criticality Analysis*—(FMECA—The Failure-Mode Effect and Criticality Analysis is a type of FMEA used to determine probable, reasonably probable, critical, and catastrophic failures. The method also provides clues for modifying the system so as to reduce the failure frequencies or to offset the consequences of these failures (Figure 49).

This type of analysis permits quantification of the FMEA by bringing into consideration quantitative failure frequency information. If the effects' criticalities are given, weight factors and combining these factors with failure probabilities, a relative criticality ranking is possible. Thus the decision-maker is provided with a priority list for eliminating failure modes of high-risk

System: Self-contained Breathing Apparatus

Component Identification	Function	Failure Mode	Failure Effect	Failure Detection	Corrective Action	Crit.*	Remarks
I. Harness and Back Plate Assembly	n/a	n/a	n/a	n/a	n/a		
A. Waist Back	n/a	n/a	n/a	n/a	n/a		
1. Metal and Plastic Plate	Rigid support of waist belt	Non-flex for long life	Waist belt comes apart	Visual inspection before and after each use for fatigue cracks	Select material with greater flex life	2	This failure will cause mission to abort. Possible cut to user from jagged edge. A substitute material for metal may be used as replacement.
2. Grommet at end of waist belt	Holds front connecting belt to metal and plastic plate	Comes apart	same	none	Design new	2	Will cause mission to abort.
3. Valve end release spring	Releases cylinder when pushed in	Plastic cover comes off after a few users	Leaves exposed sharp edges	Looseness of component	Re-fit or bond plastic to metal	3	These will come off and be easily lost, which causes a replacement problem.
4. Top cylinder bracket	Holds top of cylinder in harness	Slips loose from vibration	Leaves pressure vessel unstable	Comes loose	Provide a positive vertical location on frame for locking in correct position	3	Cylinder replacement will be faster. Will provide a no-fail, positive locking position.
5. Mid-Back Plate	Mounting for high pressure regulator	Sharp top edge	Cuts cylinder when mounting or dismounting. Potential danger to fibers	Visible wear on vessel	Needs radius surface	3	Could weaken cylinder over long use. Also destroys instruction markings on cylinder.
6. Lower back frame standoff	Mount lock for lower cylinder 2½" distance from belt to outer frame	n/a	n/a	n/a	Reduces distance by 1"	3	Makes cylinder stick out too far—reduces function in tight places (windows, attics, fire escapes, etc.).

Figure 48. Failure mode and effects analysis.

Figure 48. *Continued.*

Component Identification	Function	Failure Mode	Failure Effect	Failure Detection	Corrective Action	Crit*	Remarks
II. Demand Regulator Assembly							
A. Gasket	seal	can come off	will cause inhalation of toxic gases	visual or physical detection through inhalation	Bond gasket to regulator assembly	1	No seal could get someone into trouble. It would cause mission to abort.
B. Pressure gauge on cylinder and regulator	To provide notification of cylinder pressure and a choise that regulator is functioning properly	Regulator pressure gauge may not indicate leak between cylinder and regulator	Potential loss of air supply	Visual detection	Provide quantitative readings on regulator game to coincide with that of cylinder	3	Visual check of regulator's ability to function may not indicate small leak due to amount of variance that is built into a dichotomous gauge.
III. Face Piece Assembly							
A. Straps							
1. Lock Washer (strap retainer to face piece)	Holds strap to face piece	Retainer pops off—lets strap come loose	Makes face piece unusable	Comes off	Design a new, stronger retainer washer	2	Will cause mission to abort.

*Hazard Classification

1—injury
2—cause mission to be aborted
3—nuisance

Program ___XSAM-X___

System ___Surface Missile System___

Subsystem ___Missile System___

Revision ___ Rev. Date ___

Failure Mode Effects and Criticality Analysis

(FMECA)

Engineer ___J. Doe___

Date started ___

Date completed ___

Page ___ of ___ Pages

Item Identification				Failure Mode and Cause			Failure Mode Effects				Criticality Evaluation		
Name	Drawing Part No.	Generic Failure Rate ( ) (per 10^6 Hr.)	Function	Failure Mode and Cause	Prob. of Occur ( ) (per 10^6 Hr.)	Mission Phase	Component or Functional Assembly	Subsystem	Mission or System	Hazard	Prob. of Failure Mode Effects	Probability of Critical Effects (Col. 6 X Col. 12)	Remarks or Recommended Actions
1	2	3	4	5	6	7	8	9	10	11	12	13	14
Propellant Case	0000	0.4×10^{-5}	Serves as container for propellant during handling, transportation, storage and firing	Case cracked (exposed to sub-zero temperatures for extended period of time)	0.25×10^{-6}	Stored on the pier to await loading aboard ship	Propellant will rupture case due to weakening	Propulsion subsystem will cause damage and lack of control of the missile	Missile will cause damage to equipment and possible injury or death	IV	.5	0.125×10^{-6}	Design investigation recommended to increase stability of material of case at low temperatures

Figure 49. FMECA worksheet, completed (Naval Ordnance Systems Command; 1974).

nature. The FMECA is conducted by first describing the system in terms of functional block diagrams showing each critical function which makes up the overall system. Secondly, consideration is given to each possible failure of every critical function by listing all failure modes for each. Thirdly, a determination is made of the root cause for the failure. Finally, an assessment is made of the effects of the failure on adjoining functions and on the system output. At this stage in the analysis, the analyst can pursue either quantitative or qualitative approach, as the adequacy of accumulated data permits. Quantification occurs through the use of failure probabilities which are numerical values for the likelihood that the assumed failure mode will be experienced. Failure probabilities can be expressed as mean time between failures or failures per operating period. Qualitatively one can express failure probabilities in terms of general ranges:

1. Probable—one failure in less than 10,000 hours of operation.
2. Reasonably probable—one failure in 10,000 to 100,000 hours of operation.
3. Remote—one failure in 100,000 to 10,000,000 hours of operation.
4. Extremely remote—one failure in more than 10,000,000 hours of operation.

Before the analysis is completed, a determination if made as to the most practicable and effective means of limiting the severity of the hazard's potential effects.

The output from a FMECA will provide a listing of failure modes for each critical function, along with the corresponding failure causes, the detection and control measure that are required for each failure mode, and the hazard criticality rankings of the hazards.

Since the Failure Mode Effect and Criticality Analysis is simply an expanded FMEA, the criticisms of the FMEA presented above still apply (e.g.: treatment of human errors problems).

Systems Hazard Analysis (SHA)   Systems Hazard Analysis (SHA) combines some of the characteristics of the Preliminary Hazard Analysis and Failure-Mode Effect Analysis with provisions for considering work tasks which correspond to operational procedures. The basis behind the approach is that failures (undesired events) may be eliminated by systematically tracing through a system for hazards that may culminate in the failure situation. Table 5 (Table of Undesired Events) lists typical undesired events found in a given system that are considered potentially injurious or even catastrophic to the system's operation. These events may be responsible for accidents and system failures.

TABLE 5

Undesired Events
Fire
Explosion
Detonation
Release of toxic material
Injury to man
Death of man
Interruption of production
Loss of production equipment
Loss of production facilities
Release of pollutants

Criteria for Analysis   Many systems are similar in that their components, processes, man/machine interfaces, environment, and mission lend themselves to analysis by virtue of preestablished criteria. As a result, special criteria sheets designed to cover general hazardous elements have been developed (See Tables 6, 7, and 8). While some elements in these criteria sheets may be used to analyze other systems, special ones should be developed for the specialized needs of the particular system under analysis. It should be stressed that the invention and use of new hardware, procedures, etc., may produce new hazardous elements requiring expanded and up-dated checklists. The primary purpose of the checklists is to discipline thinking while the attempt is made to ferret out hazards in each step of the operation.

It is not intended, nor is it even suggested, that the checklists cover all possible hazardous elements. They do, however, provide guideposts around which more specific inquiry may be made and relationships drawn. In the selection of criteria to aid in analysis, care must be taken not to set standards so high that they will be self-defeating.

The Approach to SHA   The *first step* is to acquire an understanding of the system to be analyzed. Before he begins, the analyst must be thoroughly familiar with the procedures involved in the operation and the interactions between the system he is concentrating on and other associated systems and subsystems. To assist himself in this endeavor, he should draw a flow diagram that describes each step in the overall process from the time it begins through its completion (Figure 50). As is illustrated in Figure 50, four basic symbols are used to depict the stages in the flow process. Each step must be broad. Details are omitted at this stage, as they would only add to the confusion and impede progress. Drawing an operational flow diagram enables the analyst to gain

TABLE 6

Hazardous Energy Forms

Chemical Reaction
Unstable materials—violent decomposition
Reaction of materials with moisture
Reaction of materials with acidic contaminants
Reaction of materials with caustic contaminants
Inter-reaction of materials (incompatability)

Heat
Heating devices
Electrical equipment and fixtures
Electromagnetic radiation
Mechanical
Chemical reactions
Weather

Open Flames or Sparks
Electrostatic discharge
Electrical failures
Mechanical sparks
Open flame devices
Chemical reaction
Heat
Lightning

Mechanical
Impact
Friction
Stress (shear, pinching, crushing, grinding, etc.)
Static loading

thorough comprehension of the subsystems, methods, transfer operations, inspection techniques, and man/machine interactions pertinent to this system he is about to analyze.

The *second step* in a systems hazard analysis process is to define those undesired events (Table 5) that can detract from the successful operation of the system. Once the undesired events are listed, the analyst can then intelligently set out to locate those hazards in the system that can make the undesired events happen.

The *third step* will be referred to as "bounding" the system. The size and complexity of some operations may restrict the analyst to a particular segment (subsystem) at the outset. The necessity of establishing limits around a specific

TABLE 7

Typical Hazardous Conditions

Man	Materials in Process	Equipment and Facilities
1. Is exposed to: toxic materials; Irritants; Excessive or improper lifting; Slippery, uneven, or rough floors; Falls from elevated surfaces; Contact with hot materials; surfaces Rough, sharp, or cutting surfaces; Electrical shock; Mechanical hazard points (nip, shear, crushing, etc.); Noise or vibration; Thermal stress; Radiation (ionizing or non-ionizing); Weather; Fire, explosion, or detonation. 2. Physical, psychological, physiological stressors: Drugs and medicines; Alcohol; Intoxicating vapors, dusts, or fumes; Fatigue.	1. Becomes more sensitive, less stable: Reaction to contaminants; Due to crystal growth; Due to separation of ingredients; Due to side reactions; Due to increased temperature or pressure; Due to physical stimulation. 2. Is exposed to: Solid contaminants; Mechanical shock Friction; Pinching, shearing, grinding, or compressive actions; Excessive heat; Freezing; Open flames or sparks; Radiation Electrostatic discharge; Moisture. 3. Escapes from container or process equipment.	1. Exposed to: Fire, explosion, or detonation; Friction or wear; Metal fatigue; Corrosion; Vibration; Physical damage. 2. Inadvertant operation in the wrong sequence or at the wrong time. 3. Inadequate maintenance or cleaning. 4. Controls not properly set. 5. Power failure. 6. Lightning (other weather).

segment of a system gives rise to what is referred to in system analysis language as the "boundary concept." The use of boundaries enables the analyst to cut out a segment of the universe that he wishes to focus his attention on, by establishing a hypothetical line around it. Boundaries are also useful because they restrict the scope of the problem to a size commensurate with the time available and the cost of the analysis. To "bound" the system effectively, the analyst must make a subjective appraisal of the overall system prior to actually working on the problem.

The *fourth step* is to acquire an analysis format, a special format designed to facilitate the recording of data pertinent to the system under study (Figure 51). This particular format has proven its usefulness in applied situations. The Systems Hazard Analysis Format provides space for recording relevant information concerning the identity of hazards, their causes, the effects of these hazards on the system, and, finally, the corrective measures required to

TABLE 8

Typical Sources of Hazardous Energy in Sub-System Operation

I. Chemical Reaction

  A. Violent decomposition of explosives
    1. at elevated temperature
    2. at low temperature
    3. crystalline growth—components of Comp. B
      a. RDX
      b. TNT

  B. Aluminum power + moisture

  C. Comp B + acidic contaminants

  D. Comp B + caustic contaminants

II. Heat

  A. Steam
    1. Failure or pressure controls
    2. Inadvertent setting of steam controls at high pressure

  B. Electrical equipment and fixtures
    1. low voltage short
    2. unprotected light or other electrical fixture
    3. electric motor over-loaded
    4. power source—voltage drop
    5. improper for hazard present

  C. Electromagnetic radiation from
    1. motor vehicle radios
    2. train radios
    3. ham radios
    4. radar
      aircraft

  D. Mechanical heat from
    1. failure of shaft bearings
    2. inadequate clearance of moving parts

  E. Chemical reactions producing heat build-up without detonation or flaming

III. Open flames or sparks

  A. Electrostatic discharge from
    1. charge generated on man
    2. charge generated on equipment
    3. charge generated on materials

  B. Electrical failure
    1. direct short in wiring
    2. breakage of light globe or electrical enclosure
    3. water in conduit
    4. opening electrical enclosures

  C. Mechanical sparks from ferrous tools striking concrete or equipment

  D. Open flame devices
    1. maintenance work involving welding, soldering, or other open-flame or spark-producing devices

  F. Heat causing chemical reaction to occur

  G. Atmospheric electrical disturbance
    1. lightning striking building
    2. induced electrical charge from atmospheric disturbance resulting in interior discharge

IV. Mechanical

  A. Impact
    1. dropped tools or materials
    2. striking agitator shaft to remove build-up
    3. valve closing in discharge lines
    4. explosive particles impinging in dust exhaust system

  B. Friction
    1. materials spilled on floor and workers walking over them
    2. agitator blade rubbing kettle wall
    3. agitator shaft and housing
    4. conveyor drive mechanism
    5. sliding containers over a contaminated surface
    6. particles in dust exhaust system

  C. Stress (shearing, pinching, etc.)
    1. due to lack of clearance between agitator blade and kettle wall
    2. in conveyor system—gear box and drive mechanism
    3. discharge valve operation
    4. workers walking over spilled materials
    5. carts rolling over spilled materials
    6. solid foreign material in kettle, such as glass, rocks, nuts, bolts, etc.
      a. entry in explosives
      b. entry in transfer of explosives
      c. entry in kettle room from kettle appurtenances
      d. from broken windows or light fixtures

---

remedy the situation and the management system responsible for the correction. The following specific types of information required for the analysis are listed on the next page:

1. Operational step—the particular suboperation being analyzed.

2. Hazardous element—the part or substance in the equipment, environment, etc., that has natural properties which make it inherently hazardous.

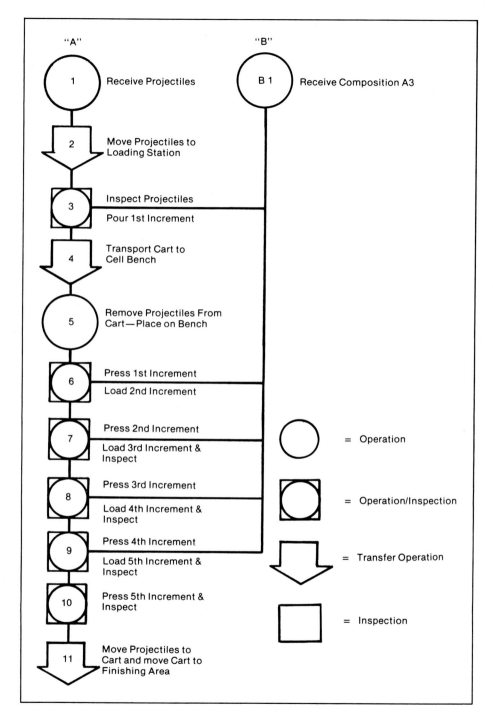

Figure 50. Flow diagram, 5″ 38 projectile pressing operation.

Operational Step	Hazardous Element	Hazardous Condition	Trigger Event	Potential Failure	Effect	Haz. Cat.	Risk	Std.	Corrective Action	Mngt. Syst.
(*) Moving projectiles from inert area to loading room	4-wheel cart (Weight = 1800 lbs. loaded)	Proximity of cart operator and other workers and equipment to cart while it is being moved	Tilting or bumping 4-wheel cart while it is in motion	Projectiles falling over in cart bed and out of cart bed to floor	Injury to cart operator and others in close proximity	II	1	OS-N	1. Compartmentize cart bed or	Ind. Engr.
	Guards missing on 4 sides of cart bed								2. Install guards on 4 sides of cart bed	Safety
								OS-I AN 2 41.1	3. Provide steel tip safety shoes. (2500 foot/lb. variety) for cart operator and others in work area	
	No adequate braking device							OS-N	4. Provide an adequate braking system for cart	Ind. Engr.
	4-wheel cart with loose or worn wheels	Wheels binding or coming off cart	Maneuvering and stopping moving cart	Loss of cart control Cart tilting; spilling projectiles on floor	Injury to operator and others in close proximity				5. Reduce the number of projectiles in cart or make the job a two-man operation	Proc. Engr.
				Cart striking work station where 1st increment of explosives is being poured, pinching and crushing the explosives	Detonation	IV	1			Proc. Engr.
								OS-D AN 01.1	6. Maintenance of cart	Maint.
(*) Bringing explosives (Comp A3) into loading room	Tote box— (Weight = 100 lbs. loaded)	Manner by which tote box is carried by two female workers	Hands of worker slipping off small handles	Dropping tote box	Back injury Foot and leg injury	III III	2 2		1. Reduce weight of explosives in tote box	Proc. Engr.
	Inadequate handles for worker to get firm grip			Pinching and crushing explosives	Possible detonation of explosives	IV	3		2. Provide larger handgrips on tote box	Ind. Engr.
									3. Instruct workers in correct lifting methods	Pers.
									4. Procedural change—using men instead of women	Proc. Engr.

Key: OS—Federal Occupational Safety Standards
AN—American National Standards Institute

Hazard category: I (Negligible), II (Marginal), III (Critical), IV (Catastrophic).
Risk probability: I (Probable), II Reasonably probable), III (Remote), IV (Extremely remote).

Figure 51. Systems hazard analysis format.

Figure 51. *Continued.*

Operational Step	Hazardous Element	Hazardous Condition	Trigger Event	Potential Failure	Effect	Haz. Cat.	Risk	Std.	Corrective Action	Mngt. Syst.
(*) Inspect projectile and load 1st increment of explosives	Composition A3 Explosives	Airborne particulates	Pouring 1st increment of explosives into projectiles via funnel	Build-up of static charge	Fire and possible detonation	IV	3	OS-G AN Z 9.2	1. Installation of local exhaust system with collector	Maint.
				Operator inhaling airborne particulates	Respiratory, eye and skin damage to workers	III	1	OS-I AN Z1 Z2 C33-3	2. Installation of conductive plate under feet of worker or install conductive floor	Maint.
					Damage to or loss of operating facility	IV	3	OS-1	3. Protective equipment a. Eye protection b. Respirator for worker pouring 1st increment Conductive shoes if conductive floor is provided c. Conductive floor is provided	Safety
								AN Z2.1 AN Z 88.2		
								OS-S AN Z 41	4. Monthly maintenance inspection to determine serviceability of conductive plate or floor	Maint.
(*) Transport cart from 1st increment of pouring operation to pressing cell bench	Projectiles loaded with 1st increment of Comp 3A	Projectiles impacting against each other in cart or	Jarring projectiles while they are being transported to pressing cell bench or	Shock delivered to projectile	Detonation			OS S AN Z 12	1. Static arrestors	Ind. Engr.
		Falling to floor			Fire			OS-N		Ind. Engr.
		Cart without adequate brakes	Running cart over uneven surfaces or jamming cart into substantial objects or structures		Personnel Injury				2. Monthly maintenance inspection of cart	Maint.
		Insufficient aisle space			Death					
					Damage to or loss of facility					

A3

A4

Figure 51. *Continued.*

Operational Step	Hazardous Element	Hazardous Condition	Trigger Event	Potential Failure	Effect	Haz. Cat.	Risk	Std.	Corrective Action	Mngt. Syst.
						IV	4	OS-N	3. Guards on four sides of cart bed or Compartmentize cart bed	Ind. Engr.
								OS-D AN 01.1	4. Provide adequate aisle space	Maint.
									5. Instruct operators on proper movement of cart	Pers.
									6. Maintenance of walking and working surfaces	
(*) Removing projectiles from cart to cell bench	Projectiles loaded with 1st increment of explosives (Weight of projectile 35 lbs.)	Projectile impacting with steel bench or with floor	Projectiles dropped while being carried to cell bench and from cell bench to vise in pressing cell	Shock delivered to projectile	Detonation Fire	IV	4		1. Use conveyor to transport projectiles from 1st increment pouring process to cell bench	Proc. Engr.
				Strain on operator	Injury to worker	III	2		2. Position cart closer to bench	Proc. Engr.
				Projectile coming in contact with operator's hands, feet, etc.	Loss of or damage to facility	IV	4		3. Instruct operator on proper unloading technique	Pers.
								OS-I AN Z 41	4. Provide safety shoes	Safety
(*) Inspecting and setting up projectiles on press vise and pressing 1, 2, 3, 4 and 5th increments of explosives	Projectile loaded with first increment	Workers in cell during pressing mode	Activating press	Projectile being double pressed	Detonation Fire Death Injury	IV	1	OS-H AN A 10.2	1. Provide blow-out walls at rear of all cells	Ind. Engr.
		Workers in joining cells while any cell is in pressing mode		Fracture in projectile case	Loss or damage to pressing cells and production equipment				2. Provide blow-out ceiling over all pressing cells	
		Pressing taking place with cell door open		Metallic object pressed with explosives						

A5

A6 A7 A8 A9 A10

Figure 51. Continued.

Operational Step	Hazardous Element	Hazardous Condition	Trigger Event	Potential Failure	Effect	Haz. Cat.	Risk	Std.	Corrective Action	Mngh. Syst.
									3. Install interlock to prevent workers from entering any cell while other cell is in pressing mode	Ind. Engr.
									4. Projectile cases to be fluoroscoped	QC.
									5. Operators instructed in the hazards of being in cell while any other cell in the chain is in pressing mode	
									6. Adequate supervision	
(*) Fully pressed projectile carried from cell to 4-wheel cart bed	Loaded projectile	Projectiles impacting with steel bed of cart or on floor or impacting with one another	Worker dropping projectile on floor in cell, outside cell, in cart bed or	Shock produced with the capacity to initiate detonation of projectile	Detonation Fire Death and injury to personnel	IV IV IV	3 3 3	OS-N	1. Provide small cart to transport projectiles from vise to 4-wheel cart or conveyor (if installed as per recommendation in Step 4	Proc. Engr.
			Allowing projectiles to impact together in cart bed	Projectile coming in contact with workers hands, feet, legs, etc.	Damage to or loss of facility and equipment	IV	3	OS-I AN Z 41	2. Safety shoes for all personnel in work area (or if conductive floor is installed as per recommendation in Step 3) safety toe conductive shoes with instep protection	Safety
									3. Instruction in proper lifting, carrying, load-unloading of ing and projectiles in cart	Pers.

Figure 51. Continued.

Operational Step	Hazardous Element	Hazardous Condition	Trigger Event	Potential Failure	Effect	Haz. Cat.	Risk	Std.	Corrective Action	Mngt. Syst.
(*) 4-wheel cart loaded with fully pressed projectiles removed to finishing area	Weight of cart —now 2100 lbs. Explosives in projectiles	Moving heavy cart	Impacting cart with obstruction on the way out of the room Loss of control of cart by operator Wheels coming off or brakes failing on cart	Undue strain on operator Projectiles falling out of cart bed.	Detonation Fire Death Injury Damage to or loss of facility	IV III IV	4 4 4	 OS-N OS-D AN 01.1 OS-N	1. Install conveyor to transport projectiles to finishing area or 2. Reduce the number of projectiles in cart 3. Provide adequate brakes on cart and maintain same 4. Provide adequate aisle space 5. Install guard around 4 sides of cart to contain projectiles or compartmentize cart bed	Proc. Engr. Ind. Engr. Maint. Ind. Engr.

3. Hazardous condition—those circumstances under which the hazardous element is placed in a situation where an accident is much more probable.
4. Triggering event—that action or situation that could trigger the hazardous condition into becoming a potential accident.
5. Potential failure—an unplanned, potentially injurious or damaging event that is caused by a human or physical action in the workplace.
6. Effect—the destructive effect on personnel, equipment materials, plant, and operation.
7. Hazard category—a category providing a qualitative measure of the hazard's most severe effect, i.e.,
7a. Risk probability
   1. Probable
   2. Reasonable probable
   3. Remote
   4. Extremely remote
8. Standard or regulation—the applicable OSHA, American National Standards Institute standards or other regulations.
9. Preventive/Corrective action—this category is reserved for listing those control measures necessary to eliminate or control the identified hazardous condition. Corrective actions will fall into engineering design or redesign of tools, equipment or apparatus, incorporation of safety devices, procedural revisions, personnel requirements, protective equipment, supervision. etc.
10. Management system—the particular management system or subsystem most directly involved in making the corrective action.

Once the Systems Hazard Analysis format is obtained, the *fifth step* involves the actual analytical procedure (i.e., completing the matrix). Each suboperation is analyzed individually, and hazardous elements in, or associated with the operation, are identified. It must be remembered that even though concentration is seemingly placed on one function at a time, each of the steps is part of the overall system under study, and not an isolated entity. Each step has effects upon other steps in the overall operation. These interfaces must be considered as the analyst picks his way through the analytical process.

The *sixth step* is to evaluate the probability of the uncovered hazards resulting in a failure situation. In most cases this decision will be a subjective estimate on the part of the analyst based on his or her experience, familiarity with the system, and professional judgement. However, he should certainly consider all available experience and test data before making the final assessment.

The *seventh step* is to list any standard or regulation that may have been, or will be violated, by the hazardous condition.

The *eighth step* concerns the recommendation of effective preventive and corrective measures necessary to eliminate or at least reduce the severity of the hazard.

The *ninth step* is to locate the management subsystem or subsystems most closely concerned with and having the capacity and jurisdiction to effect any necessary changes in the system. It is at this point that we bring the members of the staff and line organization together to pool their talents for the common good of the organization.

Utility of Systems Hazard Analysis

The most direct benefit of SHA is the information it provides for management hazard control decisions. These decisions can be made with the full knowledge of the high severity hazards associated with operations. Other potential benefits of the analysis include:

1. Identifying and locating hazardous elements, conditions, and potential accident sources;
2. Determining the significance of the hazard's potential effect on the systems operation;
3. Providing information with which effective control measures may be established, e.g., design changes, safety devices, special procedures, etc.;
4. Discovering and eliminating unsafe procedures, techniques, motions, positions, and actions;
5. Locating areas requiring further analysis;
6. Identifying possible system interface problems that may result in an accident; and
7. Uncovering special areas of hazard control consideration, such as system limitations, risks, etc.

Examples of control methods derived from a Systems Hazard Analysis are based on those mentioned in Chapter 4, pages 89–94. They are:

1. Isolating hazardous operations from other activities, areas, and personnel;
2. Providing control measures where failures would adversely affect the system or cause a catastrophic event through personnel injury, equipment damage, or inadvertent operation or movement of dangerous equipment;
3. Designing, locating, and arranging equipment components so that access to them by personnel during work operations, maintainance, repair, or adjustment will not expose them to hazards, such as electrical shock, cutting edges, toxic fumes, and so forth;

4. Avoiding undue exposure of personnel to physiological and psychological stressors, which might cause them to make errors; and

5. Installing effective standardized warning systems on hazardous components, equipment, etc., for the protection of personnel in the event of system failure.

Systems Hazard Analysis overcomes some of the limitations of the previously discussed hazard analysis methods. It focuses on system operations rather than components, making it easier to deal with the linkages among system components. The hazard information provided is often not quantifiable. However, it is in a form readily usable for management decisions. More so than some of the other hazard analysis approaches, Systems Hazard Analysis treats human error as an integral aspect of system operation.

Over the past few years the author has been experimenting with the adaptation of variations of the SHA technique to construction operations in an attempt to locate hazards with high consequence potential. Figure 52 illustrates a sample hazard analysis called Construction Hazard Analysis (CHA) which has been conducted on a specific phase of construction involving the installation of conduit in a trench. Figures 53–56 illustrate the specific job while at the same time illustrating many of the hazards spelled out in the analysis matrix in Figure 52. Applying the same step-by-step process described for the Systems Hazard Analysis (SHA) technique, construction safety personnel may find this technique a helpful aid in assisting with the hazard identification and evaluation process.

Variations of Systems Hazard Analysis

The benefits derived from the CHA include, but are not limited to:

1. Providing the basis for systematic thinking in the quest for locating hazards on the construction site.
2. Facilitating understanding of the ramifications of hazards uniquely associated with various building trades.
3. Understanding the role of human error on project performance.
4. Identifying hazardous conditions, and potential accident sources.
5. Determining the significance of the hazard's potential effect on the construction project.
6. Enabling those involved with construction safety and health to define problems sufficiently before recommending and establishing control meaures.
7. Discovering and eliminating, or at least reducing procedures techniques, motions, positions, etc., which place workers in potential accident situations.
8. Locating areas where new standards need to be developed.
9. Identifying interface problems between and among the operations of various trades on a job site.

Operational Step	Equipment and Materials	Potential Hazardous Condition	Potential Human Error	Potential Accident	Accident Probability Estimate 1	2	3	Effect	Haz. Cl.	Applicable Standard
Installing a conduit in a trench	Backhoe, Conduit, Sling, Bulldozer, Compactor, Spoil pile	Workman exposure to unstable trench walls	Failure to achieve proper trench wall sloping	Cave in of trench walls	X			Death or injury	III	OSHA P1
			Incorrect determination or evaluation of soils at the site			X			II	P-1 1926.651(h)
			Failure to recognize the effects of surcharges	Earth sliding into the trench		X		Permanent damage to workman's circulatory system	III	1926.651(e) .651(o) .651(q)
			Failure to recognize the effects of vibration				X		III	.651(k) .651(e)
			Failure to recognize previous excavations				X		III	1926.652(e)
			Failure to recognize a change in soils			X			II	P-1
	Backhoe, Conduit, Sling, Bulldozer, Compactor, Spoil pile	exposure to Workman unstable trench walls	Failure to recognize a water problem	Cave in of trench walls			X	Death or injury	III	.651(d) (e) (f) (h) (p)
			Altered design without subsequent change in side sloping	Earth sliding into the trench	X			Permanent damage to workman's circulatory system	II	P-1 .651(e) .652(b)
		Workman exposed to falling objects in trench	Failure to keep all excavated materials and equipment well back from the edge of the trench			X			III	.651(i1) (i2)

Figure 52. Construction hazard analysis format. Contributed by J. Mickie—Iowa State University.

Figure 52. Continued.

Operational Step	Equipment and Materials	Potential Hazardous Condition	Potential Human Error	Potential Accident	Accident Probability Estimate 1	2	3	Effect	Haz. Cl.	Applicable Standard
Installing a conduit in a trench (con't)	Backhoe, Conduit, Sling, Bulldozer, Compactor, Spoil pile	Workman exposed to falling objects in trench	Failure to clear the work site	Workman struck by materials falling into the trench	x				II	.651(b)
			Failure to remove all loosened soils and rocks from the trench walls		x				II	.651(j)
			Workman not wearing hardhat	Workman struck by materials falling into the trench		x			II	.650(e)
			Backfilling operation too close to the workman		x				II	.650(h)
			Workman under the conduit			x		Death or injury	III	.650(h)
			Failure to properly locate and/or fasten sling	Pipe falling on workman	x				II	
			Failure to recognize damaged equipment (sling, etc.)	Workman struck by broken cable	x				II	.650(h) .650(e)
			Workman too close to the conduit being lowered	Workman struck by swinging conduit		x			II	.650(h)

Accident Probability Estimate: (1) Low, (2) Fair, (3) High

Figure 52. *Continued.*

Operational Step	Equipment and Materials	Potential Hazardous Condition	Potential Human Error	Potential Accident	Accident Probability Estimate 1	Accident Probability Estimate 2	Accident Probability Estimate 3	Effect	Haz. Cl.	Applicable Standard
Installing a conduit in a trench (con't)	Backhoe, Conduit, Sling, Bulldozer, Compactor, Spoil pile	Bedding the pipe and making the joint; man-machine operation	Machine operator: inability, negligence, or error	Workman having his fingers pinched in joint	x			Pinched or broken fingers	—	.650(e)
			Faulty equipment		x					
			Improper placement of the backhoe (poor soil foundation)	Workman struck by the backhoe		x		Broken bones, abrasions	—	.650(h) .650(e)
				Bedding materials striking the workman				Cuts, abrasions	—	.650(h)

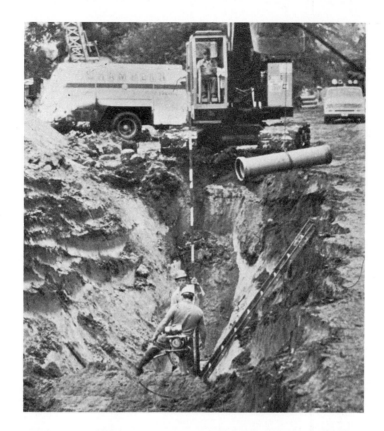

Figure 53.

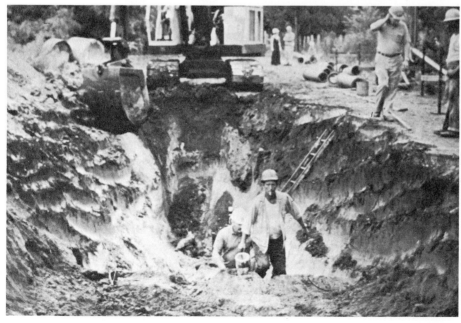

Figure 54.

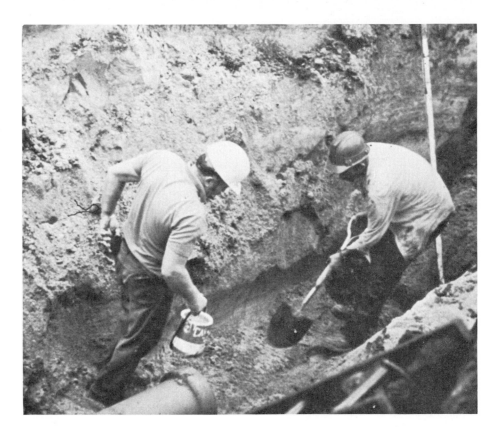

Figure 55.

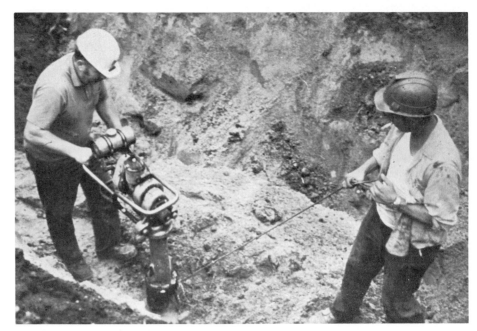

Figure 56.

A completed CHA will serve many useful purposes. Among them are:

1. To examine a prospective construction project during a prejob conference with emphasis on locating primary hazard areas and providing for effective controls.
2. To use data acquired from a CHA as an aid in teaching personnel about a particular job in terms of its operation, man-machine requirements, where and how failures can occur, what effect these failures can have on the system if they should occur, and most important, the operations which need constant monitoring to assure continued safety.
3. To investigate accidents. By reasoning backwards from the predetermined potential failures and the conditions responsible for these failures, the investigator is in a more desirable position to assess the state of the system prior to the accident and to find the hazardous elements or human failures which were responsible for the unfortunate situation.
4. To record data pertaining to a job in a logical manner, comprehensible to others. The analyst is then more readily able to convey his findings to others involved with safety and health, his management, and the union representatives.

Case Study—Construction Hazard Analysis

The analysis formats appearing in Figure 57 contain hazard data generated for a construction project which involved the consturction of an elevated concrete turbine generator pedestal deck. It was assumed that the operation would take place at an approximate elevation of fifty feet and would involve a monolithic structure. Assumption was made that the base mat and piers were already available and that other materials were stored on site. The operational steps necessary for this project were: (1) erection of the shoring support system (including tubular steel scaffold, aluminum joists, steel "I" beams, plywood deck, perimeter guardrail, stairway, etc.; (2) erection of the framework; (3) setting of reinforcing bar (including any miscellaneous imbedded metal dowels, etc.); (4) pouring of concrete (continuous operation approximately 1,000 cu/yds; (5) stripping and removal of form work (erect guardrail on deck) finishing of concrete (cut rods and protruding metals) grinding and rubbing (concrete, etc.); (6) backing off and dissembling shoring system. Upon completing the analysis illustrated in Figure 57 the construction safety engineer determined that:

1. The most probable and serious hazard, was the erection and stripping of the shoring system and formwork. Working at elevations on the sides of unprotected structures is a commonplace activity, and many workers do not take the time to tie off. Due to the nature of the work

Operational Step	Equipment and Materials	Potential Hazardous Condition	Potential Human Error	Potential Accident	Accident Probability Estimate 1	2	3	Effect	Haz. Class.	Applicable Standard
1. Erection of engineered shoring system	Crawler Crane app. 65 ton w/150' of boom and rigging	Failure of rig or equipment (slings, cable, belts, brakes, etc.)	Not properly maintained or inspected slings, cable, belts, etc. Improper/lack of signals	Dropping load on adjacent ground or people		x		Death, injury, property damage	IV	1926.550(a) and (b) 1926.51 and Tables H-1 through H-20
		Unstable placement of rig	Unqualified operator Lack of mats	Shift of load or entire rig	x			Death, injury, property damage	III	1926.550(b) (2)
			Improper placement of crane on base capable of support	Losing load and possible fall	x			Death, injury, property damage	III	None
			Working too close to excavations, trenches, tunnels, non-compacted areas	Overturning rig	x			Death, injury, property damage	IV	1926.651(q) and (S)
		Swing radius of rotating superstructure	No physical barrier or observer provided for protection to rear end of crane	Crushing individual between superstructure and cats.		x		Death, injury	III	1926.550(a) (9)
	Crawler Crane	Operating close to overhead power lines or other existing lines, equipment structures	Miscalculation of proper working area Malfunction of operator signalman or equipment	Shock hazard, fire		x		Death, injury, damage to equipment or structures from boom, cable, load contact with energy source	III	1926.550(a) (15)
			Improper positioning of crane							
		Overload and stressing crane beyond working limits	Improper calculation of load weight or use of damaged or insufficient rigging	Losing load and having it fall on adjacent ground or people		x		Death, injury, property damage	IV	1926.550(a) 1 through (7), (16) (b) 1926.251 and Table H-1-H-20
		using incorrect size shieve/cable arrangement	Not inspecting crane before lifting load	Shieve failure— cable failure			x	Death, injury, damage to crane, structure, etc.	IV	1926.700(e)
	Tubular frame shoring (joists, deck, etc.)	improper erection or foundation contact	Not following design or specifications	Failure of system, possible collapse under load	x			Death, injury, property damage	IV	1926.700(e)
		damaged equipment or material	Not inspecting equipment or material before use	Failure of system, possible collapse under load	x			Death, injury, property damage	II	1926.700(e)
		material falling off deck	Lack of protective screening	Material falling on individuals below			x	Death, injury	III	1926.451(a) (6)
		erection fall hazard	Individual not secured	Fall of individual doing erection			x	Death, injury	III	None
		working deck on open side	Lack of perimeter guarding	Fall of workmen on deck			x	Death, injury	III	1926.500(d) and (b), 1926.451(a) (4) and (5)

Accident Probability Estimate: (1) Low, (2) Fair, (3) High

Figure 57. Construction hazard analysis format.

Figure 57. Continued.

Operational Step	Equipment and Materials	Potential Hazardous Condition	Potential Human Error	Potential Accident	Accident Probability Estimate 1	2	3	Effect	Haz. Class.	Applicable Standard
		tripping hazards on deck	Tools and material not properly stored or secured	Tripping and falling of workmen on deck or to level below			x	Death, injury	III	None
	Stairways (metal erected)	Protruding rebar below	Not protecting workmen or eliminating hazard	Impalement			x	Death, injury	III	None
		Damaged equipment, improper erection or support	Faulty erection, equipment or material	Failure or collapse of stairway	x			Death, injury	IV	1926.501
		Debris, materials, tripping hazards	Tools, materials, leads, etc., not properly secured or stored	Tripping and possible fall of workmen			x	Death, injury	II	1926.501(c) (d) (e)
2. Erection of formwork	Crane (see previous notes)	Material conveyance								
	Formwork	Damaged equipment or material —improper erection	Lack of inspection or disposal of damaged material	Failure of system at high elevation; fall hazard	x			Death, injury, property damage	III	1926.700(a) 1926.701
		Workmen performing erection above deck	Not tying off when securing forms	Fall hazard			x	Death, injury	III	None
	Tie rods	Protruding rods from formwork	Not providing protective guards or cutting rods off short	Workers and tripping; falling on rods			x	Injury, death remote	II	None
	Curing Compounds (spray on forms)	Compounds highly combustible	Application of material in presence of source of ignition	Spray atomizes— highly flammable			x	Injury, fire	II	None
3. Set reinforcing steel (including misc. metals, dowels, etc.)	Crane (see previous notes)	Material conveyance								
	Reinforcing Steel	Walking hazard created by grid and tools and equipment on grid	Improper or unstable working surface	Worker falling onto or through grid			x	Death, injury	III	1926.700(b) (2)
	Welding or cutting of misc. metals	Briefly: ventilation, eye protection, fire prevention, grounding, etc.	Lack of inspection, improper or damaged equipment, use by unqualified personnel, etc.	Fire, flash, eye damage, explosion, etc.			x	Death, injury, property damage	III	1926.350 through .354
		Note: Welding and cutting operations are the subject of a separate hazard analysis								
4. Concrete pour	Pumpcrete system	Insufficient or unstable pipe supports	Lack of inspection, use of improper or damaged material	Collapse of system			x	Death, injury, property damage	III	1926.700(d) (6)
	Vibratory equipment and misc. power tools	Improper grounding, lack of G.F.C.I. or faulty equipment or cord	Lack of inspection or poor quality equipment or insufficient grounding system	Shock or electrocution		x		Death, injury	III	1926.300, .302(a) .400, .401, .402

Accident Probability Estimate: (1) Low; (2) Fair; (3) High

Figure 57. Continued.

Operational Step	Equipment and Materials	Potential Hazardous Condition	Potential Human Error	Potential Accident	Accident Probability Estimate 1	2	3	Effect	Haz. Class.	Applicable Standard
	Concrete	Skin exposure to concrete	Lack of protective equipment	Concrete burns or allergic reactions			x	Injury	II	1926.102 (eyes) None (skin)
	Concrete	Insufficient work space	Bulk pour creates congested operation due to use of too many personnel	Tripping, bumping, etc.			x	Injury, death remote		None
5. Strip and re- move form- work and finish concrete	Crane (see previous notes)	Material conveyance								
	Burning and Cutting (see previous notes)									
	Hand tools (hammers, chisels, cutting tools)	Unsafe tools or use of tool not designed for purpose	Improper inspection or use	Airborne metal particles; worker tripping over tools; using tools improper- ly, etc.			x	Injury	II	1926.301
	Pneumatic tools	Poor hose connec- tion or untrained operator	Improper inspection operation or connection	Hitting, tripping on hose; fall of workmen			x	Injury, death	II	1926.301
	Finished deck	Open sided elevated working surface	Lack of guardrail	Worker falling onto adjacent surfaces			x	Death, injury	III	1926.500(d) (f)
	Power tools (grinding)	Improper grounding or faulty equipment or cord	Lack of inspection, poor quality equipment or insufficient grounding system	Worker exposed to electrical energy		x		Shock, electro- cution	III	1926.300, .302(a, .400, .401, .402
	Finishing con- crete (sides of pedestal)	Elevated above working deck	Individual not secured or tied off	Worker falling to ground			x	Death, injury	III	None
6. Back off and disassamble shoring system	Tear down of system	Unsafe, stripping of shoring system	Disorganized and hap- hazard removal of materials	Materials coming in contact with people on property below			x	Death, injury	III	1926.701(a) (3)
		Poor storage and housekeeping of materials	Lack of direction or organization—poor workmanship	Worker tripping, striking against, etc.			x	Death, injury	III	1926.25 1926.701(a) (3)
		Stripping fall hazard	Individual not secured or tied off	Fall to ground			x	Death, injury	III	None

Accident Probability Estimate: (1) Low; (2) Fair; (3) High

involved, the most suitable way to provide adequate protection and required mobility is to use a safety belt and lanyard.

2. Placement and operation of the crane used to handle materials is a serious concern. Failure of the rig or equipment, operating too close to electric lines, overlaod, etc., can cause very serious and catastrophic accidents. The probability of such accidents is very high. With proper planning, inspection, design, maintainence, and operation, crane and material handling accidents can be effectively reduced or even completely eliminated.

3. Failure of the shoring system, either free standing or under load would also be a major concern. The magnitude of this system requires a crew of considerable size in the erection and removal stage, and an even larger force during the pouring operation. Such a failure could be the result of improper erection or support, lack of inspection, an assembly not in conformance with design or specifications, damaged equipment or material, etc., and could cause multiple deaths or injuries. The probability of such an accident is rather low, and owing to procedural safeguards and quality construction according to design, will most probably never occur.

4. Failure or collapse of the stairways can be classified in the same category as noted in 3 above, with only one slight difference. The stairway referred to here is separate from the shoring system and must be tied in to the shoring structure at piers with planking, wire, cable, etc., for proper stability.

5. Tripping and/or falling onto exposed rebar or dowels either at or adjacent to working area or at grade level below working area presents a serious impalement hazard. Eliminating the tripping or falling potential and "barricading" the hazard by use of bar caps (guards) or wood devices, etc., may control it. Further working surface protection, safety nets or belts, guardrails, etc., may also act to avert a fall and subsequent accident.

6. Welding, burning, electric, and pneumatic equipment and tools have the potential for accidental death or injury. However, when properly maintained, inspected and operated (by trained and qualified personnel) the hazardous potential is reduced considerably.

7. The primary and most prominent cause of major injuries and deaths is the potential of a worker falling from elevated work areas which do not easily and economically lend themselves to protective measures. Preventive action requires planning, expertise, knowledge, supervision, and above all, cooperation.

Deductive Analysis—Fault-Tree Analysis (FTA)

Fault Tree Analysis, a form of combined events analysis, is a deductive process that identifies the possible modes of occurrence of specific undesired events within the bounds of a given system. The Fault Tree is a graphic model of the various parallel and sequential combinations of system component faults that will result in the occurrence of a single selected system fault. See Figure 58. The objectives of FTA are:

1. The identification of failure and condition combinations which could result in the occurrence of an undesired event.
2. The presentation of these events so that their relationships can be visually evaluated.
3. The development of the event relationships in terms of Boolean Algebra so that it becomes possible to (a) express the probability of the occurrence of the undesired event in terms of the probabilities of all other events and conditions; (b) determine the relative importance of the undesired event in terms of the probabilities of all other events and conditions; (c) identify the smallest number of events which in combination could cause the undesired event; (d) establish remedial measures which would have the greatest possible effect on reducing the probability of occurrence of the undesired event.

Fault-Tree Construction

The first step in the construction of a fault tree is to define the undesired event to be analyzed. The undesired event may be taken directly from the data developed during either Preliminary Hazard Analysis or Failure-Mode Effect Analysis, or perhaps may come to the attention of the analyst for some other reason. Remember to define the undesired event as realistically as possible, while at the same time making sure that the problem is important enough to spend the time and energy to develop a tree. The second step is to acquire an understanding of the system to be analyzed. The analyst must understand the systems' operation well enough to determine how the system, including the people involved with system operation and maintenance, could fail, and cause the undesired event. The third step is to construct the fault tree by properly relating all possible sequences of events that, upon occurrence, could result in the unwanted event. Beginning with the most undesired (top) event, the Fault Tree graphically depicts the paths that lead to each succeeding lower branch of the display. This does not imply that each descending fault path has a "higher probability of occurrence," in fact, in many instances, the opposite may be the case. However, a series of lesser potential problems, each with a relatively low probability of occurrence, may trigger an event at the next higher level. This is depicted in the Fault Tree as a progression of events through the logic gates. See Figure 59.

Figure 58. (Courtesy of the National Safety Council.)

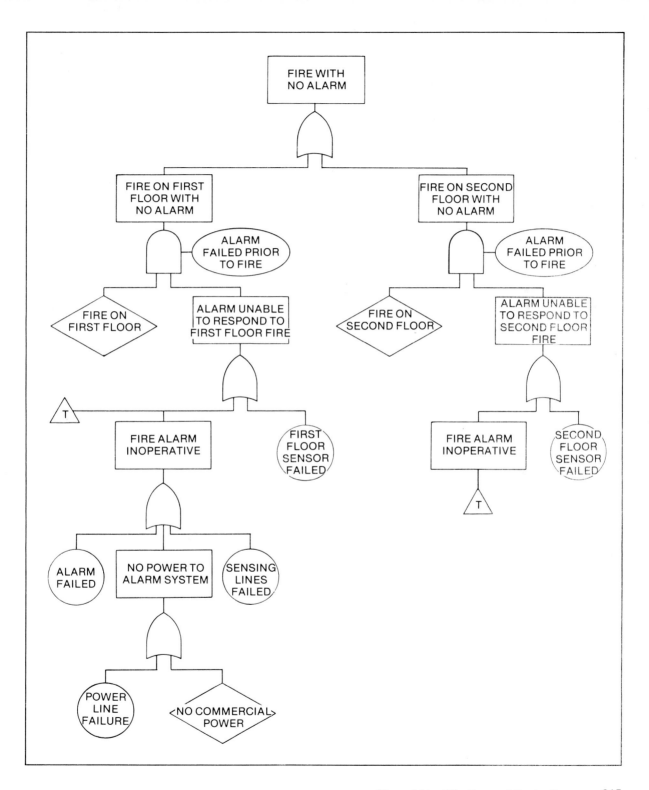

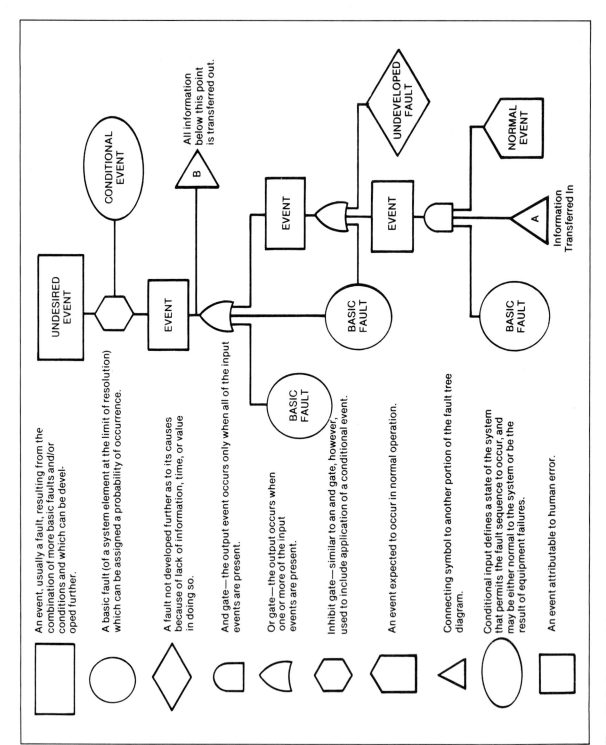

The following symbols and their descriptions appear in the figure:

An event, usually a fault, resulting from the combination of more basic faults and/or conditions and which can be developed further.

A basic fault (of a system element at the limit of resolution) which can be assigned a probability of occurrence.

A fault not developed further as to its causes because of lack of information, time, or value in doing so.

And gate—the output event occurs only when all of the input events are present.

Or gate—the output occurs when one or more of the input events are present.

Inhibit gate—similar to an and gate, however, used to include application of a conditional event.

An event expected to occur in normal operation.

Connecting symbol to another portion of the fault tree diagram.

Conditional input defines a state of the system that permits the fault sequence to occur, and may be either normal to the system or be the result of equipment failures.

An event attributable to human error.

Figure 59. Fault tree symbols.

Further Explanation of Fault Tree Symbology—Figure 59

1. The Circle—The symbol of a circle describes an independent basic failure or fault event that requires no further development. It is used to indicate a termination of further breakdown of causes because a further breakdown would not give any further analytical information. Logic flow in the Tree is stopped, not because of any lack of data, but because the failure is being considered as a basic independent event and may be predicted from a variety of data sources.

2. The Diamond—The diamond on the other hand, indicates a termination of diagramming activities because of a lack of information or data on consequences. Unlike the circle, the diamond indicates events which are not necessarily considered independent or basic, but for which no further data are available. Therefore, out of necessity ,the analyst is forced to terminate further diagramming.

3. The House—The house indicates an event that must occur in the system under normal operating conditions, but which is not actually a fault event. Examples include any phase change in a dynamic system, such as take-off, flight or landing phase of an aircraft, or production line shutdown for maintenance purposes.

4. The Triangles—Two other symbols which are useful as shorthand devices are the triangles. These triangles are used to indicate whole sections or branches of the Tree which are transferred to other sections or branches. A triangle with the apex pointing upward indicates that everything below that triangle is transferable to some other part of the Tree intact. A triangle with the apex pointing downward indicates that the elements contained below it are transferred, but they may have different numerical values. Transfer symbols are labeled with some kind of notation to aid in identification, when more than one transfer symbol is used in the same Fault Tree. For example, if we had two transfer functions, we may label one Triangle T Sub 1 and the other Triangle T Sub 2. The point from which elements of the Tree are transferred would contain the triangle labeled T Sub 1, and the point at which the elements should be inserted would likewise be labeled T Sub 1. In the latter case, the triangle would indicate that whatever followed beneath T Sub 1 should also be applied at each of these points. We can, of course, have as many transfer functions and symbols in our diagram as we wish.

Again, just as in talking about the other symbols and the gates, there are a number of more deluxe versions of event symbols, that can be used, but these are the basic ones that will satisfy most of your needs. Again, let's not get hung up on the symbolism. Any symbolism that is logical and understandable can be used. The use of standardized symbols merely aids in the communication, since it is assumed that all analysts will be using the same symbolism to connote the same type of events, conditions, and situations.

Basic Logic Gates	Three basic symbols, or logic gates, are used in constructing a Fault Tree: the **and,** the **or,** and the **inhibit** gates. The **and** and **or** gates represent the fundamental boolean functions that form the basis for all logic analysis. See Figures 60 and 61.

The decision whether to use an **and** or an **or** gate can be made by this simple rule: if the event being considered will, by itself, cause the next higher event to occur, use **or** gate. *Otherwise, determine what is necessary and sufficient to cause the next higher event and* **and** *gate.*

The **And** Gate

As shown in Figure 60 and 60a, the **and** gate performs the logic functions that require the coexistence of all gate inputs, in this case events A, B, C, and D, in order to realize an output X event. That is, in the **and** gate situation, the output of that gate, the event that is on top of the symbol, can occur only if *all* of the conditions below the gate and feeding into the gate coexist. To use our example, light E can be left on only if switches A, B, C, and D are on. If any one of those switches is off, we will not get the undesired event of light E being left on only if switches A, B, C, and D are on. Therefore, as a control strategy we know that to eliminate the possibility of light E being inadvertently left on, we only have to reduce or eliminate one of the input events from occurring. That is, if we eliminate either switch A, switch B, switch C, or switch D from erroneously being in the "on" position, then we have eliminated the possibility of light E ever being inadvertently left on. So our control strategies should focus on reducing error in any one of the input conditions. A reduction in the probability of failure of either condition A, B, C, or D will result in a reduction in the probability of failure of the undesired event. Systems which utilize a great deal of **and** types of logic gates are the most easily controlled.

The **Or** Gate

The utilization of the **or** Gate is shown in Figure 61 and Figure 61a. The **or** gate performs the logic function that requires any one of the gate inputs (in this case A, B, C, and D events) to realize an output X event. The **or** gate, then, is used to describe the circumstance in which the output event occurs, if and only if any one of the input events occurs. Again, looking at the example, consider that our circuit, unlike the previous case, consists of switches which are aligned in parallel, so that if any one switch is turned on, light E will go on. In this case, you can see that the logic gate is an **or** gate, since if either A or B or C or D are on, light E will be left on. Unlike the previous example of the **and** gate, if we eliminate failure in switch A, we have not eliminated the undesired event. For, if switch B is left on while all other switches are off, light E will still re-

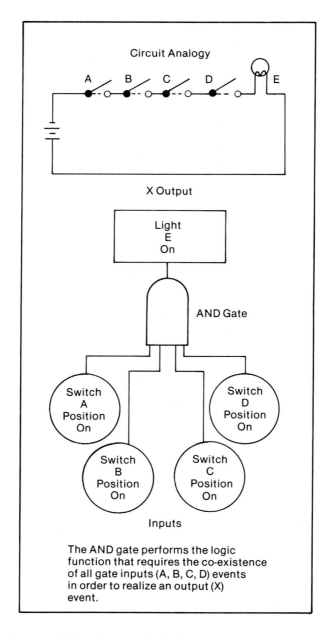

Figure 60. Use of "AND" Gate (Courtesy of the Boeing Corporation).

main on. So to eliminate the possibility of the undesired events ever occurring, countermeasures must be taken to eliminate the occurrence of each of the four branches in this case example. So control strategies, unlike the previous example, cannot be designed simply to attack one branch. You can see, therefore, that systems in which the predominate gate is an **or** gate represent more difficult control situations, those in which the predominant gate is the **and** gate.

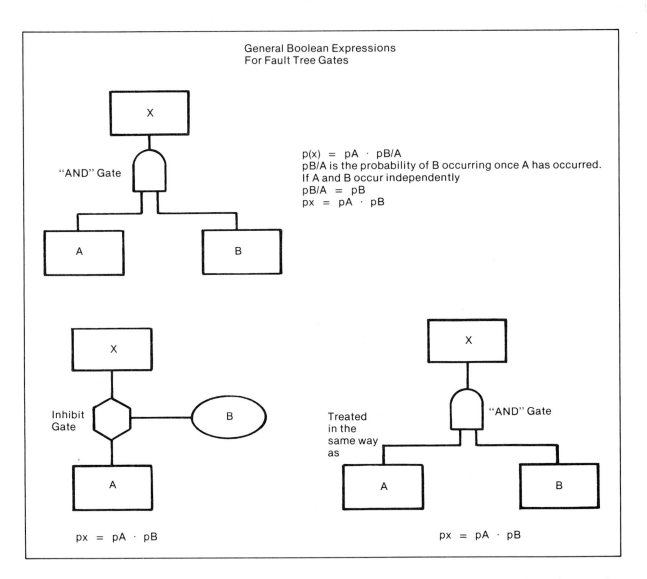

General Boolean Expressions
For Fault Tree Gates

X

"AND" Gate

A   B

$p(x) = pA \cdot pB/A$
pB/A is the probability of B occurring once A has occurred.
If A and B occur independently
$pB/A = pB$
$px = pA \cdot pB$

X

Inhibit
Gate

B

A

$px = pA \cdot pB$

X

Treated
in the
same way
as

"AND" Gate

A   B

$px = pA \cdot pB$

**Figure 60a. General
Boolean expressions for
fault tree gates.**

This is because in the **or** gate situation, every branch, *every branch,* must be eliminated to eliminate the possibility of the undesired event from occurring. Now, of course, in the real world we would have different probabilities of failure associated with each of those conditions, namely A, B, C, and D.

If we cannot eliminate all four conditions from occurring, then of course we would single out for attention that branch which has the highest degree of probability of occurrence. But in so doing, we should recognize that by totally eliminating one of the branches, we have not eliminated the possibility of the undesired events occurring.

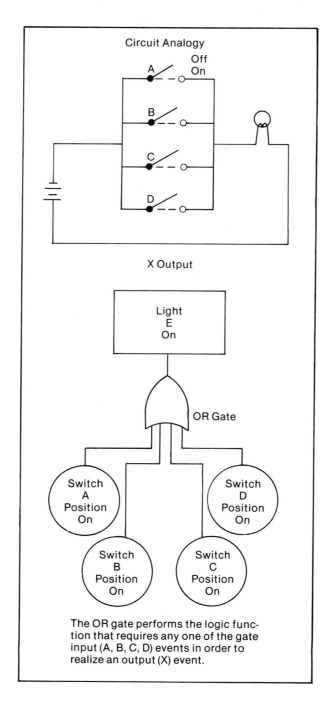

Figure 61. Use of "OR" Gate (Courtesy of the Boeing Corporation).

General Boolean Expressions for Fault Tree Gates

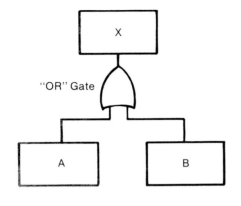

"OR" Gate

$p(x) = p(A) + p(B) - p(A \cap B)$

px = pA = + pB are very small, pA $\cdot$ pB is negligible and can be assumed to equal 0

px = pA + pB

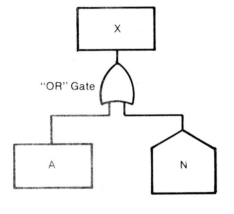

"OR" Gate

$p(x) = p(A) + (N) - p(A \cap N)$
px = p(A) + pN - pA $\cdot$ pN

If pN = 1

px = pA + pN - pA
px = pN = 1

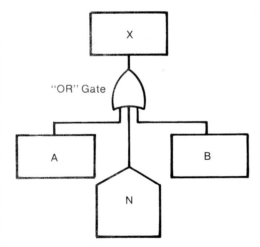

"OR" Gate

$p(x) = p(A) + p(B) + p(N) - p(A \cap N)$
$\quad - p(A \cap B) - p(B \cap N) -$
$\quad\quad p(A \cap B \cap N)$

px = pA + pB + pN - pA $\cdot$ pN
- pA $\cdot$ pB - pB $\cdot$ N - pA $\cdot$ pB $\cdot$ pN

If pN = 1

px = pA + pB + pN - pA - pA $\cdot$ pB - pA $\cdot$ pB

px = pN - 2pA $\cdot$ pB

If pA and pB are very small 2pA $\cdot$ 2pB is negligible and can be assumed to equal 0

px = pN

Inhibit Gate

A third type of gate is the inhibit gate. The inhibit gate provides a means of applying conditional probabilities to the fault sequence. If the input occurs, and the condition that is described in the rectangle is satisfied, and the output event will be generated. If that conditions is not satisfied, then no output will occur. For example, consider the following: Suppose the undesired event is an allergic reaction to a chemical, say a rash. For the rash to occur, we need exposure to the chemical. If exposure occurs, but the person is not allergic to the chemical, then a rash is unlikely. But if the exposed person is allergic, then a rash is most probable. In this case, our inhibiter would be allergies. An exposure to the chemical will still not result in a rash unless, and this is the key, the person is allergic to the chemical. In a Fault Tree, the symbol shown in Figure 62 is used.

The fourth step involves the collection of quantitative data. If it is necessary to quantify the Tree, then specific data on component reliability and likelihood or probability or occurrence need to be collected. Statistical data based on experience are used in developing probability levels. Each event in the Tree has a particular probability of occurrence. The safety of the total system is a function of the probability of occurrence of components. A simplistic example—if the probability of the light being left on is dependent upon one individual, then obviously the light will be left on only when the individual forgets to turn it out. If the likelihood or probability of that individual forgetting to turn out the light is one in a million, then the probability of the undesired event, i.e., the light being left on, is one in a million.

The fifth step is to simplify the tree-after drawing the preliminary Tree, the Tree is then rewritten in symbolic logic format. The simplified Fault Tree, represented by the symbolic logic expressions, now contains only those events that are actual contributors to occurrence of the undesired event. The reliabilities for failure rate data for each of the elements in the Tree then combine to determine the overall reliability of the system. It is from the simplified Tree and the probability of the independent events that statements about the potential benefit from reduction of various branches of the Tree can be made.

The sixth step is to evaluate the Tree-after simplifying the Tree and determining the reliability coefficients, the logic inherent in the Tree construction should be reviewed to identify those branches that are most likely to occur, as well as those branches requiring immediate action and/or attention. In this step we apply our experience and previous knowledge to interpret the feasibility and rationality of the Tree. We ask ourselves such questions as, have all the branches and possibilities been considered? Are the branches consistent with our knowledge? Is the elimination of certain events feasible and realistic, etc.?

Figure 61a. General Boolean expressions for fault tree gates.

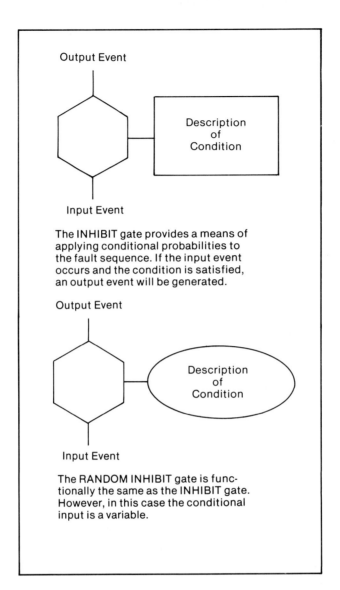

Figure 62. Use of "INHIBIT" Gate (Courtesy of the Boeing Corporation).

The seventh step is to select appropriate controls—after constructing the tree and doing our preliminary analysis and evaluation of our findings, the last step is to implement or apply those findings in some program of control. It is in Step 7 that we utilize the results of Fault Tree Analysis and identify what needs to be done to reduce or prevent the undesired event from occurring. In selecting controls, the energy transfer model which is explained as an integral part of this course is appropriate, as well as are, of course, considerations of available resources.

1. Tests and Analyses of Safety Latch on Elevator Work Cage

Case History—
Application of
Fault Tree
Analysis to
Engineering
Design
Alternatives[10]

A. Purpose

To determine: (1) probable causes for safety latch malfunctions on the Type A and Type B hooks for the elevator work cage and (2) the hazards associated with the operation of the work cage, using both configurations I and II, when using the aforementioned hooks for support.

B. Background

An elevator work cage and yoke became disengaged from the hoist cable hook and fell approximately fifteen feet to the bottom of the shaft. The occupant of the cage was saved from serious injury by his safety belt and attached lanyard. An examination of the safety latch on the hook revealed that it was worn at the pin attachment so that it could easily be pushed from inside the hook around the tip to the outside of the hook. An inspection of other work cage assemblies revealed that the majority of safety latches in use were bent, worn, or defective.

C. Discussion and Results

Tests and analyses were first conducted with Type A hoist cable hook on Configuration II, shown in Figure 63, which is replacing Configuration I, shown in Figure 64.

To provide a baseline for the tests and analyses, the following parameters were established: (1) any failure of the latch would be due to an inadvertent operation, since the latch has no normal operational function but is protected against any inadvertent operation; (2) only new latches would be used for testing.

Initially, the hooks were fitted on Configuration II to see how the hook can disengage or become damaged when in actual use. It was found that if the cage hoist cable becomes slack, and with the slight twist force that exists in all wire cables when a load is released, it is highly probable that the hook will position itself as shown in Figure 65 or Figure 66.

Tests were conducted to determine the loads that the hook is able to carry in positions shown in Figures 65 and 66. Load Test 1 in Figure 65 shows the load hung on the screw-nut assembly of the Type A hook, which attaches the latch to the hook. Under this condition, 1,000 pounds were applied to the hook before the head of the latch screw, which supported the cage, sheared off. Figure 67 shows the sheared screw and deflected latch. From inspection of latches in the field it was evident that many latches were damaged, and prob-

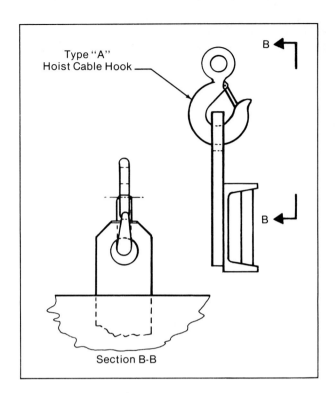

Type "A"
Hoist Cable Hook

B

B

Section B-B

Figure 63. Type "A" hoist cablehook, Configuration II.

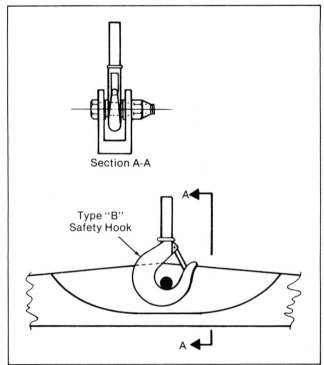

Section A-A

Type "B"
Safety Hook

A

A

Figure 64. Hoist cable hook, Configuration I.

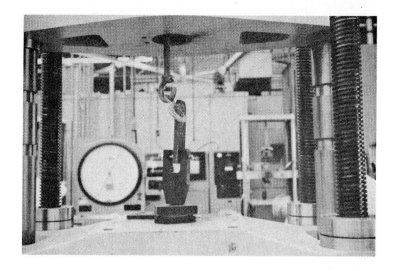

Figure 65. Load carried by the screw-nut assembly of the latch.

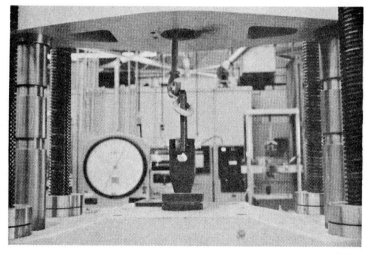

Figure 66. Load carried by the safety latch.

ably have weakened pin attachments. This would allow the screw to shear with a smaller load. The cage can be lifted with the load supported on the latch attachment and a jerk will cause it to slip from the screw-nut assembly onto the latch (Figure 66), which will deflect and quite possibly allow the hook to disengage.

Load Test 2 in Figure 66 shows the load being applied on the latch of the Type A hook. As the load was applied, the hook slowly turned and slipped into the proper lift in position at 95 pounds. The latch was slightly bent.

Load Test 3 was loaded in the same manner as Test 2, except that the load was applied on a hook produced by a different manufacturer. The hook slowly turned and slipped into its proper lifting position at 85 pounds. The pin that attaches the safety latch broke in two locations, as shown in Figure 68.

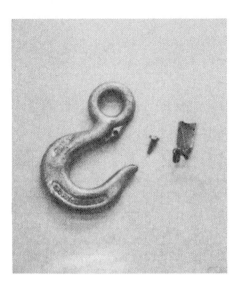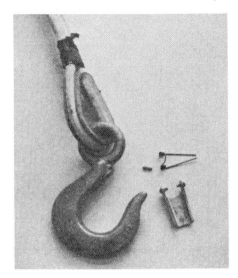

Figure 67. Head of screw sheared off and latch deflected as a result of loading shown in figure 65.

Figure 68. Latch attachment pin sheared in two locations as a result of similar loading shown in figure 66.

The latch on the hook is more substantial than the one on the previously tested hook, but the latch pin attachment was found to be much weaker.

Load Test 4 was conducted on the hook (same manufacturer as hook tested in Load Test 1 and 2) by applying a direct side thrust on the latch, as shown in Figure 69. With a slowly increasing force, the latch deflected at 65 pounds. A second test on the same hook, using a suddenly applied force similar to the effect of a workman straightening his lanyard, caused the latch to deflect.

The second sequence of studies was done by fitting the hooks on Configuration I to determine how the hook can be disengaged or the latch damaged when in use. There were no positions in which force could be applied by the work cage attachment to deflect an undamaged latch. If a hook with a defective latch is used, the work cage can be raised by the tip of the hook as shown in Figure 70, and made to disengage with a slight jerk while the cage is suspended. This was considered to be the cause of the accident under investigation.

During the test period, one latch was pushed sideways with the thumb and then straightened. After being straightened, the pin showed no damage that could be detected visually, even though it had been stressed beyond the yield point.

Load tests were also conducted on the Type C hook (see Figure 71).

The load test used was similar to the one shown in Figure 66, 600 pounds were applied to both sides of the latch and there was no apparent damage.

An explanation of the fault tree logic used in this study along with the actual fault three analysis will be found on pages 220 and 222. The fault trees identify the potential failure modes of the safety latches used on the Type A

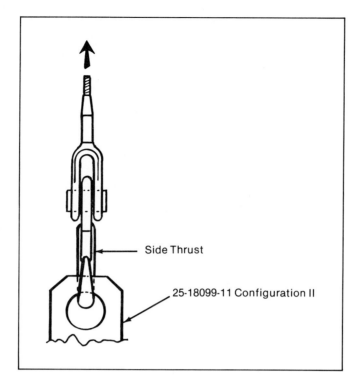

Figure 69. Direct side pressure applied to latch.

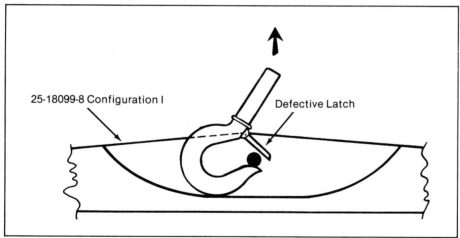

Figure 70. Load carried by tip of hook.

and Type B hooks when the hook supports the work cage. This analysis covers safety latch failure modes when the hook is connected to both the "old" Configuration I and the "new" Configuration II. It provides a numerical scale that allows comparison of the failure probabilities when these safety latches are used with either yoke configuration. This comparative failure probability scale is presented in Figure 72. The numerical values in this analysis are for

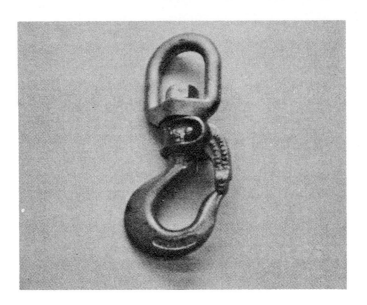

Figure 71. Recommended
type "C" safety hook

comparison within this report and to verify that these scale numbers are not reliability or probability figures.

D. Conclusions

(1) From the fault tree analysis, Figures 72 through 77, it is apparent that the new Configuration II, has a higher probability of failure than the old Configuration I.

(2) Since the accident involving Configuration I could not be duplicated in the laboratory as single operation using a new latch, the latch that failed was probably damaged prior to the failure.

(3) Insufficient maintenance is being accomplished on the latches and latch attachments in the field for one or a combination of the following reasons:

a. Maintenance procedures do not require adequate or frequent enough inspections.

b. Maintenance and operating personnel are not following the procedures.

c. Excessive maintenance is required.

(4) Sufficient forces are being applied to the latches during normal use to damage both the latches and the pins.

(5) Unless the operator inspects the hook position before each movement, it is probable that the hook can position itself on the Configuration II support as shown in Figure 65 or Figure 66. Then lifting or supporting the cage can cause latch damage or failure.

(6) With the Configuration I support and a defective latch, a failure can occur when the cage is lifted with the hook positioned as shown in Figure 70.

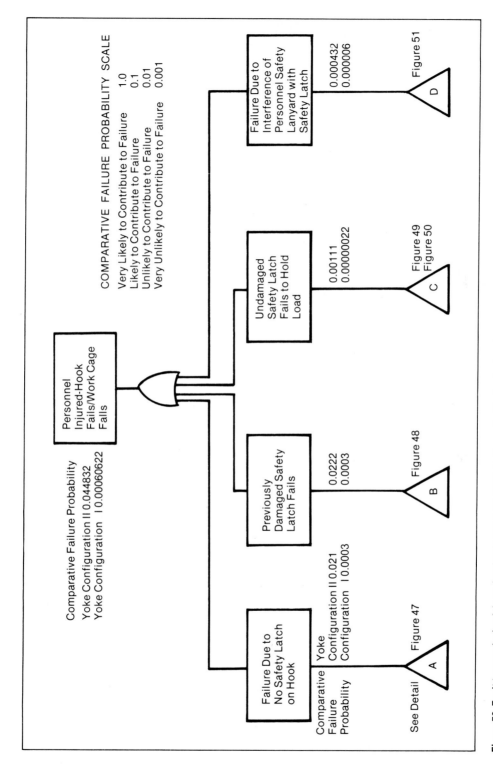

Figure 72. Fault tree analysis of the safety latch on the type "A" hook used with standard work cage.

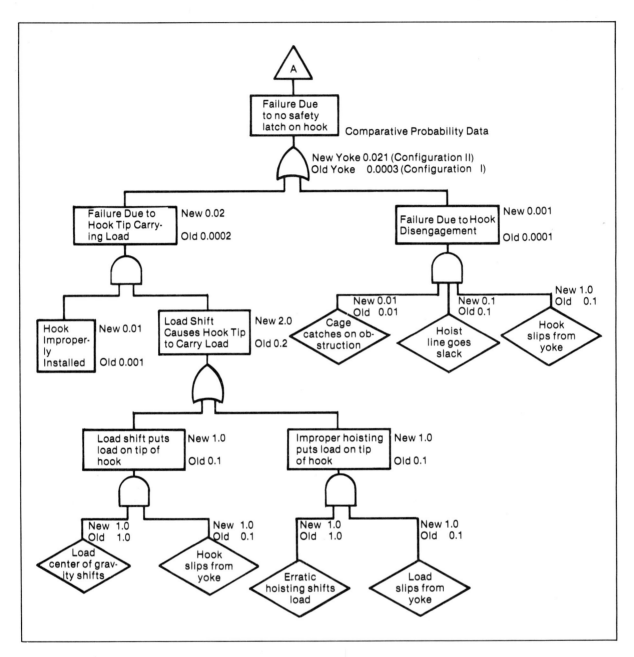

Figure 73. Fault tree
analysis failure due to no
safety latch on hook.

Figure 74. Fault tree
analysis previously
damaged safety latch
fails.

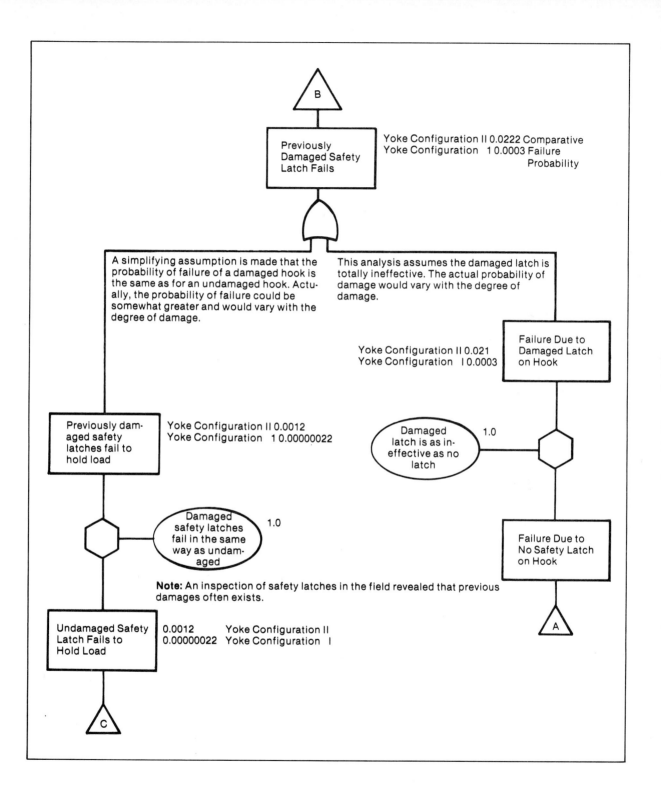

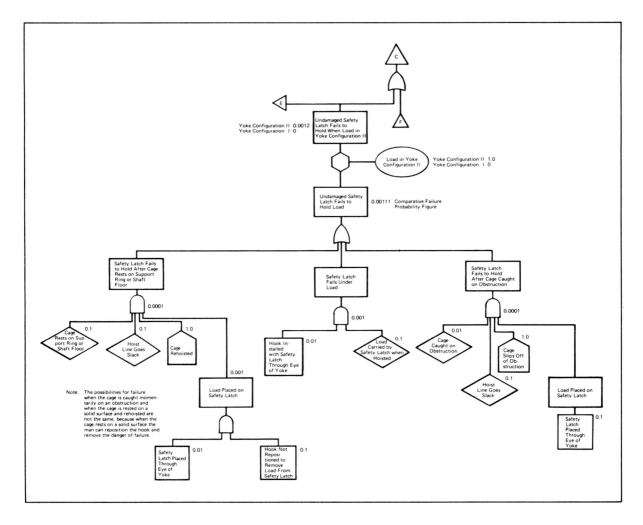

Figure 75. Fault tree analysis undamaged saftey hook fails to hold load (in yoke Configuration II).

(7) A high latch damage rate is apparent from the field reports.

(8) Damaged latch pins and latches can be straightened without leaving apparent visual evidence of the damage, thus permitting the operator a false sense of security.

(9) The present Type A and Type B hooks and latch do not provide sufficient assurance of proper connection between hook and yoke to be used for support of personnel in standard work cage.

The comparative failure probability scale numbers associated with basic faults on the fault tree indicate the comparative probability that an event will contribute to a failure. These assignments are the result of judgements based on available information. When applied to an **and** gate, the input event comparative numbers are multiplied to produce the comparative probability of an output event. (For example: Two input comparative probability numbers, 0.1

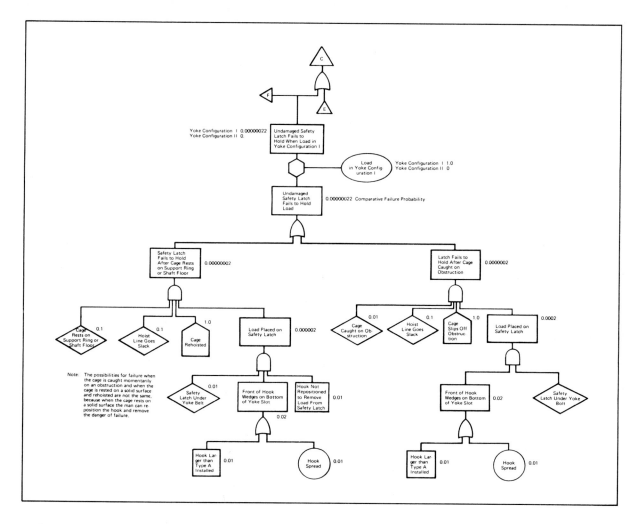

Figure 76. Fault tree analysis undamaged safety latch fails to hold load (in yoke Configuration I).

and 0.1, produce an output comparative probability of 0.01.) When applied to an **or** gate, input comparative probabilities are added. (For example: Inputs of 0.1 and 0.1 produce an output comparative probability of 0.2) At the top of the fault tree, a comparative probability of 0.0001 is less likely to contribute to a failure than a comparative probability of 0.01.

Qualitatively assessing the data in the fault tree is apparent that:

(1) It requires at least three basic failure events to cause the undesired event when yoke is in Configuration I.

(2) It requires at least two basic failure events to cause the undesired event when yoke is in Configuration II.

Note: Events occurring with high probability have been assigned a probability of 1.0. Other event probabilities have been estimated in Type I and Type II configurations.

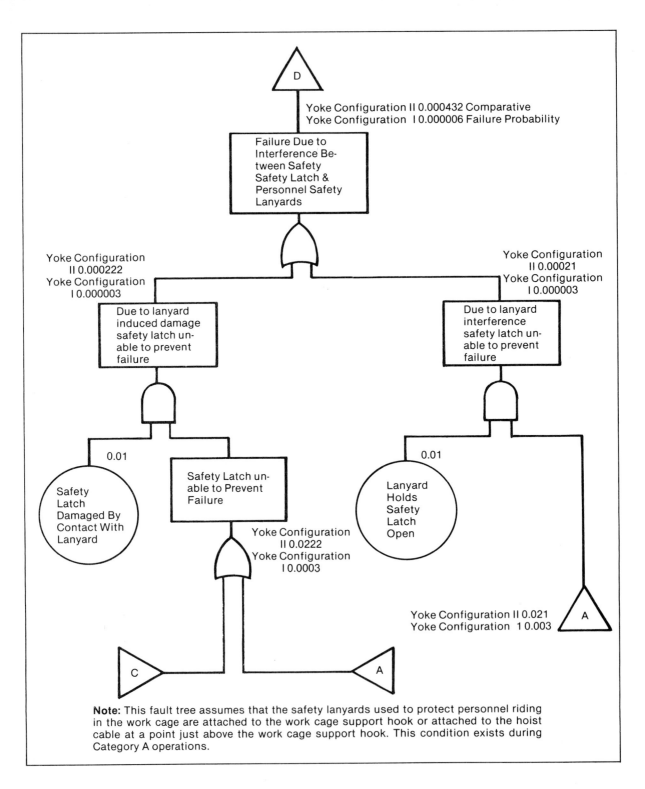

Note: This fault tree assumes that the safety lanyards used to protect personnel riding in the work cage are attached to the work cage support hook or attached to the hoist cable at a point just above the work cage support hook. This condition exists during Category A operations.

Simplified Utilization of Fault-Tree

In recent years, many hazard control specialists have attempted to utilize Fault Tree analysis to assess production and construction operations. The model which appears in Figure 78 demonstrates one possible use of the technique to locate potential failures in the construction industry. In addition to locating primary failures associated with the undesired event of the crane block falling, the data has provided a wealth of additional information relating to inspection, education, and training.

Uses of Fault Tree Analysis

Generally speaking, the Fault Tree technique's strength lies in the fact that it is a planning tool which enables the analyst to examine as many things which could go wrong with a systems operation as are possible, within human constraints. Using known data, the analyst can identify the single and multiple causes capable of inducing the undesired event. Secondly, Fault Tree is able to demonstrate the need for and utility of control measures which when adequately applied to specific tree paths, can cope with potential failure situations. Thirdly, the data developed in a tree serves to specify training and inspection requirements necessary to reduce the possibility of system failure. also, as an educational tool the Fault Tree allows for the rapid transfer of hazard data from person to person, group to group, with fewer possibilities of communication loss. Furthermore, the tree data is invaluable in educating safety inspectors and operational personnel in the critical areas of a particular system's operation, while demonstrating the capability and limitations of provided control measures. Lastly, Fault Tree can be used as an investigative tool. By reasoning backwards from the accident, the investigator may be able to reconstruct the system and those elements which, prior to the accident situation, were responsible for the undesired event.

Limitations of Fault Tree Analysis

Among the primary limitations of Fault Tree Analysis as a popular hazard analytical tool is that it can be, as previously stated, expensive. Of course the expense is directly related to the size and complexity of the system, the degree of detail necessary, and the need for data processing. However, the most important limitation of all is the fact that before Fault Tree Analysis is attempted, those conducting the analysis must have a thorough knowledge of the system's operation. The Fault Tree in Figure 78 (crane Block Failure) was con-

Figure 77. Fault tree analysis failure due to interference of safety lanyards.

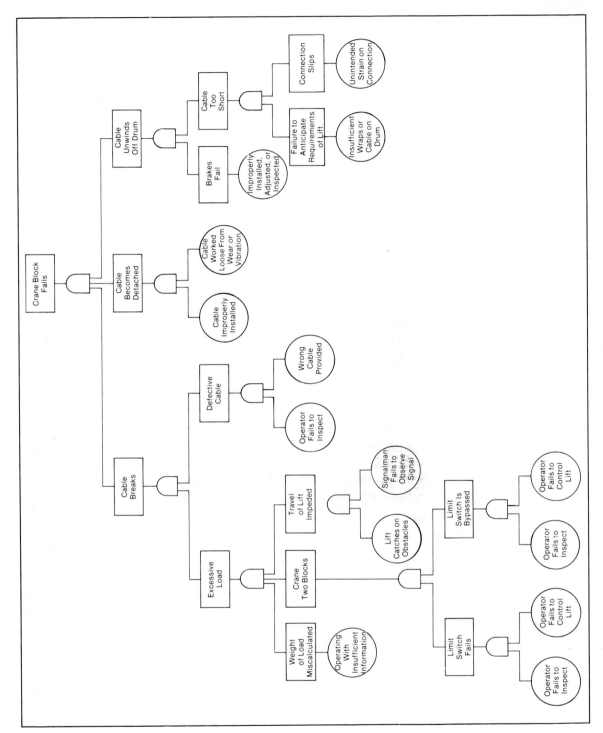

Figure 78. This tree is an extension of that developed by Mossa, M., "Professional Safety," Nov. 1976.

structed by a group of Operating Engineers who, being knowledgeable of the materials handling and crane operation process, were able to list the important failure possibilities which, if not rectified, could result in the situation of the crane block failing.

When to Choose the Combined Events Type Analysis

There are three general conditions which, if they exist, may entice a hazard control specialist to utilize the Fault-Tree method in locating and evaluating hazards associated with a particular system. They are:

1. When it is suspected that certain failure combinations could cause major system damage or injury;
2. When effects of single failures are predictable. This information is often known after the Preliminary Hazard Analyses or one of the severity grading type analyses are utilized to make a first-cut evaluation of the system's hazard potential;
3. After system designs or design alternatives have been finalized. The primary reason behind this point is that Fault-Tree analysis can be expensive in terms of both time, energy, and dollars. It must be judiciously used at a time when the basic system configuration has been decided on and all initial changes have been made.

Output from Hazard Analytical Techniques

The chart below, Figure 79, is presented to illustrate what data can be expected to be acquired from the various hazard analytical methods mentioned throughout this chapter.

Information	P.H.A.	FMEA	FMECA	SHA	Fault-tree
Absolute Probablistic Information	No	No	No	No	Yes
Relative Hazard Level	No	No	No	No	Yes
Relative Consequence Level	Yes	Yes	Yes	Yes	Yes
Other Qualitative Information	Yes	Yes	Yes	Yes	No
Other Management Information	Yes	Yes	Yes	Yes	Yes
Input for Other Analyses	Yes	Yes	Yes	Yes	Yes

Figure 79.

Use of Analytical
Trees in the
Reduction of
Occupational
Accidents and
Illnesses*

Introduction

If one wishes to undertake an effective program designed to reduce occupational accidents and illnesses, two basic criteria should be observed:

1. The supporting analytical program should provide quantitative evaluation of hazards and risks to a maximum practicable degree.
2. The supporting analytical program must control the probability of safety related oversights and omissions to a minimum practical level.

The first criterion arises because, as indicated in Figure 80, the hazard control program must interface with operating and program considerations in evaluation and control of the risks and costs associated with total organizational activities. While a strictly quantitative evaluation of hazard considerations on a dollar equivalent or time (schedule) equivalent basis is not always possible or even desirable, the hazard control program's analytical methodology must provide a method for indicating probabilities and consequences of undesirable events associated with operational and project activities. This is necessary to permit necessary management trade studies and decision.

The second criterion has to do with two sorts of oversights. The first of these is the oversight which omits consideration of certain operational activities. That is to say, certain operational activities are not formally identified and, therefore, escape from the hazard control system. The other type of potential oversight has to do with inadequacies and oversights lying in the analytical and control systems which are associated with hazard control and risk management for identified field activities.

An analytical method which is particularly appropriate to satisfying these two basic criteria involves the use of analytical tree.

The analytical tree provides a method which:

1. May be used in a qualitative sense for prevention of oversights and omissions.
2. May be used in a quantitative or semi-quantitative sense for evaluation of safety risks associated with all types of operational activities.
3. May be readily scaled to any desired level of detail.
4. Interfaces readily with other modern management methods (Management by Objectives, planning trees and networks, management acceptance networks, PERT and other forms of work flow charting, etc.).
5. May be easily learned and used in elementary form by most types of technical and nontechnical personnel within an industrial organization.

*Contributing author: Dr. R. J. Nertney, E. G. and G. Idaho, Inc., Idaho Falls, IO.

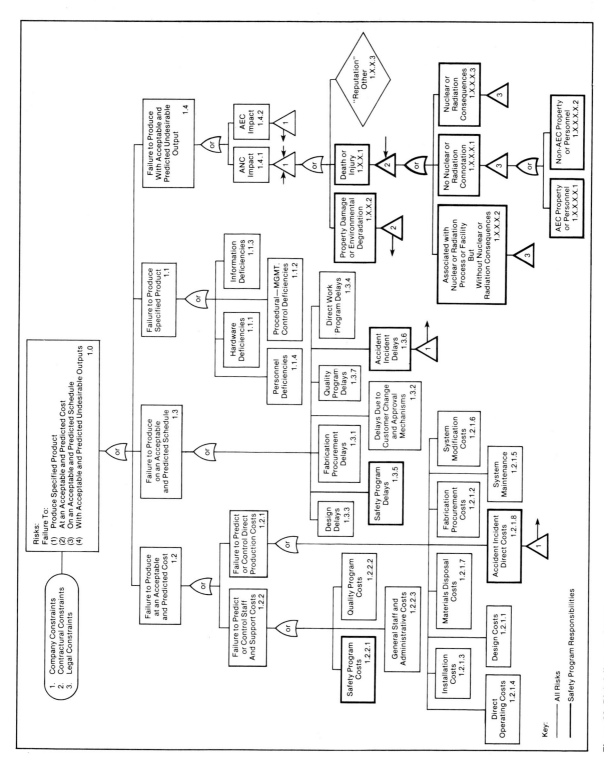

Figure 80. Risk failure mode tree.

The Atomic Energy Commission's System Safety Program, MORT (The Management Oversight and Risk Tree), as developed and applied within Aerojet Nuclear Company, illustrates the use of analytical trees, and this discussion of the trees will be, in part, within the context of the MORT program. As will be seen later, the utility and practicality of using tree type analytical methods are highly dependent on the nature of the entire technical and management control programs within which they are utilized. This is, of course, true of any of the systems safety methodology.

Positive Trees

Detailed discussion of positive analytical trees and networks exist in the literature (Ayres, 1969; Johnson, 1973; Lanford, 1972). These discussions are often associated with forecasting techniques. Since risk projection is essentially a specialized form of forecasting, the forecasting methods are ordinarily directly applicable to the hazard control program.

The example chosen relates to a situation which often faces the hazard control specialist, and the line manager. A job or process is awaiting release. The question is whether the process is, in fact, ready and whether or not necessary releases should be authorized.

The positive tree at the upper left of Figure 81 forms the basis to determine whether a process or job is ready for release. The "objective" then is to ascertain whether or not all aspects of the process are indeed "ready."

If the process is to be "ready," the involved personnel must be ready, **and** the plant and hardware must be ready, **and** the procedural (management control) system must be ready.

One may then proceed to develop the lower structure of the tree. For example, the question must be asked, "What personnel are involved?" This leads to development of a tree tier or "layer" which would specify operators, maintenance personnel, hazard control specialists, management-supervisory personnel, etc.

The next question which must be asked is, "What is meant by a state of readiness?" This leads, in turn, to a tier or layer of the tree which is based on evaluation of the life cycle of events which make an individual "ready." That is to say:

Selection	(Have color-blind individuals been selected to read color-coded information displays?)
Basic Skills	(Is the welder a craft qualified welder?)
Special Skills	(If the welding involves exotic materials, is the welder exotic material qualified?)
Job and System Readiness	(Are the personnel trained to *this* job and *this* system?)

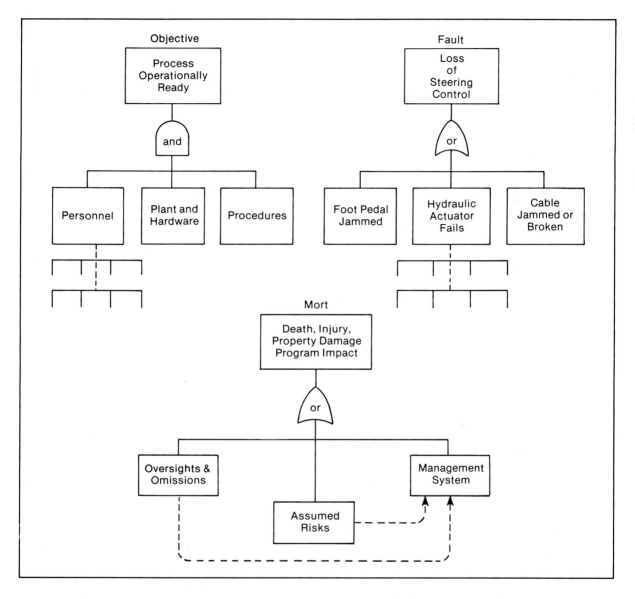

Figure 81. Types of analytical trees.

Here and Now Readiness (Are the personnel ready *today*? Are there problems associated with over-work, illness, drug or alcohol problems, etc.?)

The other branches of the tree are developed in the same way. Plant and hardware lower tiers are developed, based on required configuration and quality controls ranging from the setting of specifications through procurement, inspection, protection of inspected materials to point of use, etc.

The procedures branch includes not only detailed operating procedures, but the entire organizational control structure up to and including basic policy statement; e.g., Is this job or project covered by policy statements: If policy statements exist, is the job or project in compliance: If relevant policy statements do not exist, should they?

In order to maintain continuity, the total system will function more effectively if similar trees are used in the job planning process, as indicated in Figure 82. In this situation, one may:

1. Structure the tree indicating, in successively greater detail, those things which must be done to make the top objective come true.
2. Utilize the tree to structure work flow and PERT type charts.
3. Structure a "readiness matrix" indicating "who" must do "what" to provide a state of readiness.
4. Utilize the matrix to maintain task completion status up to the time of release.

It must be remembered that all of this discussion of the analytical trees is highly dependent on their use in context in the overall management system. This subject will be addressed in terms of other organizational functions later in this discussion.

In the broad sense, the positive analytical trees are based on organizational objectives and are developed using **and** and **or** logic gates. **And** gates develop the tree through statements of the necessary and sufficient conditions to achieve the next tier conditions. **Or** gates are utilized to indicate alternative and/or redundant means of achieving the objective.

As indicated earlier, these positive trees may be developed at broad strategic levels, lower tactical levels based on accomplishment of missions and tasks of limited scope, or both. The tree can include administrative and management activities, hardware functions, or both.

Basically, four types of positive trees are utilized:

1. The Contingency Tree—In ideal concept, this tree indicates *all* alternative means of achieving the top objective and provides *all* lower tier necessary-and-sufficient conditions required to achieve all alternatives. In real life, of course, it is impossible to indicate "all" alternatives and only the principal alternatives are charted.

2. The Decision Tree—This is a contingency tree from which the "or" options, prohibited by constraint systems, have been removed. This leaves only the "or" decisions which the internal management system is authorized to make.

3. The Relevance Tree—This tree indicates the relative importance of lower tier tasks in fulfilling the top objective and thereby provides guidance in allocation of resources and establishment of controls. "Relative importance" may be evaluated in terms of such indices as potential cost or time impact, or

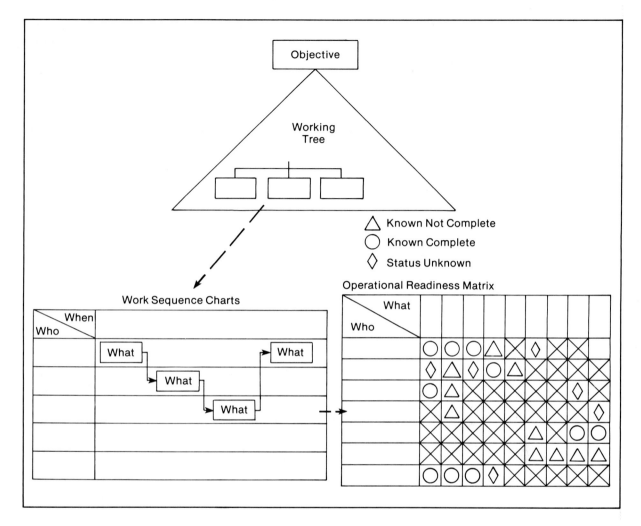

Figure 82. Use of trees in the job planning process.

in terms of more subjective "importance" scales. Generally speaking, both the probability of failure to accomplish the task, as well as the potential consequences, must be considered.

4. The Working Tree—This tree indicates the chosen method of accomplishment and eliminates all **or** gates except those remaining for purposes of redundancy or to provide future implementation options. This positive tree is the dual image of the associated fault tree in the sense that "success" and "failure" statements are inverted as are the **and** and **or** gates.

Application of the Trees

The Atomic Energy Commission's MORT System Safety Program (Johnson, 1973) makes probably the most extensive and broadest use of tree type analytical methods. This program utilizes both fault and positive analytical trees in both the quantitative and qualitative senses. The MORT program is scoped to cover the entire spectrum of safety program considerations ranging from conventional shop and laboratory safety to complex nuclear systems. It further is designed to relate hazard analysis of jobs and tasks to analysis of the management system which are designed to control safety performance.

The MORT program is designed to:

1. Result in reduction of safety related oversights, errors, and omissions.
2. Result in risk quantification *and* referral of residual risks to proper organizational management levels for appropriate action.
3. Optimize allocation of resources to the safety program and to organizational hazard control efforts.

The analytical trees are utilized in both the qualitative and in a limited quantitative sense in implementation of the MORT program.

In the quantitative sense, probabilities are assigned to the lower tier tasks and functions and may be propagated and combined to yield probabilities of success in achieving the top objective for the positive trees or the probabilities of the top failure event occurring for the fault tree.

The probabilities of success or failure generated in this manner may then be combined with the consequences of failure to yield quantitative risk statements associated with the task or process under analysis. An important point in performing such evaluations is that the interbounds of the study be fine enough that the initiating or primary events at the lowest tiers of the trees are independent components for which data exist (or may be obtained).

In design of the MORT programs and its associated training programs, emphasis is placed both on construction of trees developed for one's own programmatic needs, as well as use of a set of MORT readimade trees which may be used for program design, program evaluation, or accident-incident investigation. The latter include trees associated with configuration control, independent safety review, accident-incident analysis, etc.

The lower tree in Figure 81 represents one of the readimade trees provided by MORT and is the analytical tree from which the MORT program derives its name.

As indicated in Figure 81, the MORT tree is a negative or fault tree developed in two major branches. The first branch of the left deals with specific hazard control program inadequacies which can lead to the undesirable effects associated with accidents and incidents. The major branch on the right deals with the inadequacies in the management system. The center branch, assumes risk in conduction operations. The quantification and formal acceptance characteristics of the MORT "assumed risk" must be emphasized: these are not the familiar "calculated risks"—which are seldom supported by "calculations."

The MORT tree is developed to some two hundred lower tier safety program elements whose purpose is to prevent the undesirable consequences indicated at the top of the tree.

As indicated by the dotted lines, the "specific oversights and omissions" and "assumed risk" branches are coupled to the management system in the lower tiers of the tree. This leads not only to analysis of specific hazard control program elements, but to analysis of the deficiencies in management control system which permits the specific deficiencies to improper acceptance of risks to occur.

This coupling between specific hazard control program elements, company risk assumption, and the organization's management system indicates a fundamental consideration in use of the analytical trees. The ultimate benefits of use of analytical trees within the system safety and hazard control program are dependent, to a high degree, on the extent to which similar or compatible methodology is used in the organization's other activities (Millikin & Morrision, 1973).

In particular, maximum benefits will be achieved if formal trees are used as analytical and design models and are utilized as follows:

1. Planning and Forecasting—Use of morphological planning trees and networks.
2. Management Review and Acceptance—Formal risk acceptance trees and networks.
3. Engineering and Technical Support—Formal fault tree and Failure-Mode and Effect (FMEA) processes.
4. Implementation—Formal "Management by Objectives" (MBO) implementation trees.

This sort of coherent interrelationship is indicated schematically in Figure 83. In one organization where the MORT methodology is used, EG&G Idaho, Inc., system safety personnel conduct active programs to encourage development and use of compatible methodologies in the interface activities.

This experience indicates that the use of the analytical trees in reduction of occupational accidents and incidents should be considered in three types of application:

1. In the qualitative sense, for prevention of oversights and omissions.
2. In the projection of future risk and of decision making relative to risk acceptance and resource allocation, for relatively stable systems.
3. In the projection of risk for new systems or existing systems following major changes.

The methodology for qualitative application of tree analytics is sufficiently developed for practical and effective use. The benefits to be achieved in

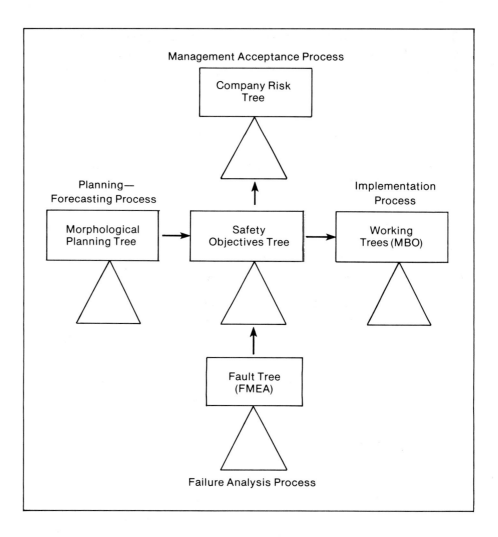

Figure 83. Safety trees—
other activities.

prevention of oversights and in identification and elimination of "soft spots" in the system under analysis make this mode of application not only feasible and desirable, but highly useful in any well-managed organization.

Risk projection and resource allocation, making use of relevance trees, risk projection techniques, and intuitive (but structured) forecasting techniques, represent a somewhat closer approach to state-of-the-art limits. In this case, experience indicates that such efforts are both feasible and practical in the quantitative sense for relatively stable systems. This endorsement must be accompanied, however, by a caution that we live in a changing world and that one must be constantly alert for changes which can render his projections invalid.

The final application of tree analytics for purposes of risk projection in new systems or systems which experience major changes presents the most serious problems at present state-of-the-art.

The benefits of such application include:

1. Logical rigor.
2. Visibility and the consequent ability to engage in systems modeling exercises.
3. Ability to combine human and hardware reliability considerations in a single and analytical model (Homes and Narver, Inc., 1967; IEE Transactions on Reliability, 1973; Swain).

While adequate models exist for quantitative use of analytical trees in risk projection and control (Hammer, 1972; Nielson, undated; Rasmussen, 1973; Vesley & Narum, 1972; Vesley, 1969), serious limitations exist which restrict use of the models in the general sense. The most serious of these are:

1. Inadequacies in hardware reliability data stores.
2. Inadequacies in human factors data stores.
3. The resultant degree of expertise required to make use of existing data stores.

Because data stores are limited in scope and in one-to-one applicability, available data must be modeled to actual system conditions. This, in turn, means that if one is to produce valid risk projections, he must utilize the highest quality data and information systems. It further means that one must utilize advanced state-of-the-art expertise both in the areas of hardware reliability and hxman factors data interpretation and in the handling of uncertainties in the subsequent risk projection process. If this is not done, the apparent rigor of the analytic process can be seriously degraded through the subjective and nonrigorous interpretive links with the data stores.

The result of this situation is that *strictly quantitative* application of analytical trees to projection and control of hazards in new and/or changing systems is presently limited to:

1. Key subsystems.
2. Large complex systems for which failure consequences justify development of sophisticated data and information systems *and* the retention of highly specialized staff expertise.

Such application leads to a situation in which systems having serious failure consequences can become the principal contributions to such central data stores as GIDEP (Government Industry Data Exchange Program, 1972). This in turn, can lead to concentrations of data relating to particular system types, utilizing special, high reliability components operating under restricted environmental and operating conditions. This can seriously limit the utility of apparently massive data blanks to the casual user.

One must also use extreme care in accepting published reliability data obtained from a single source. A recent study of data in 62 major reliability data stores has indicated variation of up to a factor of 10 in quoted reliability of similar components (Thomas, personal communication, 1974). This variation is presumably due to some combination of quality controls, environmental conditions, and operating conditions.

Summary

In summary,

1. Use of qualitative trees is feasible and practical in prevention of safety program oversights and omissions;
2. Use of analytical trees in conjunction with risk forecasting and resource allocation in establishing hazard control for relatively stable systems is feasible and practical;
3. Reliability data stores limitations leading to severe requirements for staff expertise presently limit the scope and depth of fully quantitative application of analytical trees in risk application and control; and
4. Effectiveness and utility of the analytical trees in the safety program is dependent, to a considerable degree, on the extent to which other organizational activities utilize similar and compatible methodology.

Bibliography

Boeing, "Support Systems Engineering," Fault Tree for Safety; D6-53004, November, 1968.

Department of Defense. Requirements for Systems Safety Program and Association of Subsystems and Equipment. (Military Standard 882). Washington, D.C. 20305, July 15, 1969.

Firenze, R. J., "Systems Approach to System Safety Evaluation," National Safety News, National Safety Council, 44 N. Michigan Ave., Chicago 60611. Vol. 101, No. 2, February, 1970, pp. 50-54.

Haasl, David F. (From a seminar on Systems Safety). University of Washington, Seattle, WA 98105, August, 1969.

Meister, D., and Rabideau, G., "Human Factors Evaluation in System Development," John Wiley and Sons, Inc., New York, p. 21.

McCormick, E. J., "Human Factors Engineering," McGraw-Hill Book Company, 330 W. 42nd Street, New York 10036, 1964.

Optner, S. L., "Systems Analysis for Business Management," Prentice-Hall, Inc., 70 Fifth Avenue, New York 10011, 1968.

Peters, G. A., "Systematic Safety," National Safety News, September, 1975.

Quade, E. F., "Analysis for Military Decisions," The Rand Corporation, Santa Monica, California, 1964, p. 4.

Recht, J. L., "An Introduction to System Safety Analysis," National Safety News, December, 1965, February, April and June, 1966.

Rickenbacker, E. V., "Rickenbacker," Prentice-Hall, Inc., Englewood Cliffs, New Jersey, 1967.

"Risk Management Guide," EG&G Idaho, Inc.,/ERDA 76–45/11 SSDC-11, June, 1977.

"Safety Information System Guide," EG&G Idaho, Inc.,/ERDA 76–45/9SSDC-9, March, 1977.

"Standardization Guide for Construction and Use of MORT-Type Analytic Trees," EG&G Idaho, Inc./ERDA 76–45/8 SSDC-8, February, 1977.

Notes

1. E. F. Quade, Analysis of Military Decision, The Rand Corporation, Santa Monica, California, 1964, page 4.
2. D. Meister, C. Rabideau, Human Factors Evaluation in System Development, John Wiley and Sons, Inc., N.Y., page 21.
3. D. Meister, G. Rabideau, Human Factors Evaluation in Systems Development, John Wiley and Sons, Inc., New York, page 21.
4. Meister, loc. cit.
5. Meister, loc. cit.
6. E. F. Quade, "Analysis of Military Decisions," The Rand Corporation, Santa Monica, California, 1964.
7. David F. Haasl, (from a seminar on system safety), August 1969. University of Washington, Seattle, Washington.
8. E. V. Rickenbacker, "Rickenbacker" Prentice-Hall, Inc., Englewood Cliffs, New Jersey, 1967, page 228.
9. W. Hammer, "Handbook of System and Product Safety," Prentice-Hall, 1972.
10. This section is reprinted in part from a study conducted by R. I. Fujimoto and J. W. Neurauter with permission of the Boeing Company Strategic Missile Systems Division Aerospace Group Seattle, Washington.

Application of Ergonomics in Hazard Control 7

This chapter is designed to introduce ergonomics, and the design of optimum man-machine systems. Its purpose is twofold: First, it will provide an introduction to ergonomics, through the discussion of its history, basic terminology, and application to the work environment. Secondly, it will serve to give the reader a "feel" for the place of ergonomics in the design of efficient, and productive work environments.

The tasks which human beings perform create certain requirements. The ability of the worker to meet these requirements is often the critical factor in the success or failure of his job. If human abilities and limitations along with machinery and equipment limitations are considered in advance, and the machines, equipment, and the physical surroundings are designed with human performance in mind, the probability of successful task performance can be noticeably increased.

Ergonomics, as defined in this chapter is *the study of man's relationship to his work*. In practice, the ergonomist is concerned with the design of work (design in a broad sense) insofar as it involves the interaction of people, machines, tools, and the working environment, and takes into account the anatomical and physiological capabilities and limitations of man.

The purpose of applying these factors to workplace design is to improve the performance of workers in operating and maintaining their machines and equipment without unduly taxing the worker in the process.

This chapter is not intended to be an exhaustive analysis of behavioral parameters involved in perception, discrimination, decision-making, manipu-

Permission to use the information contained in this chapter was granted by Prof. Richard G. Pearson and Prof. Mahmoud A. Ayoub of North Carolina State University and the American Institute of Industrial Engineering.

lation responses, etc., but rather is concerned with a description of how some of these factors are involved from a practical standpoint in the design of more optimum workplaces.

Background   Ergonomics is probably as old as the human race itself and can be traced back as far as primeval man where evidence illustrates that he protected himself from the elements by seeking refuge in caves, and used fire to cook and preserve his food. For all practical purposes, we can say that man has been a practitioner of ergonomics ever since he invented tools to extend and reinforce the range, strength, and effectiveness of his limb movements. History tells us that tool designs were fashioned so to protect the limb in use from damaging contact with hard materials, while at the same time, fitting well into the gripping hand.

The configuration of early tools indicates that prehistoric toolmakers were considering the surface anatomy of the human hand. Since then, a sound knowledge of the form and function of the human body has formed an essential part of the professional know-how of designers and makers of tools, machinery, and workplace equipment.

Early in this century, Frank Bunker Gilbreth, having conducted extensive studies of man at work, virtually invented and introduced scientific "motion study" in industry. His activities in the field of "efficiency engineering" were so extraordinarily successful that this great pioneer was also the first proponent of ergonomics as we know it today. Since ergonomics is concerned with the efficiency of human performance and thus consequently its inefficiency— there is a real justification for application of ergonomics to problems of occupational safety and health. The very fact that accidents and disabilities are observed within industry constitutes sufficient rationale for consideration of the ergonomics approach to problems of injury and work-related health problems. The ergonomics approach that is now evolving in the United States combines consideration of performance, safety, and health criteria in a total systems approach to the design of work and the workplace.

A second rationale for considering the ergonomics approach is inherent in the fact that the old approaches to safety problems have not been very successful. Swain, Reference (1), provides a cogent critique of past emphasis on motivational campaigns and on the identification of accident-prone workers, and concludes that these play a lesser role in job safety than what he calls "work situation" factors. In Swain's approach the goal is to provide the worker with a "safetyprone" work situation through design (or redesign) of the task and workplace, in order to prevent accidents from occurring. Such an approach is essentially embraced in our later discussion under "The systems approach."

To demonstrate the effectiveness of a good work situation design, it is necessary to conduct a systems evaluation. This may involve a number of indices which can be related to the identification of accident-conducive situations, e.g., accidents, near-accidents, incidents, medical data, and hazard reports. More will be said about these topics later. The important point to be made here is that a total approach to safety involves both design (prevention) and evaluation—the latter providing feedback for the improvement of the system. While the same concepts are involved, whether a new industrial plant or an existing (old) plant are to be evaluated, it should be noted that "after the fact," corrective approaches to job safety do exist.(1)

The validity of the ergonomics approach is, to a large extent, represented intrinsically by the kinds of problems which justify the existence of the field. That is, problems in performance and safety (e.g., inefficiency and accidents) are everywhere around us—many, as noted above, being a function of poor or improper engineering design in the first place. Solutions then become obvious, after the fact, as one or more causes are identified. Insofar as human efficiency is concerned, the ergonomics data bank does have much to offer. While difficulties may be encountered in the translation of laboratory findings into usable design data, the application is straightforward in many situations. When displays are illegible, ergonomics data can suggest a number of ways to provide legibility. When control errors and confusion are common, ergonomics data have much to suggest in the way of control coding, location, mode of operation, etc. Such data are available in a number of sources and guides (2), (3), (4).

The Systems Approach

The term *approach means a conscientious, "organized" effort to design an effective system, such as a production plant, giving due consideration to the interaction among worker, machine, and environment.* From the ergonomics viewpoint, prime attention is given to human performance and safety considerations (criteria). A cardinal principal of ergonomics is that, since everything is designed ultimately for man's use or consumption, man's characteristics should be considered from the very beginning of the design cycle. Based upon the objectives of the system, certain functions are identified early in this cycle and these should be allocated to man or machine on the basis or relative capabilities (e.g., application of force, data logging, decision-making). As human functions are identified within the system, ultimately tasks come to be structured out of the specified interrelationships between worker and machine. It is at this point that the ergonomist must endeavor to ensure optimum performance (and safety) at the man-machine interface. Blueprints are studied, plant layout is evaluated, and full scale mock-ups of individual work stations may be constructed. Is information needed by the worker going to be available to him in proper and effective form? (Are controls located in an efficient manner? What about height of the work surface?) These are but a few of many questions that can be asked.

Once tasks are specified, the human skills specific to each can be delineated. For example, assembly of small parts requires finger dexterity, crane operation requires good depth perception, and so on. Such information is then passed on to personnel specialists responsible for manning the system once it is operational.

With the plant in operation, the ergonomist then turns his attention to evaluation of systems effectiveness. While the ergonomist is interested in traditional management criteria of effective production (productivity, defective products, scrap), his focus is more directed on human error per se, as reflected in individual performance, errors, near-accidents, and accidents. The results of systems evaluation provide data which can be fed back to the designers, staffers, and managers of the system, for their utilization in improving the system. Thus, a loop is completed between design analysis and evaluation—a process in which the ergonomist should continually participate, for the effectivenesss of the system and, especially, for the well-being of the workers.

As a function of the ergonomics-systems approach, there should be no need, "when things go wrong," to ascribe blame to mysterious circumstances. The only ingredients of system error are those designed into the system in the first place, and these ingredients are the elements which must be subject to thorough systems evaluation.

Equipment Design

Ample historical evidence exists that worker's limitations have typically received little attention during the design of equipment for his use. Thus, managers have commonly been in the position of adapting the worker to fit the machine. With regard to equipment having injury potential, the approach has too often been to instruct, train, or motivate the worker to avoid the hazard—rather than to design the hazard out of the system in the first place. "Fitting the worker to the task" runs contrary to the basic principle of ergonomics. Numerous studies have shown how minor changes in equipment design produce significant improvements in performance, in contrast to efforts involving training or motivation.

Undesirable Design Characteristics

Certain design practices which increase the probability of human error (and hence accidents) have been identified through the analysis of accident data, case studies, and laboratory research. For example, designs which violate "population stereotypes" are a common source of error. Population stereotype is defined by the characteristic response in a given situation by a particular group of users. Examples include the association of the color red with "stop" or "danger," the forward movement of a control to increase power, the clockwise turning of a rotary knob to increase electrical current flow, and the clockwise turning of a knob to decrease fluid flow in plumbing applications.

When relationships between controls and their associated displays, indicators, or machine responses are not logical or clearcut, there is again an increased probability for human error which can be attributed to poor design. Wherever practicable, controls should be placed close to the displays which they affect, Figure 84A; if separated, at least a similar geometric arrangement should be used so that it is clear which control goes with which display, Figure 84B. To aid in the identification of subsections of large display panels, lines may be used to segment the panel, and color coding may be used as a further supplemental cue to relate controls with displays; in the display systems of very large operations the use of sensor lines coupled with color coding is recommended to indicate relationships, Figure 84C.

Insofar as similar equipment or work stations are involved in tasks performed in an industrial plant, every effort should be made to select equipment and to design workplace layouts to avoid the problem of having interference. This requires standardization in equipment design and installation practice. If

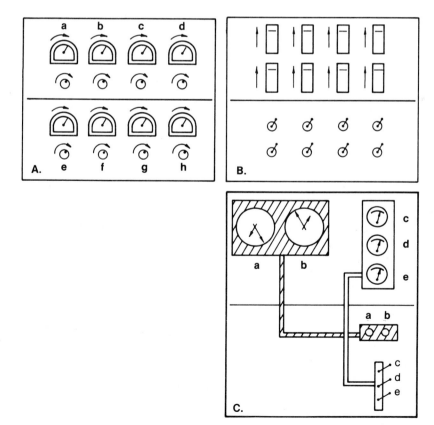

Figure 84. Accepted practice in display and control layout.

designs vary from one work situation to another, errors can be expected since the worker who learns a task in situation A finds difficulty in adapting to situation B. Thus, "old" habits interefere with performance in the new situation. This is particularly true with regard to display-control relationships where standardization is lacking.

The limits of human sensory acuities and discrimination abilities should be considered by designers. In terms of vision, hearing, and tactual (touch) sensitivity, there is much data from sensory psychology that can be applied. What can be heard, seen? How large a display? What distance? What colors should be used? How much information can be displayed at 30 inches for a given diameter panel meter? How many knob shapes and sizes can be discriminated effectively by touch alone? Design data are available, (2), (4), to designers.

Human Physical Limitations

Human physical structure can be related in many instances to the proper design of equipment. Two areas of study that are adjunct to ergonomics are relevant—anthropometry and biomechanics. *Anthropometry deals with the measurement of various physical features of the body, including linear dimensions, circumference, and weight. Biomechanics on the other hand, deals more with the mechanical aspects of human motion, including consideration of range, speed, and strength of body movements.* Again, accident data make it obvious (after the fact) when work situation designs fail to give proper attention to these areas, their concepts and data. For example, failure to take into account anthropometric characteristics (human body size and shape)—especially with regard to sex, age, and cultural differences—can lead to work inefficiency and job dissatisfaction, and thus, ultimately, to worker error. Accidents can also result as a by-product of physical straining of individuals. A physically-overloaded individual can have difficulty in reacting to, and coping with hazardous events. In severe cases of physical loading, disorganization of the established patterns of motor acts may result: reaction time increases; motion path and its characteristics become erratic, and in most cases unpredictable. Based on an analysis of 427 accidents in a machine shop, Branton, (5), concludes that a direct correlation does exist between variability in hand motion (especially unintentional motions) and accident occurrences. Since equipment, task, and protective measures are usually designed based on a set of well-learned and organized motor acts, physical loading-induced changes in these acts can constitute a conflict which, if not resolved through providing rest periods, change in task design, or other means, will ultimately produce accidents.

Detection of Error-Producing Designs

Ideally, designs which are conducive to human error should be eliminated in the development of an industrial plant, i.e., during the task analysis stage as discussed previously. Certainly, at least inferences should be drawn at this point concerning where equipment designs are incompatible with human capabilities. This may be done by searching for limitations in existing, operational systems, or in simulated or prototype systems (either with real equipment or with full-scale mockups.) Other sources of data include information on malfunctioning systems, accident data, incident data, critical incident studies, and workers' unsatisfactory reports on equipment operation, (1), (6), (7).

A number of useful ergonomic checklists are available for the designer to use, in evaluating his efforts in considering the human element in equipment design, (3), (8). While such checklists are mainly intended for use in evaluating systems under development, they can also be used with operational systems.

Much of what has been written so far regarding ergonomics design assumes that an efficient worker is a safe worker. But there are countless industrial work situations involving hazards where efficiency per se is not enough. In these, the worker still needs to be warned of equipment failures, to be prevented from inadvertently activating equipment which could injure him, or to be alerted to his own inattentiveness. The very nature of many industrial equipments/tasks preclude their being totally safe, e.g., power presses, welding, drill presses, lathes, grinding wheels, power sanders, saws of all kinds, and conveyor belt systems. In short, it is necessary to acknowledge that certain tasks require a man-machine interaction carrying with it inherent hazards without which the tasks could not be performed. Fortunately, ergonomics practice also has application in such situations, involving many of the approaches already discussed as well as others.

Hazard Control in Job-Workplace Design

Displays and Controls

To provide cautions and warnings to the worker in the interest of workplace hazard control, some sort of visual or auditory displays may be useful. The principal requirements are getting the attention of the worker, and telling him what is wrong, or what he should do. Because of the nature of man and industrial tasks, ideal solutions are difficult to achieve. When several visual indicator lights are used to indicate the status of a system, the operator may adapt and "tune out" their presence. A recommended alternative is to use one conspicuous master warning light to indicate trouble, and then a remote, supplemental panel with signals (such as annunciator displays) to identify the locus of malfunction, or to suggest a course of action. One limitation of warning lights is that they must be located within a reasonable range of the worker's visual field of attention. Another problem is that workers find flashing lights to be a source of annoyance. When the visual channel is overloaded, or illumination precludes optimal use of visual displays, auditory signals may be used. They have the advantage over visual displays of being omni-directional—the worker doesn't need to face the display source. Their use is limited, however, when too many different auditory signals must be received and discriminated among or when background noise is high. The latter is a particularly critical problem today which demands attention. For example, workers may be required to wear some type of ear protection against high noise levels, yet be alert to the auditory warning devices of moving vehicles within the plant. Thus, solution to a health problem here can run counter to that involving a safety problem.

Common control error problems needing hazard control consideration include: control confusion (especially in blind reaching), and accidental activation. Controls should be designed so that the worker receives feedback which tells him which control he is operating, and which also provides confirmation of control activation. Thus, controls can be selected that are different in size and shape to facilitate tactual (touch) discrimination—particularly critical in blind reaching. Spacing is important to prevent accidental activation—even more so if gloves are worn. Push-buttons with snap action, and which illuminate when depressed, provide three modes of feedback—visual, auditory, and tactual. Controls may be recessed or enclosed barriers to prevent activation by bumping while reaching for another control or by being caught by a shirt cuff. Critical controls may be protected with hinged covers or even locked in position.

In designing the workplace with hazard control considerations in mind it is obvious that important critical displays and controls should be located in positions that permit optimal viewing and response. This is often easier said than accomplished in practice—but it should be a design goal. Consideration should be given to human reaction time, accuracy requirements, and force that must be applied, e.g., which limb should be used, which muscles are to be involved? Inevitably, conflicts will exist and trade-offs will have to be made.

Machine Guarding and Maintenance

Protecting the worker from the hazards of moving machinery is a major safety problem. Interlocks are useful, as are approaches which require the arms and legs to be in specific positions before the machine can be safely operated, e.g., each hand on a control in order to activate a powerpress of shear. Contemporary approaches to the design of machine guarding wisely involve application of anthropometric data; the height, width, or depth of a barrier may be related to reach/mobility characteristics of the human torso, arm, and hand. The amount of spacing in wire grids can determine (limit) the degree of penetration of fingers, hands, arms, and feet.

A report by Singleton, (8), frequently cites maintenance activity as a major factor in workplace accidents and injuries. Often these are seen to occur when machine guards are not replaced following maintenance, an occurrence common with workers on piece rates. An indirect effect here, the workers simply don't want to take the time to clean and adjust their equipment, or report its faults. Singleton endorses more attention to design for maintenance, noting that a guard, ". . . which is difficult to remove is usually also difficult to replace; for this reason it is often not replaced." Again, good ergonomics data for maintainability design do exist, (2). Application emphasis is on ease of access, anthropometric considerations, task reliability, and error-free replacement. The latter is a critical safety consideration; often components are reinstated in damage to equipment and worker injury. The solution is to design for "one-way" installation, e.g., asymmetrical arrangement of aligning pins on connector cable plugs.

While environmental factors are typically regarded as a source of health-related problems, they also have potential effects on human efficiency, thereby increasing the probability of accidents. This is particularly true with regard to noise and heat stress. A major deficiency in the area is knowledge concerning the interaction effects of two or more stressors in combination, such as heat, noise, and vibration. An obvious inconsistency is the tendency by plant engineers to treat noise and vibration as separate problems and introduce control methods accordingly. Also, there is need to recognize that the solution to one stressor may contravene other workplace design objectives, e.g., installation of sound-absorbing baffles hung from the ceiling which compromises previously-effective illumination. It is also important to note that some noise (and perhaps vibration, too) is useful as a cue to the worker regarding the use and efficiency of his equipment, e.g., the feedback property of drill press operation noise. Elimination of such noise may be to the detriment of efficient task performance.

Environmental Stress

The characteristics of the task and work schedule are relevant to safety insofar as these related to work efficiency. Monotonous, boring tasks are hardly conducive to sustaining of attention. Then, too, there are distractions from outside the workplace and from petty irritants within it that can compromise performance. A sudden glance away from the task and a fingertip is lost, or an eye is pierced by a flying fragment. The job design objective here is to optimize human efficiency through task variety and optimal loading of the human at-

Task Stress

tentional and information processing mechanisms, (9). Too much load stress (too high a work pace) is undesirable, particularly when combined with environmental stressors such as noise.

Biomechanical Hazards

The literature of ergonomics contains numerous examples of how the interface between man and machine, if not controlled, can be hazardous to one's safety and health. In many instances, the interface may subject both man's anatomy and physiology to excessive and highly concentrated stresses and strains. Persistence of these stresses can lead to the occurrence of an array of health disorders and occupational diseases.

For example, the task in some occupations might force the individual to maintain an awkward posture during extended periods. Such awkard postures, when imposed (through faulty equipment design, or workplace arrangement) over a number of years are apt to deform the anatomical system of the human body and ultimately lead to permanent occupational deformities. This is quite commonly the case in tasks requiring the operator to stand on one leg (the other being used for control operation) or to bending and leaning required in maintenance tasks it is not surprising that these are a common source of disability involving the human anatomical structure. Apart from awkard postures per se, the stress also includes static loads from extension of body mass (head, arms), and loads from tools used and from equipment being lifted into or out of place.

A paper by Van Wely, (10), suggests a correlation between improper work postures and diseases of the musculo-skeletal system (muscles, tendons, joints, and bones). For instance, static loading of the cervical vertebrae—a posture prone to the meat packing industry—has been found to be conducive to lesions of the spine Similarly a report by Podzimek et al, (11), describes a phenomenon in shoemakers who work in unnatural positions (head inclined to side, operator standing on one leg). Known as "lasters' back" the disability is described by ". . . projecting right shoulder-blade, protuberance of the backbone erector to the right of the right shoulder. . . ."

The potential for disability can also be a function of an interaction between the physical and mental demands of a task. Draus, (12), for example, argues that undue amounts of mental stress affect the flexibility of the muscular system adversely, thereby setting the stage for backache episodes.

Hazards of Manual Materials Handling

Manual materials handling activities (lifting, carrying, pushing, and pulling) constitute a major source of spinal disorders and back problems. Despite modern-day increases in automation, mechanization, and miniaturization relative to problems of industrial materials handling, injuries from manual handling of objects have not decreased as one might expect. A recent review,

(13), of industrial back injury problems emphasizes the seriousness and extent of this situation. Brown shows that 32 percent of lifting injuries resulted in sprains of the low back, 12 percent resulted in hernias and six percent in slipped discs. Brown further notes that 60 percent of all reportable injuries were caused by lifting objects which were beyond the "physical capability" of the worker. At the same time, it is important to note that abnormality of the spine can compound the frequency and severity of back accidents; e.g., spine disorders can increase the potential for materials handling accidents by as much as 300 percent, (14). Such injuries, at a cost often exceeding $1,000 per case, represent a considerable financial burden to industry, not to mention the misery, anguish, and suffering which victims, their families, and society have to sustain.

The question of what constitutes lifting stress, beyond consideration of the mass of the object, is one that is in need of definitive research. For instance, most previous studies have addressed themselves to the study of sagittal (involving "middle plane" of body) lifting instead of unconstrained lifting (lifting which involves trunk rotation). Further, the problem of studying lifting under the combined effects of physical and mental loads has not received adequate attention.

Hazards of Hand Tools

Hazards associated with the design and the use of hand tools may not be as severe or as well-pronounced as those from other hazards, yet hand tool-related ailments do exist in industry, Figure 85. In this regard a worker who is crippled by repeated long-term usage of a poorly designed tool has just as much right to receive protection (as well as compensation) as the worker who is adversely affected by the breathing of toxic gases. Recent rulings by the courts in liability cases consider hand tool ailments as occupational diseases for which compensation claims should be awarded. As part of the process of extending man's functional capabilities, the use of tools which fail to take into account man's biomechanical attributes may impose stresses and strains of various characteristics on the anatomy and physiology of the human body. These stresses and strains, if not controlled, can ultimately be a source of trauma and disability. The manifestation of such design-related disabilities requires time and repeated exposure.

Tichauer, (15), (16), discusses many of the anatomical features of the hand and forearm as related to tool design. In particular, the mechanism that generates muscular power during working operations is analyzed. He cites the experience of redesigning an ordinary ratchet screwdriver to include a better biomechanical advantage. It is ascertained that the conventionally-shaped handle puts severe physical stress on the distal phalanx of the index finger. In addition, manipulating the tool with an extended wrist causes the pinching of

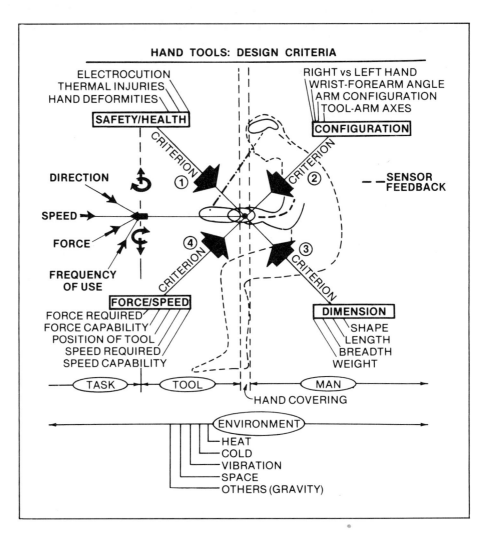

Figure 85. Design criteria
for hand tools.

the median nerve and other structures passing through the carpal tunnel. Since this type of operation is performed frequently, a further undesirable condition of static loading also exists. In another case involving the application of an ordinary paint scraper under frequent use, it was found that many of the women performing the task complained of "numbness and coldness in their fingertips"; and in fact several required surgery for superficial cases or symptoms of gangrene. A simple redesign of the tool handle allowed the external stresses to be applied more evenly across the surface of the hand. Thus, the complete solution to the problem was attributed to the change in the hand tool design.

Hand tools which vibrate have unique, adverse effects on man's physiology. For example, swelling of the tissues in the hand may result after less than an hour of exposure. In addition to swelling, the operator may experience a decrease in cutaneous (skin) sensitivity; hence, the nerves in the hands are affected and in turn cause numbness of the fingers, (17). In the case of hand tools operating (vibrating) at high frequency, especially those whose power source is either an electrical motor or compresses air, adverse effects have been noted in the cardiovascular system and, in particular, the blood vessels in the fingers—this being apparent by the whitening and numbing of the fingers, (18).

In terms of the human benefits which can be realized from applying biomechanics to tool design, Kaplan, (19), enumerates the following: minimizing the physical output by the human, reducing or eliminating muscle strain, and providing safer products. It is emphasized that most of the power generated by an individual emanates not so much from the hand, as it does from the entire body; therefore, to maximize this power transfer, the most effective linkages must exist between the hand and the tool being used. Thus an effectively designed tool not only eliminates possible injury, but also increases the amount of power a person can generate from the tool/hand combination.

Despite recent strides which have been made in the application of biomechanical principles to hand tool design, it is still unfortunately true that most hand tools in use in industry are selected from production models which emphasize "cosmetic" features. In contrast, the pioneering and extensive efforts of Western Electric Company to the applications of biomechanics to tool design and usage are an exception, as illustrated by the following two examples.

Damon, (20), explains how excessive forces and unnatural configurations may lead to discomfort and, in time, to physical deformity. Tenosynovitis (inflammation of the tendons in the wrist) and ulnar deviation are both covered. One poor design cited is a form-fitted tool handle grip which prevents the fingers from coming together during normal grasping and detracts from the normally available strength. Also this type of grip usually fits only the hand size from which it was "modeled," and thus will cause discomfort when used by the majority of the population.

Long, (21), describes and illustrates some of the results achieved by Western Electric when it instituted a biomechanics program. One significant study which involved women operators using straight hand pliers in a continuous operation revealed that many women experienced "trigger finger" from having to force the jaws of the pliers open after each usage; the problem was the muscular tension which resulted from the operator's hand gripping tightly the bare metal handles. The addition of plastic grips was found to provide a cushioning effect which served to eliminate tension on the hand. Another design change involved reducing the handle size which enabled women to grip the tool more securely, thereby helping to prevent excessive strain which has a tendency to cause ganglion formations in the fingers. Due to the angle through which the wrist must bend with ordinary straight pliers, offset pliers were designed; these pliers helped to eliminate ulnar deviation. Finally, other features added were the extended handle length to keep the end of the handle from digging into the soft tissue of the palm, and a thumb rest atop the tool for a greater gripping strength.

Hazards of Seating Devices

Man spends a great deal of his life sitting down. Over the years, seating devices have evolved considerably in shape, in style, and in their mode of use; however, their main purpose remains centered on assuring human comfort and well-being. Figure 86. Comfort is a subjective feeling which is a reflection of a host of variables; the bodily structure of the worker, the task, the workplace environment, etc. When one considers the complexity of these variables, one is apt to discover that there are as many definitions of comfort as there are sitters and chairs. Behavioral analysis of sitting postures indicates the existence of posture preferences which vary with angular relationship of seat elements to each other and to the floor of the room.

In seeking comfort while using seating devices, man may subject his anatomy and physiology to a number of heatlh hazards: hazards which are caused by placing restrictions on posture, and stresses of various design attributes on the cardiovascular and nervous systems; and hazards that result from poor orientation of seat pan, from mismatch between back and rest and spinal curvature, or from awkward task—or workplace—induced postures. Manifestation of these hazards may vary from transient effects (tiredness, irritability, and increase in frequency of postural change) to permanent damage of the spine.

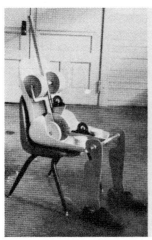 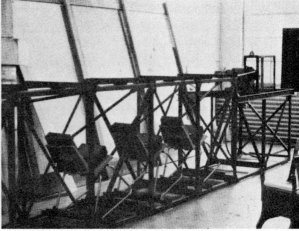

Figure 86. Details of chair testing. (Courtesy of Dr. Anco Prak, Professor of Furniture Manufacturing and Management, North Carolina State University.)

Failure to preserve the natural curvature of the spinal column may greatly contribute to the aches and pains reported by sedentary workers. Also, unfavorable positions of the trunk as well as other body segments can contribute to pain and discomfort in the hand-arm complex—a complaint frequently received from sedentary workers, particularly typists, (22). Based on a careful X-ray analysis of sitting posture of 3,000 subjects (1,500 of them suffering from back problems), Keegan (23), concludes that the most important cause of low-back pain in sitting is the decrease of trunk-thigh angle and consequent flattening of the lumbar curve. In a follow-up paper, Keegan, (24), presents a critical analysis of 31 seats. He demonstrates how knowledge of anatomy and physiology (biomechanics) can be orutilized to assess and rank seats f comfort and suitability for the intended task. Excessive use of soft materials (in lieu of properly designed and manufactured cushions) is known to cause scoliosis, with consequent muscle spasm and pain.

Containment of health hazards of seating devices (through biomechanics) can reduce muscular (static) fatigue, increase productivity and conserve the sitter's time and energy. In contrast, a poorly-designed seat can cause poor morale, decreased efficiency, and suboptimal work performance. (4). Tichauer, (25), contends that a properly designed chair could add as much as 40 productive minutes to each working day.

In addition, to health hazards, accidents involving seating devices are known to occur. These result mainly from faulty design, material failure, manufacturing-induced failures, and improper use of the seating device. In an analysis of accidents at two firms over an eight-year period, Beaver, (26), emphasizes the financial burden which industry sustains from chair accidents; one of the firms studied incurred over $186,000 in losses. He found that women were involved in about 68 percent of all chair accidents analyzed, and outranked men in sustaining the largest percentage of all chair accidents investigated. It was also reported that women incurred a higher incidence of back injuries from chair falls.

In some cases, improper seating may be a contributory antecedent factor in accidents. Tichauer, (25), maintains that when discomfort from sitting prevails, workers simply "take a walk." This temporary absenteeism from the workplace may result in unnecessary exposure to potentially hazardous situations, and hence accidents may occur.

To analyze the seating problem properly, one must first identify the critical areas of interface in the man-chair system. These areas are of two main types: anatomical interface areas (contact of shoulder, upper back, and trunk with chair); and physiological interface areas (chair contact with lumbar spine, pelvis, ischial tuberosities, upper legs, and thighs). Next, the other relevant factors affecting the man-chair system must be considered; examples of some of these modifying factors include environmental aspects (heat, noise, vibration, ventilation, etc.), requirements for "personal space," the nature of the required task to be performed in the seated position, and attention to and provision for the comfort of the chair occupant.

Systems Evaluation

As inferred earlier under "The Systems Approach," systems evaluation should be a continuous process during the design, development, installation, operation, and maintenance of an industrial manufacturing system. Once the system is in operation, health and safety criteria should be considered important indices in assessing systems effectiveness, and should play an important role in providing data relevant to identifying where functions are being compromised and what design ingredients have failed. It is the authors opinion that adequate methodology exists in the area. The main problem is a lack of qualified people in industry to conduct quality systems evaluations.

A recent review of some of the problems and approaches involving accident and incident investigation and analysis concludes with a recommended "action program" involving different types of data for the intelligent solution of safety problems, (27); such a program involves accident and near-accident data, and performance appraisals of workers based on those dimensions of behavior which typically are specified by task analysis, (1), (6).

A well-designed system can, of course, be compromised in practice by poor hazard control practices. For example, reports by O'Connor and Pearson, (28), and Swain (1), point up the hazards of punitive actions taken against workers involved in accidents, i.e., a worker is afraid to report errors, thinking he is at fault when, in actuality, equipment deficiencies or procedures are to blame. Both Pearson, (27), and Swain, (29), are also critical of safety contest and "zero defect" approaches to efficiency and safety. Again, it should be obvious that where rewards for not having accidents are emphasized, workers will suppress data to avoid embarrassment and/or loss of an award. If such data were not suppressed, its availability could have valuable input to the systems evaluation-feedback process.

Concluding Remarks

In reflecting upon the major elements relative to the application of ergonomics practice to industrial accident and injury control the following points are to be emphasized.

1. The improper design of equipment, tasks, and the workplace can be related to "situationally-caused" errors. This emphasizes the need to "design for man" at his workplace. There is a reasonable body of ergonomics data available for application. There are, however, problems in translation of basic research findings from the behavioral sciences into useful applications.

2. Major reductions of the incidence of occupationally-related disabilities can be obtained by designing tasks for performance within human tolerance

limits. The reductions achieved will be a function of the position of task stresses along the continuum formed by tolerance limits. In the case of lifting, two work tolerance limits may be defined: acceptable and permissible. For example, the weight to be lifted is controlled by two limits: the upper limit, the permissible strength output that an individual can maintain under the specified levels of the task conditions without sustaining injuries or health hazards disorders; and the lowerlimit, the acceptable strength output that an individual can provide without unduly straining his physiological system. Other work tolerance limits can be defined in the same manner.

It should be appreciated that there are a host of human variables (age, sex, etc.) which control and affect the behavior of the selected limits, and criterion measures. This means that if criterion measures are not written in terms of individual characteristics, a sizable "safety" factor should be taken into consideration in their specification.

The process of determining the optimum interface between man and his machine is not a simple one, as it may first appear, since some criteria measures require different responses from the human body. For example, if speed and precision for a tool are system goals, the size of the tool should be kept to a minimum. On the otherhand, if a large force is desired, a bulky tool may be deemed necessary.

3. A major source of system error can be related to on-the-job decrements in human efficiency. That is, such error can be predicted to a degree from evidence of declining efficiency. Personnel specialists and ergonomists possess effective approaches for maintaining efficiency: reinforcement and feedback strategies; ergonomic design of tasks taking into account task variety, speed stress, and load stress; job enlargement and enrichment strategies; and scheduling of work-rest cycles.

4. In contrast to system errors attributed to decrement in human efficiency those attributed to attentional lapses are generally random and unpredicatble. The source of distractions which lead attention astray exists not uncommonly within the worker's head—such as worries about his family, financial problems, competition from fellow workers, the attitude of his boss, etc. Ergonomics is concerned with this problem of sustaining attention to the task at hand and does offer suggestions to the designer and "crutches" for the worker. That is, one approach is to make the task more challenging, even perhaps by giving the worker more to do. A second approach involves the use of design strategies which force attention and require specific sequences of responses in order for the task force to proceed, e.g., use of annunciator panels, warning lights, interlocks on controls, auditory signals, knowledge of results feedback, etc.

It is fair to conclude that, with regard to this area of human frailty and susceptibility, there exists a considerable challenge to the field of ergonomics.

Bibliography

1. Swain, A. D., "A Work Situation Approach to Improving Job Safety," Sandia Laboratories Report SC–R–69–1320, Albuquerque, New Mexico, 1969.
2. Van Cott, H. P. and R. G. Kinkade, "Human Engineering Guide to Equipment Design (revised edition)," U.S5 Government Printing Office, Washington, D.C., 1972.
3. Grandjean, E., "Fitting the Task to the Man," Taylor and Francis, London, England, 1969.
4. Woodson, W. E., and D. W. Conover, "Human Engineering Guide for Equipment Designers," University of California Press, Berkeley, California, 1964.
5. Branton, P., "A Field Study of Repetitive Manual Work in Relation to Accidents at the Workplace," International Journal of Production Research, Volume 8, 1970, pages 93–107.
6. Chapanis, A., "Research Techniques in Human Engineering," John Hopkins Press, Baltimore, Maryland, 1959.
7. Meister, D., and G. F. Rabideau, "Human Factors Evaluation in System Development," John Wiley & Sons, Inc., New York, 1965.
8. Singleton, W. T., "The Ergonomics of Safety and Design," University of Aston, Birmingham, United Kingdom, Applied Psychology Department A. P. Report 34, July, 1971.
9. Pearson, R. G., "Human Factors Engineering," Industrial Engineering Handbook, H. B. Maynard, Editor, McGraw-Hill Book Company, New York, New York, 1971.
10. Van Wely, P., "Design and Disease," Applied Ergonomics, Volume 1, 1970, pages 262–269.
11. Podzimek, K., M. Zenman, and B. Kvaniscka, "Design Development of Some Shoemaking Machines," Occupational Safety and Health Series 14, Volume II, Ergonomics in Machine Design, International Labour Office, Geneva, Switzerland, 1969.
12. Kraus, H., "Clinical Treatment for Back and Neck Pain," McGraw-Hill Book Company, New York, New York, 1970.
13. Brown, J. R., Manual Lifting and Related Fields: An Annotated Bibliography, Labour Safety Council of Ontario, Ontario Ministry of Labour, Ontario, Canada, 1972.
14. Connell, M. A., "Bony Anomalies of the Low Back in Relation to Back Injury," Southern Medical Journal, Volume 61, 1968, pages 482–486.
15. Tichauer, E. R., "Some Aspects of Stress on the Forearm and Hand in Industry," Journal of Occupational Medicine, Volume 8, 1966, pages 63–71.
16. Tichauer, E. R., "Ergonomics: The State of the Art," American Industrial Hygiene Association Journal, Volume 28, 1967, pages 106–116.
17. Suggs, C. W., "Vibration of Machine Handles and Controls and Propagation Through the Hands and Arms," Fourth Annual International Ergonomics Congress, Strasbourg, France, 1970.
18. Teisinger, J., "Vascular Disease Disorders Resulting from Vibrating Tools," Journal of Occupational Medicine, Volume 14, 1972, pages 129–133.
19. Kaplan, A., "Coming to Grips," Industrial Design, Volume 15, Number 3, 1968, pages 34–39.
20. Damon, F. A., "The Use of Biomechanics in Manufacturing Operations," The Western Electric Engineer, Volume 9, 1965, pages 11–20.

21. Long, E. D., "Human Productivity and Tool Design," Proceedings of the 17th Annual Convention of AIIE., 1966.
22. Kroemer, K. H. E., "Seating in Plant and Office," American Industrial Hygiene Association Journal, Volume 32, 1971, pages 633–650.
23. Keegan, J. J., "Alteration of the Lumbar Curve Related to Posture and Seating," The Journal of Bone and Joint Surgery, Volume 35–A, 1953, pages 589–603.
24. Keegan, J. J., "Evaluation and Improvement of Seats," Industrial Medicine and Surgery, Volume 31, 1962, pages 137–148.
25. Tichauer, E. R., "Ergonomics Aspects of Biomechanics," The Industrial Environment—Its Evaluation and Control, National Institute for Occupational Safety and Health, U.S. Department of Health, Education and Welfare, Washington, D.C., 1974.
26. Beaver, J. H., "When is a Chair Safe?" American Society of Safety Engineers Journal, Volume 14, Number 1, 1969, pages 16–17.
27. Pearson, R. G., "Accident Data Analysis," Symposium on Safety Methodology, Human Factors Society, Washington, D.C., October, 1973.
28. O'Connor, W. F., and R. G. Pearson, "ATC System Error and Appraisal of Controller Proficiency," FAA Office of Aviation Medicine Report, AM 65-10, Washington, D.C., March, 1965.
29. Swain, A. D., "Design Techniques for Improving Human Performance in Production, Industrial & Commercial Techniques, Ltd., London, England, 1972.

The Process of Accident Investigation 8

In Chapters 4 and 6, we addressed the importance of identifying and evaluating existing and potential hazards in the workplace, before these hazards culminate in accident situations. This prescriptive approach, in essence, stipulates that if we can locate, assess properly, and counter accident potential situations before they culminate in accidents, then perhaps we won't lose as many people, we won't absorb the losses associated with inefficiency and reduced capacity, and overall, we will maintain effective operations.

While the idea behind this approach is sound, and has in fact proven itself to be a critically desirable element of any hazard control program, there will be times when we won't find and eliminate problems before accidents occur. The fact we must own up to is that our methods are not invincible, and our best ideas and recommendations may not always do the job. There is a reason behind this situation. The knowledge available to the hazard control specialist may have been inadequate or incomplete at the time of his initial inquiry.

Time, not knowledge, is the forcing factor for all decisions.[1] It can easily be seen that, at the time the hazard control specialist makes his assessment and recommends a corrective action, he may be doing so with less information about the result of his recommended improvement than he would like. Another reason may be that the state-of-the-art in technology may not offer adequate solution alternatives to counter accident potential effectively. In situations, like this, given the fact that accidents are rare events, one *could* occur, and losses must be accounted for. Perhaps, this is the price an organization has to pay to stay in business and, in certain cases, the price workers must accept, to have a job.

Special appreciation to the U.S. Department of Energy for its permission to use information included in this chapter.

Nobody wants accidents to happen but the reality of the situation is that the complexity of industrial systems, coupled with the countless number of accident potential situations existing among the worker/machine/environment components of these systems and the lack of sufficient experience data to counter all hazards associated with these components indicates that our best efforts may often be off the mark.

So, like it or not, accidents will happen, and the hazard control specialist will be right there to learn as much as he can about the problem which precipitated the accident, in order to take action to avoid similar situations from occurring.

The process of investigating accidents, if handled properly, can add a significant dimension to the overall system of hazard indentification even though it is done after the fact. The data acquired from an accident investigation is fed into and becomes part of the updated hazard identification and evaluation arm of the total hazard control program. If accident investigations are set-up and conducted properly, the organization often reaps big rewards from what appears to be a total loss situation.

The purpose of this chapter will be to consider the intent behind the accident investigation process, the techniques involved, and the constraints which must be dealt with during the process of acquiring accurate, and valid data for informed decision-making.

The Approach

Accident investigation is spoken of as both a science and an art. Certainly it contains elements of both. A controlled method or system is essential, and a clear understanding of the techniques to be used allows investigators to develop a "feel" for what needs to be done and how far to pursue each course of action. The main point the investigator must keep in mind is that the investigative process is not one of fault-finding of some person or some group. Instead, the main thrust of the effort is concentrated on locating facts and understanding the causal factors involved in the undesired event under investigation.

The essential points for the investigator to remember are that he must: decide what organizational procedures and analytical techniques will be used as soon as possible after the accident occurs, and follow his plans until it becomes evident that a change in strategies is necessary: have specific tasks assigned to individuals and ensure that each task is accomplished; explore every possible cause of the accident until it is either ruled out or proven to be an actual cause; recognize the limitations of his own knowledge of technical subjects, and call on specialists if necessary; maintain perseverance in his probing for causes and control to avoid jumping to what appears to be an obvious conclusion; record all evidence accurately; corroborate, when possible, and evaluate all statements and testimony.

An examination of accident report forms used by many organizations reveals that a certain percentage of those organizations considers the accident investigative process and the resultant accident report as merely an exercise to satisfy a legal and administrative purpose. In some cases, the reporting method is designed with so many built-in inadequacies that accurate and reliable data is nearly impossible to accrue from the investigative process.

It has been, and in some instances still is common practice to investigate only serious or lost time accidents, expressing a "Why take the time?" attitude toward minor accidents. When a minor accident or incident occurs, the report is completed only because it is expected or required. The lack of investigation into minor accidents has resulted in input data loss for the management system. The loss of valuable accident data, may result in future operational problems in the form of delays, increased costs, accidents, etc.

Minor accidents or incidents should be investigated, even though an actual loss or injury may not have occurred, to:

1. determine the potential for loss or injury, and
2. learn how the potential for loss or injury can be prevented in the future.

With the use of only a little imagination, the benefits to be derived from investigation of minor accidents can readily be determined. It is much simpler, and of much greater benefit, to correct minor problems in the system before they cause serious accidents, than to correct them after a serious accident occurs. For these reasons, all accidents should be investigated and evaluated to provide information for informed management decisions.

Keep in mind that the investigation itself should have as its primary purpose the determination of sufficient facts to enable the hazard control specialist to come to a conclusion as to the cause of the occurrence. Without an adequate identification of cause, neither the hazard control specialist nor any supervisor or management member would be able to recommend or adopt a particular course of action for future hazard control.

The First Line Supervisor

Even though accident investigation is the responsibility of all levels of management, the first line supervisor has knowledge that makes his role as a member of the accident investigation team a very important one.

Many people question the first line supervisor's responsibility to investigate all accidents taking place in the area of his responsibility. There exist many good reasons why the supervisor should investigate. Some of the more important ones are as follows:

Supervisors are most aware of the worker/machine/environment relationships in their assigned areas. They know their workers, e.g., their job experience, personal characteristics, their shop jargon, etc. They know the equipment, how it is operated, its unusual features, and its peculiarities. They also know the environment in which the man and machine must function in. While this knowledge does not ensure that first line supervisors will make good accident investigators, it does provide an essential source of knowledge. With experience, training, and guidance, the first line supervisor will be able to apply his unique knowledge and provide valuable information for the management decision-making process. Allowing the first line supervisor this participation in accident investigation increases his sense of involvement and responsibility. Not providing the first line supervisor this opportunity tends to undermine his sense of involvement in the management system, and more importantly, his sense of accountability for accidents.

Most supervisors need to learn more about accident causes and prevention. The act of investigating accidents provides the first line supervisor the chance to learn more about potential hazards, accident causation, accident characteristics, and accident reduction methods. Everyone has a fear of the unknown, and it is this fear that keeps many first line supervisors from becoming routinely involved with hazard control. However, as the supervisor develops awareness, he will become more active in accident investigations and understand the importance of investigating even minor incidents. This resultant will increase involvement, awareness, and understanding, which in turn will pay dividends in reduced accident frequency and severity.

Nearly all corrective actions found necessary to prevent the recurrence of accidents, e.g., retraining, changed operating procedures, material changes, etc., are administered by the first line supervisor. The uninvolved or disinterested supervisor, usually, does not follow through on corrective action because he does not understand why it is necessary. If, however, he is directly involved with the accident investigation and provides input for management's use, he will understand "why" and feel a sense of responsibility toward follow-up and completion of corrective action.

The above reasons for involvement of the first line supervisor in accident investigation, though not inclusive, are substantial and should convince all concerned of the need for his involvement.

Higher Management's Role

Top management and department heads must be involved with the investigation of serious accidents, that is, those that result in lost work-day injuries or major property damage. However, its interest in minor accidents is a plus in management's favor. Active participation by management accomplishes several things.:

1. It conveys the personal interest that management has in hazard control.
2. It provides a second, more general, source of knowledge to support the accident investigator.

Management should routinely review, and periodically participate in, minor accident investigation, to emphasize the importance of investigating all accidents. It is important to remember that the accident investigation report is a tool used to provide the minimum information necessary for making informed management decisions.

It is also necessary for management to become involved with the corrective action dictated by the investigation. Management should routinely follow-up to determine the status of effectiveness of corrective action, and to provide the stimulus necessary for the effective functioning of the overall hazard control effort. A lack of management concern or involvement will be reflected in the worker's and supervisor's attitudes, resulting perhaps in a negative bias toward the investigative effort.

The Role of Lawyers

Including a legal advisor as a member of the accident investigation team will often pay dividends. Today, perhaps more than any time before, with many avenues for liability hovering over the head of an organization, having a lawyer assist in the definition, ascertainment, and analysis of the facts, interview of certain witnesses and review of the final accident report, may prove to be worth every penny spent.

The Role of Physicians in Investigations

A physician's assistance should be obtained when medical and human factors may have played a causal role in the accident. Investigators should also work with medical officers to develop advance plans for investiagtion appropriate to local conditions. Medical and human factors should be evaluated by a medical investigator, as part of any accident investigation, for a number of reasons:

1. *To assure the completeness of investigation.* No accident investigation is complete, despite detailed study of technological, engineering and management systems, unless human and medical factors are also evaluated. Human failure continues to rank high in accident causal factors. Many times it is not detected or the significance of its role in accident causation and control is not fully appreciated, due to a superficial medical/human factor evaluation.

The Role of
Specialists in
Accident
Investigations

2. *To rule out human failure in accident causation.* Human failure may be designated a primary or contributing cause of an accident or incidemt. It may be found in many forms and in many systems. Too frequently, the medical and human factor evaluation is limited to looking for obvious operator error or operator incapacitation. Attention should also be given to possible contributing human failure factors in procedures, practices, and in the area of equipment design. Special attention should be given to the design of controls and monitoring and warning systems to minimize the possibility of operator error in reading and interpreting instrument signals, and in control input responses. Are warning and monitoring signals designed with boldface, unambiguous, and fail-safe features? Are control systems too complicated? Are critical controls distinctively designed and functionally located? Do monitoring procedures induce boredom and fatigue?

3. *To establish cause and time of death.* This information is always important to an accurate reconstruction of the sequence of the accident events. In some accidents, it has altered the direction of the investigation and the determination of the causal factors.

4. *To establish mechanisms of injury.* This information is also necessary for accurate reconstruction of the sequence of accident events, and for the determination of causal factors. It is also essential for the evaluation of the adequacy and effectiveness of safety and health protection procedures and equipment.

5. *To identify victims.* In addition to the humane and legal considerations, the location and identification of victims' remains are very essential for the accurate reconstruction of events and the determination of causal factors. In accidents involving severe destruction of remains, the medical investigator plays a major role in identification. He can determine the need and arrange for special biomechanical and forensic pathology studies.

6. *To help in reconstruction of the accident scene and events, and in the determination of causal factors.* From the foregoing, it is evident that establishment of the time and cause of death, location and identification of victims, and the mechanisms of injury will be of substantial help to the investigation team, in its efforts to determine the causal factors.

In the evaluation of human factors, the medical investigator should play a major role. A truly complete human factors evaluation must look at all aspects of the man/machine interface, and this requires a team approach. The team should include capabilities in the areas of operations and maintenance, engineering and design, and occupational medicine.

7. *To help evaluate adequacy and use of safety and health protection procedures and equipment, and emergency escape procedures and equipment.*

It is important to establish the relationship between the injury, the structures, protective devices and emergency escape procedures. The physician can accurately assess the nature and degree of injury and assist in determining the source and nature of the forces that inflicted the injury. He can also determine whether injuries are premortem or postmortem. Upon examination of the structure, the physician may be able to identify obscure or small amounts of tissue or clothing and to correlate these findings with the injuries.

8. *To apply special biomedical techiniques, as needed.* Here the medical investigator will determine what special biomedical studies, if any, are needed. In order to make proper judgments, he should be well informed on the progress and courses of the overall investigative effort to date. Participation in periodic investigation committee progress briefings is an excellent method of keeping the medical investigator informed. Examples of special studies that might be needed include blood and tissue toxicological studies for specific toxins, alcohol and drug determinations.

9. *To establish physical/mental fitness for subjects' assigned jobs at time of event.*

10. *To help evaluate adequacy of plans, procedures, equipment, training and response of rescue, first aid, emergency medical care, and follow-up medical care elements.*

11. *To evaluate adequacy of worker's medical/physical standards and the screening, selection, and preplacement process.*

12. *To help evaluate impact on other employees, plant and site environments, the general environment, and the general public at large.*

13. *The physician can also evaluate the effectiveness of measures aimed at early detection of medical conditions, mental changes or emotional stresses, etc.* Early detection can trigger preventive measures by supervisors and others. Again the physician can provide instruction of nurses and supervisors, including good communications between those key groups.

Medical records: Medical records related to the accident investigation should be treated on a confidential basis as privileged information. This includes personal medical records, pictures, autopsy reports, and toxicological reports.

In general, it has been found advisable to exclude complete medical reports, pictures, autopsy reports, etc., from the official accident report, and to include instead a brief overall summary report prepared by the participating physician. Where an illustration is essential to understanding the report, a drawing may be better than a medical picture.

Only those portions of the medical records deemed necessary to the development of a complete and accurate accident investigation should be incorporated into the official accident report. The remainder should be returned to medical files.

Other Specialists (Depending on the Nature of the Event)

1. Human factors. Specialists
2. Design specialists
3. Relevant engineering specialists

The Accident Investigation Process

Some General Thoughts

It is universally agreed that immediate on-the-scene accident investigation provides the most accurate and useful information. The longer the delay in interviewing the injured and witnesses, and appraising the scene of the accident and so forth, the greater the possibility of obtaining incomplete and inaccurate facts.

The investigator must not permit conditions at the accident scene to be altered in any way (unless further injury or property damage could occur) until the area is completely surveyed, photographed, essential measurements taken, and adequate knowledge of the circumstances surrounding the accident are obtained.

Witnesses tend to forget accident details very quickly, particularly under the impact of emotional shock, and they may begin to fill in the gaps with mentally fabricated "facts." It is important to realize that mental fabrication or filling the gap is human nature and given sufficient time lapse or time opportunity to collaborate with others a witness may, without knowing it, provide inaccurate information which will have adverse effect on the conclusions drawn from the investigation. The sooner witnesses and personnel involved are interviewed, the more accurate will be the information.

Prompt accident investigation also expresses a feeling of concern for the safety and well-being of employees, and others involved and will provide invaluable in obtaining cooperation from accident victims and witnesses.

It should be remembered, that interviewing and fact-finding must begin only after medical treatment is provided the injured, and further property damage is prevented.

How to Investigate

Performing an actual accident investigation is not as simple a task as one may first think. When conducting investigations, especially of minor accidents, it can be very difficult to look beyond the incident at hand, determine the true loss potential of the occurrence, and develop practical recommendations to prevent recurrence. For these reasons, many aids have been developed to assist the investigator in determining essential facts for a complete and thorough accident investigation.

When conducting the actual on-site investigation, all factors related to contributing accidents and conditions, as well as direct accident causes, must be considered. A major weakness of many accident investigations is a failure to establish and consider all factors that contributed to the accident.

The first line supervisor, as part of the management team, often conducts the initial on-site accident investigation. As previously indicated, management either through its omission or commission, is responsible for every accident. It should, therefore, be apparent that in finding the human, situational, and environmental factors that contribute to accidents, management errors will often be detected. As a matter of human nature, few people are readily willing to admit their own errors or to criticize their cohorts or upper management. It is, however, as in all phases of successful management, essential to future success that past errors be recognized and corrected.

In this light, investigators must not think in terms of obvious defects only, but, must be ready to acknowledge as contributing causes, any factors that may have, in any way, contributed to an accident. Investigators must be prepared to challenge contributing factors that have been considered acceptable in the past. The investigator cannot obtain too much information; what may at first appear to have been a simple, uninvolved accident, may in fact have numerous contributing factors which become more complex as factors are determined and analyses completed.

It is important to recognize that there will be more than one contributing factor present in all accidents. For this reason, care should be taken to avoid the mistake of focusing investigative efforts on only one factor or cause.

Often, comment is not made in accident reports on hazards noted during an on-site investigation because, in the opinion of the investigator, they are not correctable, are acceptable, or constitute part of the job. Of course, recommending corrective action is secondary to determining the problem and assessing the facts. Without having determined all of the facts, the recommended corrective action will most often not produce the desired end result. A contributing factor should be considered and commented on, even though the investigator may believe the hazard impractical to modify, minimize, or eliminate. What is considered impossible today, may be practical tomorrow, commonplace next month, and antiquated next year. Practical is a relative term, and it is the purpose of the investigator to determine facts and report them to management with recommendations to prevent recurrence. All factors contributing to accident causes should be identified and acknowledged, as well as recommendations of corrective action, if the on-site investigation is to be complete.

The hazard control specialist, as head of the investigation team, takes on many responsibilities, including the responsibility for the safety of the members of those assisting him with the investigation.

Safety During the Investigation

The hazard control specialist must consider that:

1. In many cases the scene of an accident is more dangerous than it was prior to the accident. For example:
   a. Electrical equipment may be damaged, and the investigator must be assured that it cannot be energized while he is examining it.
   b. A building may be damaged following a fire or explosion to the extent that there may be question regarding its habitability.
   c. Radiation sources or toxic material may have been released from their confinement barriers.

   For cases such as these, the hazard control specialist should provide safeguards, and should brief the team on hazards, communications, and emergency equipment. Additionally, it is appropriate that each member of the investigative team be given a written pass for entry and work in the accident area.

2. A second problem area relates to actions that the investigative team may wish to take after an accident. Clear lines of authority should be established and delegated to the team. If this is not done, confusion will exist, and there may be the possibility of loss of evidence, further damage to the facility, or injury to the investigator. It is human nature for the organization that has been involved in an accident to want to put everything back the way it was before the accident. The team must be very alert to make sure that such actions are done in an approved manner. Extreme care must be taken in approving such actions as:
   a. Restoring electric power and other utilities.
   b. Recovering damaged equipment.
   c. Moving motor vehicles.

3. The hazard control specialist also may have to consider emergency preparedness plans to help ameliorate any second accident that might occur. If the investigation is being conducted at a remote location, he will need to know about the availability of medical service. An investigation in a facility contaminated with radioactive or toxic materials may require the use of respirators or air breathing equipment. Emergency rescue capability will need to be reviewed. The ability to detect and suppress a fire should be considered for such a location and at other investigation sites where fire might present special problems. These problems should be reviewed with those who are to supply the emergency service, and a clear assignment of responsibilities made between the leader of the investigation team and these people.

4. If the investigation team has been working in contaminated areas, the hazard control specialist should see that proper health measures are taken before the team is dismissed (blood-urine samples, whole body counts, etc.)

Physical evidence is sometimes handled in an uncontrolled manner. This has invalidated such evidence and made it difficult to find cause. If the evidence were needed in a legal case, e.g., an employee's suit against a machine manufacturer, the fact that it was lost or impaired would not only embarrass the employer, but could place him in an unfavorable light in a court of law. Tags and receipts for evidence should always be used.

Maps, Diagrams, Drawings, and Charts

At the beginning of an inquiry, the recording of measurements of transient evidence is essential. The following techniques for recording evidence have each proven their worth when used with a knowledge of their capabilities and limitations.

Maps   Overall, small-scale maps of longer distance and directions, as well as large-scale maps of the immediate scene, may be desirable. It is on the latter that witness locations will normally be shown.

Drawings   These should be simplified pictures of reality, such as manufacturing or construction prints, perspective drawings, cutaway drawings, etc. The initial effort will record only transient evidence on a sketch roughly to scale. Drawings can often be highlighted or captioned to call attention to significant detail. In order to save time that can be directed elsewhere, do not measure locations of permanent, fixed objects. They can be located on copies of drawings at a later time.

Charts   These may include photographic reproductions of records (e.g., temperature and pressure), trend analyses or types and classes (commonly seen as "statistics"), and organization charts. For statistical charting, the best advice is: consult a good statistician. However, two of the author's phobias must be mentioned:

1. Do not use broken scales on charts. Possible exception. If a variation of 1 or 2 percent in a factor is significant (i.e., a causal factor), a broken-scale chart to highlight the detail may be useful. Also, if a single value would compress the scale so as to eliminate useful detail, simply chart it at the top with an arrow pointing up.
2. Do not connect discontinuous data with a trend line—use a bar chart. Possible exception: When two or more profiles are being compared.

The investigator, in the preparation of his report, should not use more diagrams, drawings, and charts than absolutely necessary. Unneeded charts can slow and sometimes muddle understanding.

Photographic techniques   Certain basic qualities make up good pictures that are factual and accurate representations of the accident scene. Photographs can easily misrepresent a scene and lead to false conclusions or findings about an accident. Some misrepresentations occur unknowingly, while others may be purposely contrived. By reviewing the attributes of good pictures here, the investigator will be made aware of possible misrepresentations in the photographs that are examined.

1. Show enough of the scene to provide good orientation. Several pictures may have to be taken in sequence to provide this orientation. An overall shot, medium and close-up may be required.

2. Use proper perspective. The use of wide angle and telephoto lenses alters the perspective and causes distortions. Normal focal length lenses should generally be used.

3. Use proper lighting. The angle and type of lighting greatly affects the appearance of the subject. While no one lighting arrangement is correct for all conditions and subjects, the lighting should be examined for uniformity and to see that it does not produce an abnormal appearance.

4. Use the correct camera settings essential to good pictures. The three basic settings of shutter speed, aperture, and focus must be applied correctly in order to obtain a correct representation of scene. Shutter speed must be fast enough to stop action in the photograph. The aperture, along with allowing enough light to pass through the lens, also controls how much of the near and far portions of the picture will be in focus. The focus setting used in conjunction with the aperture setting controls the focus range of the picture.

5. Keep the camera level for easy orientation and reference.

6. Use known objects in the scene as size references wherever possible. In overall scenes, the presence of a person may be sufficient. In close-up photos of rubble or damaged areas, a hand or portion of a 6 foot rule may be best.

7. Use color film for maximum information content. While black and white film is cheaper and easier to print, the color information in color prints is often essential to understanding and analyzing an event. The color record must be properly done, however, otherwise it will be misleading. The use of neutral gray cards in some photos is desirable.

8. Identification and labeling of the photographs is essential. Figure 87 shows a log sheet that may be used by a photographer at the time of taking the picture. After the pictures are printed, captions should be used to point out pertinent details and to eliminate all ambiguity about whether the picture was taken at the time of the accident or was staged later. Photographs are usually date-stamped on the reverse side, but if this information is pertinent to the analysis, it should be included in the caption.

Photographer_____

Location_____

Camera type_____

Lighting type_____

Film type_____

Date of accident_____

Time of accident_____

Film Roll No._____

Picture No.	Scene/Subject	Date of Photo	Time of Photo	Lens f/	Direction Camera Pointing
1.					
2.					
2.					
3.					
4.					
5.					
6.					
7.					
8.					
8.					
9.					
10.					

Figure 87. Photographic log sheet.

9. While every accident is unique and will have its own set of features that are important, there are some general guidelines about what to photograph:
   a. Location of major identifiable pieces.
   b. Collision debris—dirt, etc.
   c. Pools of liquids
   d. Gouges, scratches, collision points, and damage
   e. Temporary view obstructions, especially from view of operator or other key person
   f. Mobile equipment
   g. Material storage
   h. Scaffolds, jigs, racks, temporary rigs
   i. Close-up of failed elements
10. If there is a fire associated with the event, pictures taken during the event are very useful. Photographs should include:
   a. Flames. They indicate what material is burning, how fire started and progressed through the structure.
   b. Smoke. Also indicates what material is burning by smoke color.

  c. Structure.

  d. Specatators. Many times if arson is involved the arsonist will stay around to watch the fire. If a series of fires are started, he may be in all photographs.

11. It should be reemphasized here that even though official photographers may not be on hand to photograph a fire, amateurs or press pictures may be available and used.

12. After the fire is out, there are several key areas to photograph that may assist in the analysis.

  a. The most charred or burned area.

  b. Any combustible materials—matchbooks, papers, paint thinners, kerosene.

  c. Spectators around the accident location.

Camera Equipment The choice of camera equipment either by a photographer or the investigator, if he is taking his own pictures, will affect the quality and the cost of the photographs. For most investigations, a roll film type camera such as a Hasselblad or 35mm single lens reflex camera is preferred. The major considerations are:

1. Modern films, such as Vericolor II, are very good and capable of rendering minute detail and color balance on small image formats.

2. A large number of pictures can be taken with very little weight to carry around-an important consideration when taking pictures in the remains of an explosion or rubble from a fire.

3. Roll films are lower in cost per picture than large format sheet films.

4. 35mm and 2 1/4 × 2 1/4 format cameras have short focal length normal lenses that have inherently better depth of fields than lenses used on 4 × 5 or 8 × 10 cameras.

5. Lens construction on smaller cameras allow for larger apertures that minimizes lighting requirements. 4 × 5 and 8 × 10 view cameras require much higher lighting levels because of their longer focal lengths and smaller apertures.

Should the investigator be forced to acquire his own pictures, an Instamatic camera with Kodacolor II film and automatic flash could be used. Limitations would be in the poorer lens (image) quality and fixed lighting arrangement. In some instances, quick reference pictures taken with a Polaroid either black or white or color may be used. This is generally not a good choice because of the effect of heat on the unexposed film. The colors of the print material are not reproduced faithfully, and an incorrect analysis could be made from the interpretation of the color. The polaroid picture also serve as back-up should the roll film be lost, damaged, or for some other reason is spoiled during its developing process.

The person conducting an accident investigation is placed in a position of fairly heavy responsibility. How he approaches the investigation, handles people, collects evidence, etc., are significant factors in enabling him to reach accurate conclusions. In order to become an outstanding accident investigator (or even a competent one), it is necessary to develop certain personal attributes. The technical or mechanical skills will be readily grasped; i.e., knowledge of standards, report writing, interviewing, etc., and these skills will fall into place and become semi-automatic once one has developed in himself the following necessary qualities.

Attributes of an Accident Investigator

Objectivity

It is not at all rare for investigators to adhere to broken hypotheses (useless preconceived ideas), turning a blind eye to contrary evidence, and not altogether unknown for them to deliberately suppress contrary results. The best protection against these tendencies is to cultivate an intellectual habit of subordinating one's opinion and wishes to objective evidence, for once an opinion has been formed, it is difficult to think of alternatives.

Imagination or Conscious Thinking

1. Dewey[2] analyses conscious thinking into the following phases. First comes awareness of some difficulty or problem which provides the stimulus This is followed by a suggested solution springing into conscious mind. Only then does reason come into play to examine and reject or accept the idea. If the idea is rejected, our mind reverts to the previous stage and the process is repeated. The important thing to realize is that the conjuring up of the idea is not a deliberate voluntary act. It is something that happens to us rather than something we do.
2. The thinker may not be sufficiently critical of ideas as they arise and may be too ready to jump to a conclusion, either through impatience or laziness.
3. Probably the main characteristic of the trained thinker is that he does not jump to conclusions on insufficient evidence, as the untrained person is inclined to do.
4. Imagination is of great importance, not only in leading us to new facts, but also in stimulating us to new efforts, for it enables us to see visions of their possible consequence.

Intuition

The word "intuition" has several slightly different usages, so it is necsssary to indicate that it is here employed as a sudden enlightenment or comprehension of a situation, a clarifying idea which springs into the consciousness, often, though not necessarily, when one is not consciously thinking of that subject. The most characteristic circumstances of an intuition are a period of intense work on a problem accompanied by a desire for its solution, abandonment of the work perhaps with attention to something else, then the appearance of the idea with dramatic suddenness and often a sense of certainty. Often there is a feeling of exhilaration and perhaps surprise that the idea had not been thought of previously.

Reason (logic)

Reason is for our purposes the analysis of investigation procedure. An appropriate golden rule would be, "give unqualified assent to no propositions but those the truth of which is so clear and distinct that they cannot be doubted."

Observation (the power of)

Observation is not passively watching but is an active process. The making of detailed notes and drawings is a valuable means of prompting one to observe accurately. Powers of observation can be developed by cultivating the habit of watching things with an active, inquiring mind. In carrying out any observation, you look deliberately for each characteristic you know may be there, for any unusual feature, and especially for any suggestive associations or relationships among the things you see, or between them and what you know.

Curiosity (inquisitiveness)

If one attribute characterizes the good investigator more than any other, it is an insatiable curiosity. Curiosity is defined as a desire to learn or know about things that do not necessarily concern one: inquisitiveness. Inquisitiveness is defined as the inclination to ask questions or seek information.

There may be many other attributes one could conjure up, such as a high intelligence, internal drive, willingness to work hard, tenacity of purpose, sound judgement, patience, etc., as further prerequisites for success in accident investigation. Any training, therefore, involves more than being "told how." Practice is required for one to learn to put the precepts into effect and develop a habit of using them. People whose minds are not disciplined by training often tend to notice and remember events that support their views and forget others. Tactful and searching inquiry is necessary to ascertain exactly what they have observed—to separate their observations from their interpretations.

The investigator by the very nature of his task, must deal with many types of personalities under strained conditions. Therefore, he must attempt to use as much empathy as possible during the interrogation process. If he puts himself in the shoes of the witness or injured, and tries to imagine how he might act under the trying circumstances, perhaps his approach, line, and manner of questioning might be more properly shaped to increase its overall effectiveness.

Dealing with People Under Strained Conditions

The actual conduct of the investigation will vary with the local situation and with the skill, imagination, an ingenuity of the investigators. Accordingly, only a few general comments will be made:

Conduct of the Investigation—An Overview

Initial Actions on Arrival at the Site

It is highly important that the senior investigator get to the scene of the accident as soon as possible after it has occurred. Prompt notification of the senior investigator and team members and provision of rapid transportation to the scene are essential.

The initial site actions generally required are to:

1. establish appropriate security and isolation of the areas involved;
2. assess the extent of damage and personal injury;
3. evaluate operatimg conditions just prior to the accident;
4. make a preliminary estimate of the accident cause;
5. obtain the confidence and cooperation of those involved, in order to proceed in an orderly and efficient manner;
6. evaluate any remaining hazards;
7. develop a formal plan for the conduct of the investigation.

Among the specific things the investigator will have to do during the first few days will be: to make contact with local and company authorities; visit the accident site; and gain an understanding of the scope and nature of the investigation. Rather than rushing out and examining evidence immediately, he should allow time for briefings by those in the operating organization. The investigators' attitudes toward those in the organization where the accidents occurred at this stage are important, for this is the point where cooperation between the two groups must be established. It is quite possible that the success or the failure of the entire investigation may depend on the first hours of contact.

Isolation of the Affected Area

The immediate accident area should be closed off. The need for security is twofold: It reduces the likelihood of further injuries to personnel, and it prevents the removal of equipment and debris from the accident area, thereby assuring that valuable evidence is not inadvertently destroyed. A procedure should be worked out with the facility by which the investigation team leader controls the release of equipment involved. He should also have control over damaged areas of the facility until the investigation is completed. A procedure should also be established whereby subsequent to evaluation the investigating team can release equipment and areas to the facility. In so doing, the facility personnel more readily will be able to perform its cleanup and plan for future utilization of equipment recovered. As for key areas and components involved in the accident, it would be wise to retain control until the technical evaluation is completed. For no matter how thoroughly the evidence is documented, an "in situ" examination of the remains may rapidly disprove an otherwise completely plausible explanation of the accident cause.

Examination of the Physical Remains

Upon completion of the immediate firefighting or other damage suppression activity, the scene should be left undisturbed to the maximum extent possible, until the investigation team arrives. Where equipment has to be removed to eliminate remaining hazards, a record (and if possible photographs) should be made of such actions. Photographs will prove useful both as a record and a basis for analysis. By including a photographer with the first few people to enter the accident area, the investigators insure that a record is made of much valuabl evidence. Although the investigators must be prepared to take their own pictures, having a photographer available during the entire fact-gathering phase of the investigation will permit rapid development of good quality photographs and relieve the investigators of this task. Each photograph should be numbered, and the position of the camera and its direction of vision indicated in a map or sketch. As stated earlier, color pictures often provide information not discerned in black and white. When pieces of equipment are photographed, it will be helpful to include something of known size, to show the relative size of the object photographed. A Polaroid camera may be particularly useful in the absence of a local photographer.

The investigation should be conducted so as not to destroy the evidence. The accident area having been previously isolated for hazard and/or security reasons should be entered only by those with a definite purpose. Such entries should be preplanned with attention given to remaining hazards. A record should be kept of any materials or equipment removed from the area.

Significant clues may sometimes be hidden in small components or pieces that seem relatively unimportant at the outset of the investigation. While moving wreckage, extreme care must be taken not to lose or destroy equipment parts.

The investigation of the circumstances surrounding the accident is a methodical accumulation of small bits of information which eventually form a pattern. The wreckage contains valuable evidence which, if correctly identified and assessed, will provide factual evidence necessary for the determination of the cause. The investigators should draw upon the intimate knowledge local people have of their equipment and how it is put together and operated. In particular, little differences that distinguish it from similar pieces of equipment should be identified. Prior to the disassembly of any items of equipment, the investigator should have a thorough understanding of component characteristics and function, and should develop a detailed plan for disassembling the components. Key or unexpected evidence destroyed in a careless, unplanned disassembly cannot later be recovered. A permanent photographic record of the disassembly operation will frequently prove of value.

Interviews

Interviewing a person who had an accident as well as witnesses who saw the accident occur can be a very difficult assignment. The individual being interviewed usually possesses some kind of fear that creates a reluctance to provide the interviewer true and complete facts about the accident. The individual injured may be embarrassed, afraid of disciplinary action, or afraid for any number of reasons. A witness may not want to provide information that will place blame on friends, co-workers, or possibly himself. To obtain the necessary facts during an interview, the interviewer must first develop a rapport with the individual being interviewed which will help eliminate or reduce his fear. Once such a rapport has been established, the following five-step method should be used during the actual interview:

1. Discuss the purpose of the investigation (fact finding not fault finding).
2. Have the individual relate his version of the complete accident with minimal interruption.
3. Ask questions to clarify facts or fill in any gaps.
4. The interviewer should relate his understanding of the accident to the individual
5. Discuss methods of preventing recurrence.

Establishing rapport with the individual prior to beginning the actual interview is the most important step. Discuss with the individual the purpose of the investigation and specifically the purpose of the interview. The objective of this first step is to clear the air and establish lines of communication that will best fulfill the purpose of the investigation, fact-finding.

The second step is to have the individual relate his complete version of the accident. If the individual being interviewed is one that was injured, ask him to explain where he was, what he was doing, how he was doing it, and what happened. If practical, have the witness explain the sequence of events which occurred, at the time of the accident. While the witness is on the scene, he will be able to relate facts that might otherwise be very difficult to explain. Another technique might be to ask witnesses to explain exactly what they saw, and to include what they heard to be fact although they did witness it firsthand. During this step the inverviewer should not interrupt, unless absolutely necessary, except for clarification of something that was said.

After the individual has related his version of the accident, ask questions necessary to further clarify facts or fill in gaps that may exist. Ask only one question at a time, do not ask leading questions, and ask only questions that are pertinent to the investigation.

After all questions have been answered, the interviewer should review the injured or witness's version of the accident, as the interviewer understands it. Through this review process there will be ample opportunity to correct any misunderstanding that may have occurred and clarify, if necessary, any area of the accident details. The last portion of the interview should consist of a discussion concerning methods of preventing a recurrence. Ask the individual for his thoughts, ideas, and opinions on how to prevent recurrence. By asking for his ideas and discussing them with him, the interviewer will show sincerity and place emphasis on the investigative purpose—fact-finding—as initially discussed at the beginning of the inverview.

Important points to be remembered and practiced by interviewers:

1. Conduct interviews as soon after the accident as practical.
2. Delay interviews with the injured until he has received medical treatment—no matter how minor his injuries. If the injured feels that his best interests are being placed second to "some report"— he is not apt to cooperate.
3. Avoid making people feel they are informers.
4. Be diplomatic.
5. Put witnesses at ease.
6. Explain the purpose of the investigation; fact-finding, not fault-finding for disciplinary action.
7. Establish rapport.
8. Avoid the implied answer or leading question.
9. Avoid the long complicated question. Keep questions as simple as possible.

10. Give the person the opportunity to present relevant information in its entirety, without interruption. If possible, avoid "yes" or "no" answers.

11. Interview one person at a time.

12. Provide good facilities for the interview when possible. However, in some instances it may be better to interview the witness in the environment where the accident took place—seeing the "real world" again may jog the witness's memory and enable him to provide information which might have otherwise been lost.

13. Let one person at a time ask questions.

14. Explain to witness that you will be taking notes and review the notes with him as they are being taken.

15. Tape recording witness testimony can be controversial and must have witness consent. Generally people tend to "freeze" up when they know they are being taped and may withhold valuable information, refusing to commit themselves because of possible incrimination.

16. Don't argue with witnesses.

17. Inconsistent statements should be discussed and clarified.

18. Never intimidate or induce witnesses.

19. Review all facts and other information with the witness, at the end of the interview.

20. Ask for ideas from the witness which might help prevent a similar accident's occurrence.

The locating of accident witnesses often requires an extensive search of the accident site area; the following potential sources are intended as a guide in supplementing the investigator's ingenuity in locating witnesses. **Locating Eyewitness**

1. Residents in the vicinity as well as workers in adjacent or nearby areas to the accident site may have information regarding: time of accident, engine sound, duration of sound, fluctuation of dynamic level, unusual noises, local weather, relative speed heading, initial condition of wreckage, rescue operations, etc.

2. A newspaper office, often contacted by the witness who believes he possesses significant information, is often a good place to look.

3. A plea via local news media may encourage the reticent or transient witness to contact the investigator.

4. Contacting temporary area personnel such as letter carriers, delivery men, public utility employees, repairmen, etc., may produce people who were in the area at the time of the accident.

5. Expeditious arrival at the accident site facilitates the questioning of sightseers and the curious regarding what attracted them to the accident. Those spectators may also know of other witnesses who have departed the site.

6. Rescue personnel can often provide significant occupant evacuation information prior to rescue operations.

7. One witness may lead to another. Ascertain whether or not the witness was alone at the time of the observation. The reticent or introverted witness may be reluctant to volunteer information, and as a consequence may never be found without the aid of his more talkative companion.

Witness Location Significance

A witness location chart, to be used in conjunction with the written statement, should be prepared for clarification purposes. The exact spot from which a witness makes an observation may explain why his statement differs from that of other witnesses in the vicinity, e.g.:

1. A witness downwind of the accident may often hear engine or other sounds not audible to the upwind observer.

2. Sound is deflected and distorted by walls or buildings and may cause the witness erroneously report direction, sound origin, or dynamic level.

3. Noise level at the point of observation may account for a witness missing significant sounds noted by other observers.

4. The witness looking toward the sun sees only a silhouette, while the witness with the sun at his back may note color and other details.

5. A witness located in a group may be influenced by the power of suggestion. An outspoken member of the group might exclaim, "Those two trains missed a collision by inches!" when, if fact, the lateral separation was 100 ft. The type of individual who hates to be critical of others concurs that the trains passed in close proximity when in reality his initial impression was that there was adequate separation.

Sensory Illusions—Factors That Inhibit the Portrayal of Accurate Information

Most investigators are aware of sensory illusions and their effects on worker actions. These same illusions and their influence on witnesses should be considered by the interviewer. The following examples of sensory illusions will serve to create an awareness of their existence and their potential influence upon witness observations.

1. Consider the observer susceptibility to illusions. The rotating versus the oscillating object. (The experiment with the rotating trapezoidal window is an excellent example.)[4]

2. Consider the relative motion illusion, particularly with reference to velocity, when the observer in motion views a vehicle also in motion. It is incumbent upon the investigator to consider speed and direction in which the witness was moving, in relation to the direction of the

observed vehicle. The apparent speed of a vehicle will be higher when the vehicle and observer are moving in opposite directions.

3. Understanding that visual illusions resulting from false information fed to the brain may account for erroneous witness observations. The accident investigator must evaluate before accepting credibility, e.g.:

   a. Flicker vertigo: In rare cases, people suffer adverse effects such as nausea, vomiting, disorientation, or unconsciousness, resulting from the effect of a flickering light.

   b. Autokinesis: Staring at an isolated light at night can produce a false sensation that the light is moving nondirectionally.

4. Understanding that the absence of shadows at night makes size and distance estimates difficult.

   a. Night vision limitation imposed by the physical structure of the eye.

   b. Refraction error caused by a wet windshield.

   c. Illusion of being closer to signal lights on bright, versus lights on dim.

   d. Erroneous estimate of attitude when there is an up or down slope to the track.

   e. Reduction in night perception after a bright day on the beach or ski slope.

   f. Fatigue, inadequate oxygen, smoking, and distraction of bright lights in the cab also decrease night vision.

5. Understanding that the possibility of illusions may distort the perception makes is advisable that witnesses be selected from various points of observation. This tends to provide a more comprehensive coverage of the occurrence. This is not to say, however, that an average of witness observations is to be assigned greater credibility than a competent witness whose observation deviates from the majority.

6. The Interviewers should pay particular attention to the local observer who, in many cases, is more apt to note occurrences significant or unique to local surroundings than is the transient to whom the same occurrence would hold little significance.

Prompt arrival at the accident site is probably the accident investigator's finest investigation aid. It affords the opportunity of examining the wreckage before excessive disturbance, and permits questioning of witnesses before they reflect on their observations. The investigator is urged to visit the accident site, survey the situation, and decide upon certain questions which he feels witnesses could answer. Witnesses forget as time elapses. They are influenced by association with other witnesses and other people. They read newspapers, listen to the radio, and watch television; news media has its effect on them. The witness, like the fisherman, may embellish his story when he finds listeners less atten-

Expediting the Interviewing of Witnesses

tive than when he originally told the story. The best solution for remedying these witness frailties is to interview the witness promptly.

A memory experiment associated with time lapse was conducted by a group of psychologists and revealed the following facts of significance to the witness interviewer:

1. Interviews taken immediately following an occurrence contained maximum detail, and were generally more complete.
2. After a two-day delay, the information was more general, with fewer specifics, but the main or more vivid points remained.
3. After a seven-day delay, a few of the more vivid elements remained, but there was conderably more conjecture, analysis, and opinion injected by the witness. Certainty to events observed also declined with time.

Witnesses, when contacted promptly, are usually appreciative of the need for accident investigation and the promotion of safety. Some witnesses may consider the interview an imposition and become indignant and impatient when asked to recount their observations. This sort of witness is unfortunate to encounter, but preferable to the one who complains about the complacency of the accident investigators, because he was never contacted. The intelligent witness is aware of voids or blanks in his statement (which the trained interviewer, incidentally, realizes exist in all observations) and endeavors to eliminate them through the application of logic or reasoning. The longer a witness has to reflect on his observations, the more likely he is to modify or supplement the facts, in the interest of coherency. Maximum witness reliability can best be achieved via prompt interviewing.

Occasionally, subsequent evidence dictates that certain witnesses be requestioned. The requestioning of a witness does not necessarily indicate that the interviewer was remiss in the conduct of the initial interview. Instead, the investigator may employ this technique with the witness who appears to rationalize and analyze during the initial interview. The investigator must separate fact and analysis by observing whether or not the more vivid areas of suspected conjecture and mere opinion were analyzed differently from when the witness was first interviewed. By this means, the investigator would attempt to separate fact and analysis, and verify witness reliability. Requestioning a witness may also be in order to confirm technical group findings.

A Successful Interview

The information derived from the witness interview is often directly proportional to the skill of the investigator in establishing rapport. The Witness Group spokesman is responsible for the success or failure of the interview.

The interview should not resemble a surprise party. Make prior arrangements to interview the witness at a time and place convenient for him, under conditions conductive to maximum cooperation and recall. Optimum results are obtained by appointing a spokesman for the Witness Group who is responsible for: introducing the witness to members of the Group, showing credentials, allaying any qualms the witness might have relative to submitting a signed statement, answering any questions posed by the witness concerning the need for and the use of the signed statement, general control of the Witness Group, and establishment of rapport.

Rapport consists primarily of placing the witness at ease, and assuring him that he is not going to be grilled, or given the third degree. Setting the stage and placing the witness at ease should include explaining the objective of accident investigation—**accident prevention.**

Initially, encourage the witness to tell his story in his own way, without questions, comments, suggestions, or interruptions. Periods of silence in this phase, while the witness collects his thoughts, have been found to encourage the witness to expound more fully and to avoid omissions. The investigator's ability to be a good listener and to keep the interviewee talking is essential in this phase.

Prior planning on the part of the interviewer is necessary, to direct the interview in a systematic line of questioning. Predetermined questions concerning suspect areas should be asked of all witnesses.

This does not mean "use of a prepared list of questions," but rather, explore areas of greatest importance based on the technical knowledge of the interviewer. Prior planning has the advantage of:

1. Reducing the number of bare "yes" or "no" responses common to the prepared questionnaire.
2. Containing the interview within areas relevant to the occurrence.
3. Reducing the tendency of the interviewer to ask leading questions.
4. Avoiding the rigid stereotyped interview.

Aids to Interviewing

Successfully interviewing the accident witness is primarily an application of empathy. Show the witness the same consideration that you would appreciate if the situation were reversed. The experienced interviewer adopts a certain style or technique in interviewing witnesses that he found effective. The following suggested interviewing tips for the novice interviewer will also serve as a review or checklist for the experienced witness interviewer:

1. During the initial narration of the witness and only with the consent of the witness, it is advisable for the interviewer to take notes. The note taking should be unobstrusive. Even with the consent of the witness discretion should be used, and note taking should cease if it proves distracting. Notes should not be so extensive that the witness becomes

absorbed with what the interviewer is doing. Explain the witness that the notes are used to suggest areas in his narration that may require further explanation.

2. Frequently the witness has difficulty putting into words what he observed. In cases such as this, explanatory sketches or diagrams are valuable supplements to the witnesses statement. They should not be construed, however, as substitutes for the narrative statement. When there doubt in the mind of the investigator concerning the exact meaning of a statement, check the answer. The simplest method is to rephrase the answer and get the witness to confirm it.

3. Courtesy and consideration should be afforded the witness at all times. Be patient with the witness if he has difficulty in remembering details. Normal witness observations are expected to have periodic voids. If the witness is indefinite in a given area, allow him to record his statement that way. Do not insist that the witness give a straight "yes" or "no" answer.

4. Attempt to have the witness confine his comments to his observations. Avoid hearsay or areas not within his personal knowledge. If the witness reports that someone else described the accident to him, take the name and contact the person at a later date. Get the full meaning of each statement of the witness. Analyze each answer carefully for suggestions or leads to further questions.

5. After the witness has completed his narrative, the investigator usually will have some specific questions to ask relative to areas that appear in his notes. Keep questions simple: avoid jargon, slang, or terminology that could be foreign to the witness.

6. Use the straightforward and frank approach in questioning the witness, as opposed to the shrewd or clever technique employed by an attorney. The investigator is interested in obtaining information from the witness and not in tricking him or trapping him into an unguarded statement.

7. Avoid arguing with the witness concerning moral responsibility of the crew, operator, or public. Witnesses have been known to regard the interview as a medium for voicing their opinions on things that annoy them. Attempt to keep the witness confined to his observations relative to the accident.

8. Do not assist the witness with terminology, when he experiences difficulty in describing a technical matter. The statement should be in the words of the witness and in terms that he understands.

9. Percentages and fractions, when used by a witness in describing an event, should be translated into exact descriptions. There is a tendency to exaggerate percentages or fractions of the whole, e.g., "That train goes through town too fast about 90 percent of the time."

10. The wording of the question is very important. The following example illustrates how answers are affected by rewording the question. "Should the United States do all in her power to promote world peace?" Of the people questioned, 97 percent answered yes. The question was reworded: "Should the United States become involved in plans to promote world peace?" In this instance only 60 percent answered yes. Apparently the connotation of the word "involved" made the difference.

11. Qualifying the witness is important in establishing observation credibility. Witness vocation and job experience observation credibility. Witness vocation and job experience should be established. When a mechanic describes the sound of an engine as surging or backfiring, his observation should be more reliable than a similar observation of a person totally unfamiliar with the operation of this type of equipment.

12. Compare the individual to the collective witness interview. The collective witness interview allows witness # 2 to hear the statement of witness # 1. In hearing the statement, witness # 2 could possibly take information that is mentioned by witness # 1 and use this information to fill blanks in his obseravation. Many times the collective witness interview will result in one witness contradicting and correcting another. In the collective witness interview, one witness may be influenced by the statement of another. Feeling that a witness knows more about a specific issue will cause another to alter his original observation to conform with the statement of the first witness. Conformity of witness observation is not necessarily what the accident investigator desires.

13. Use of a tape recorder is a matter of individual interviewer preference, and as stated before may be undesirable. However, if tape recorders are used, consideration should be given to certain associated circumstances and requisites:
   a. A signed written statement is most desirable.
   b. Tape must be transcribed and forwarded to witness for signature.
   c. Witness must edit transcription.
   d. Some witnesses concentrate more on the microphone than on their observation.
   e. Environment may not be conducive to recording.
   f. Mechanics of operating the tape recorder may be a disadvantage, e.g., changing tape in the middle of an interview; faulty recording due to inexperienced operator or mechanical malfunction.
   g. Witness should be provided with a copy of his statement.

14. Courtesy during the interview is emphasized. Courtesy is as important in concluding the witness interview as it is in conducting it. Thank the witness for his cooperation and time in providing the information and

preparing the signed statement; bear in mind that the statement was voluntary, and perhaps given during the time that the witness may have allotted for something else. The investigator should leave a phone number and address where he can be reached, should the witness recall additional information that he failed to included in his statement.

15. It is occasionally necessary that the interviewer assist certain well qualified, observant witnesses with the organization of their written statements. A few minutes spent here will aid future readers in grasping the full significance of the information. Valuable witness interviews have been wasted because an investigator has failed to obtain a recorded statement in an understandable manner. Application of the following suggestions may help avoid this problem.

   a. Assist the witness with the mechanics of organizing the written statement. Suggest the use of an outline if the witness appears to have difficulty in organizing the report and collecting his thoughts.

   b. Encourage the witness to use drawings, sketches or photographs if they will help clarify the written statement. Drawings, sketches or photographs are merely supplements to the report and do not take the place of a written statement.

   c. Assist the witness in organization only. Do not aid the witness with technical terms; his statement should be written in his own words.

   d. Witnesses tend to minimize or omit observations which, to them, have little significance. The investigator's background should guide him as to the significance of the information to be included in the statement of the witness. Frequently, relatively insignificant information becomes vital to the cause of the accident, once the pieces of information have been put together by the experienced interviewer.

   e. A witness will occasionally omit information from his written statement that he included in his oral description of the accident. It is the responsibility of the interviewer to catch these omissions and insure that they ars inserted in the written report.

   f. A professional approach to witness interviewing requires that the witness be provided with a copy of the statement. This is a common courtesy which should be afforded the witness. The copy may bring to mind additional observations, relative to the accident, when he has an opportunity to reread his statement at his leisure.

There are as many variations in witness types as there are types of people. To better evaluate the observations of the witness, it is advisable that the interviewer have some knowledge of what factors influence some of these types.

Injured Witness

When questioning the injured witness, attempt to keep the Witness Group small. Obtain the permission of the attending physician prior to interviewing the injured witness. The witness might be under sedation, in a state of shock, or in a condition where no coherent statement could be expected. The investigator should be cautioned, however, to listen to seemingly incoherent statements or ramblings of the injured witness; these ramblings may contain a clue as to the cause of the accident. Limit questions to the essentials; screen and plan them carefully. This could be the only opportunity to question the injured witness. Insure that the investigator is accompanied by amother member of the Witness Group for verification of witness observations.

Child Witness

Children may be the most objective observers. Unlike the adult witness who analyzes what he sees and may alter his observation in favor of logic the child will generally report what he sees, regardless of how improbable it may be. Discretion must be used, particularly in questioning young children (4–7 years). They sometimes live in a world of fantasy as real as actual life. The astute questioner should be able to separate fact from fantasy.

Children are particulary susceptible to leading questions (A leading question is defined as a question which contains the answer.) Most children are quite impressed with the fact that an adult is asking them questions, and they are even more impressed when the adult listens to the answers. In order to retain the adult's attention, the child may attempt to please by giving the answer he thinks the interviewer wants. Here the leading question is particularly dangerous, since the interviewer has already given the child an indication of an acceptable answer.

Illiterate Witness

The interviewing of the illiterate witness may present a delicate situation. Many people who are illiterate prefer to keep it a secret. Should this situation exist, question the witness individually to avoid any possible embarrassment. If facilities are available, it is preferable to have the illiterate witness dictate his statement. However, the interviewer may write the statement for the witness and read it back to him for verification. The interviewer should be a witness, along with another member of the Witness Group when the illiterate makes his signature.

"Know-Nothing" Witness

The "know-nothing" witness fears involvement, and even though he has witnessed the occurrence, prefers to remain the background and not get involved. This type can sometimes be approached by stressing the need for his assistance, or by appealing to his humanitarian nature.

Prejudiced Witness

The prejudiced witness may hate the way the particular job he does has been designed, consider it dangerous, and feel that it should be changed. This individual may be encouraged to give a statement by sympathizing with him and listening to his complaints.

Intoxicated Witness

The intoxicated witness should be listened to, but his statement should be taken later. Individuals often say things under the influence of alcohol that they would not say if sober. Confront the witness with his remarks the following day, when he is sober.

Suspicious Witness

The suspicious witness guards his privacy and resents any intrusion by the public. He is suspicious of investigators, hates publicity, and in all probability would prefer not to give a written statement. This witness may be encouraged to give a statement by stressing the importance of safety and by convincing him that his help is needed.

Talkative Witness

The talkative witness is usually the type of individual who is delighted to be the center of attention and will talk for hours concerning his observations. Impress upon this witness the need for a businesslike interview, the importance of safety, and your obligation to contact other witnesses. The boasting witness also falls within this category. Impress upon him the need for facts and that any stretching of these facts might mislead investigators as to the actual cause of the accident.

Timid Witness

The timid witness requires moral support and encouragement. This witness is frequently insecure, discounts his own importance, and fails to see why any information he has would be of interest to anyone else. This category often includes the foreign-born witness. Allow the witness to write his statement in his native language, permit him to dictate it to a translator, if he prefers. Allow him to write his statement in private, gain his confidence and be empathetic.

Disinterested Witness

The disinterested witness is usually uncooperative and may be indifferent to the investigation process. This type of witness is best dealt with by flattering him into believing his information is needed, if other accidents are to be avoided. Stressing the witnesses ability to add significant inputs into the total investigation activity should be stressed.

Various factors tend to influence witness observations. It is advisable that the interviewer have some knowledge of these factors, to better understand why witnesses report as they do.

Factors Affecting Witnesses

1. Witness reporting reliability is partly dependent upon intelligence. Reliability is not as apparent in observing as it is in the area of ability to recall, and in the organization of thoughts. The less intelligent witness tends to have difficulty in recalling specific details simply because they failed to interest him. He will also have difficulty in organizing his thoughts and presenting his observations in a coherent manner.

2. No witness should be overlooked on the basis of apparent lack of intelligence or because of his age.

3. No significant variation has been found in contrasting the accuracy of adult female and male observations.

4. Emotion and excitement tend to produce decided distortion and exaggeration, especially in the verbal description of an occurrence. Emotion will tend to influence the description of an accident where there is personal involvement. Accuracy depends on the observer's mental state at the time, and partly on the complexity of the situation.

5. Exaggeration tends to creep into the interview after a witness has repeated his observations several times, or has been given time to reflect on the events. He can be compared to the fisherman who in describing the fish that got away, adds a few inches to the length of the fish each time the story is told. Witnesses tend to fill in blanks or voids in their observation after they have had time to apply logic and reason. They temper their statements in the hope that their observations will be accepted by the interviewer.

6. A common witness failing is "transposition." The witness reports all the facts, but places them out of sequence with the actual occurrence. The experienced investigator should pick this up and attempt to have these areas clarified when the witness prepares his written statement.

7. Omissions are common in witness statements simply because the witness does not consider certain information important. Omissions concerning details of an observation have been found to be most common in the free narrative type report. The eyewitness is asked to prepare a statement of observation without the benefit of such questions in specific areas as: describe engine sound, vehicles involved, weather, etc. Omissions are more common in the free narrative type statement than in the completion type.

8. The "closed-lead" type statement, as contrasted with the "open-lead" asks witness to comment on specific areas of observation. The closed-lead type witness questionnaire covers a broader area of observation than does the open-lead, but it also leads the witness to comment in areas where he had no previous impression. Additions are more common in the closed-lead questionnaire, since the investigator has given the witness a clue to what information he desires. A combination of the open-lead and closed-lead type statement is recommended for accident investigation. This subject will be dealt with later on page 317.

9. When a number of witnesses reflect general agreement in describing an occurrence, the circumstances may, in general, be considered correct. Exercise caution, however, since psychological experiments show that there is a strong tendency for the same errors to appear in testimony of different individuals.

10. Witnesses tend to be particularly astute and perceptive in areas of observation in which they are personally involved.

11. Witnesses who have sustained a frightening or traumatic experience often have difficulty recalling even the most vivid events. This may be a result of the natural tendency of the mind to dispel or push unpleasant thoughts back into the subconscious, as a protection against uncomfortable and upsetting memories. Many times, for example, the operator of an automobile will recall nothing more than that "prior to the collision, everything seemed to be normal."

12. In establishing witness credibility, the investigator should be aware of the interviewer's tendency to interpret ambiguous answers in accordance with his own particular beliefs, opinions, or prejudices. For example: The temperance advocate, when interviewing a group of skid row occupants, attributed their misfortunes and current social status primarily to their excessive use of alcohol. A psychologist who was unbiased interviewed the same group; he attributes their situation to alcohol in less than 50 percent of the cases.

13. The interviewer should be aware of the Witness tendency to underestimate long distances or periods of time, but to overestimate short distances or periods of time.

The gathering of the witness evidence comprises about 50 percent of the witness phase of the accident investigation. The success of the witness phase hinges on the remaining 50 percent, the ability of the investigator as an analyst to apply his technical knowledge to the seemingly unrelated observations of lay witnesses and to emerge with possible contributing and causal factors.

The purpose behind analyzing witness statements, as opposed to accepting them at face value, is to:

1. Translate layman observations into possible causal factors.
2. Disentangle order and logic from apparent confusion.
3. Corroborate facts by coordinating witness information and other findings.
4. Evaluate witness credibility.
5. Evaluate the witness as a potential court hearing participant. Never underestimate the value of any detail in questioning a witness. A slip-shod job in the witness phase may overlook a suspect area, delay the cause finding, or even mislead investigators to the extent that the cause remains undetermined.

Sample dialogs of the incorrect and correct ways to interview:

Incorrect Method

Investigator: O.K. Bill, tell me how you got hurt! Start as far back as you can remember. I have to write it all down.

Bill: I was putting the bronze casting on the 4-wheel truck and I dropped it when . . .

Investigator: You dropped it! You mean it slipped out of your hands? Didn't you have a tight grip on it, like you should?

Bill: Well, Yeah, I did but . . .

Investigator: Well, how could you drop it then? You know if you had been more careful, these things wouldn't happen. Were you wearing gloves?

Bill: No, but I usually do.

Investigator: That's what they all say. Haven't you heard enough about wearing gloves?

Bill: (Pensive look—doesn't answer)

Investigator: See what happens from not listening. Well, O.K. Be more careful in the future. Safety is important. Do you understand that?

Bill: (Nods grimly).

Investigator: O.K. Go back to work now and remember to be more careful and watch what you're doing or you will be seeing me and your doctor again.

How do you think Bill felt at the end of this interrogation? Do you think that Bill will think twice about reporting a minor injury again? The investigator's major short-coming was that he acted and sounded like he was disgusted because had had to make out a report. He put the man on the defensive right at the start. He interrupted and didn't let the man finish. He was impersonal and abrupt. At no time did he express sympathy for the man's injury. He even terminated the interview on a sour note. To top it all, he never acquired a complete understanding of the accident. Now the the next interview:

Correct Method

Investigator:	How's the foot Bill? Did you get proper care at the dispensary?
Bill:	Yes sir, thank you—they did a good job. All I have is a bruised toe.
Investigator:	Well, Bill, I would like to take a little of your time to go over what happened. Before you tell me, I would like to tell you why I think it is important to check out even a minor injury producing accident like you just had. Quite simply, by going over such accidents carefully, often a lot can be learned to prevent similar accidents from occurring. Please don't take the questions I'm about to ask you personally and don't worry about admitting that you did something wrong. It will in no way be used against you. What I learn from you may prevent an accident from happening to another guy.
Bill:	I think I understand, and I will do the best I can do help.
Investigator:	O.K., Let's go over to where you were when the accident occurred. (Arrival at scene.) Bill, will you explain what you were doing, and how you were doing it when the accident happened. Take you time and try to remember as many things as you can which occurred just before the accident.
Bill:	Well, I was transporting the bronze casting to the 4-wheel drive truck to transport it to ths polishing section. And, you know how sharp the rough edges of a new casting can be, besides the fact that is is heavy and greasy, I lifted the casting from the table and began to move it to the 4-wheel car when I slipped, lost my grip on it and dropped it on my right foot.
Investigator:	Bill, old buddy, you were fortunate. That casting weighs about forty-five pounds. You could have broken some toes.
Bill:	You're darn right—a couple of broken toes would really put me out of service for awhile.
Investigator:	Was there water, grease, or any other substance on the floor in the vicinity of your work station—like this spot of oil (pointing to the spot).

Bill:	There is always oil on the floor. That lathe there leaks oil onto the floor every now and then. We try to mop it up when we see it.
Investigator:	What do you think is causing the oil to leak?
Bill:	I think the automatic oil feed system provides more oil than the machine can use at one time, and the overflow runs onto the floor.
Investigator:	Well, Bill, as I understand it so far, as you were placing the casting on the cart, you lost your footing, slipped, and dropped the casting onto your foot. Is that right?
Bill:	Right on the money, but remember if it wasn't for the oil on the floor I never would have dropped it.
Investigator:	There is no question about it, Bill! We will get the lathe fixed immediately. Perhaps manufacturing engineering may have to redesign the oil lubricating system.
Bill:	It needs a sheet metal container underneath the lathe to catch any oil runoff.
Investigator:	Hey, that's a heck of an idea for an immediate solution, and perhaps as back-up to whatever change engineering makes.
Bill:	It won't take too much.
Investigator:	O.K. Bill, I appreciate your cooperation and your suggestion. One thing more, please wear your safety shoes from now on. With all the heavy parts you lug around every day, its possible that something else will hit your foot. The shoe can mean the difference between no injury, a minor injury, or one which will lay you up for more time than you can afford.
Bill:	(Grinning) All I can say is I will—And thanks.

The preceding example suggests one way to interview if you are after cooperation. In this case, the investigator was friendly but at the same time created an image of competency. He showed interest in the employee's injury. He took the time to tell Bill what he was doing and why. He conducted his interview at the scene—not in an office far removed from where the accident occurred. He listened without interrupting, was not sarcastic, and didn't appear to blame Bill for the accident. He carefully and expertly guided the man into making practical suggestions for the correction of the hazard. In conclusion, he was able to enforce the wearing of protective footwear without undue criticism.

Actually, all accident investigations don't go as smoothly as the one in our example. However, by using the general guidelines offered in the second interview, there is no reason why a person cannot conduct effective accident investigation, acquire the data he needs to pinpoint the causation behind the accident under consideration and encourage worker participation at the same time.

During the accident investigation process, many questions must be considered and answered. However, due to the infinite number of accident-producing situations, contributing factors, causes, etc., it is impossible to provide a complete list of questions that will apply to all accident investigations. Although more detailed questions will be discussed later, for now the following factors should be considered:

- What was the injured person doing at the time of the accident?
- Was the injured doing the job to which he is normally assigned?
- What were fellow workers doing?
- Was the proper tool or machine being used for the job?
- Was the employee trained for the job?
- Was the employeee following approved procedures?
- Is the job or procedure new to the workplace?
- Was the employee being supervised?
- Did the injured receive instructions concerning the hazard which caused the accident?
- Was supervision adequate?
- What was the physical condition of the area when accident occurred?
- Was the employee familiar with area?
- What immediate or temporary action could have prevented the accident?
- What long term or permanent action could have prevented the accident?
- Had corrective action been recommended in the past but not followed?

During the course of any investigation, the above questions should all be answered to the satisfaction of the investigator. Many other questions will come to mind as the individual accident is being investigated questions which should be answered and included in the report. Some of them will be discussed later.

In Chapter 6 we discussed the utilization of hazard analysis techniques to identify and evaluate hazards before they culminate in an accident situation. However, hazard analysis techniques, although not popularly advertised as such, are useful in reconstructing and analyzing accidents. Perhaps the following case will demonstrate this point.

CASE: Power Rotary Mower Accident

A worker living somewhere in the midwest decided to rent a seven and one-half horse power rotary mower to clear a piece of property prior to construction. See Figures 88 and 89. Upon obtaining the mower from his local rental store, he was given very basic instructions in its starting and operation and was told to "be careful." The worker returned to his property with the rental machine and began the land clearing operation when, before he knew what hit him, he

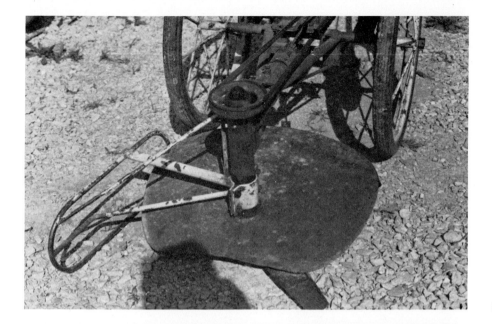

Figure 88.

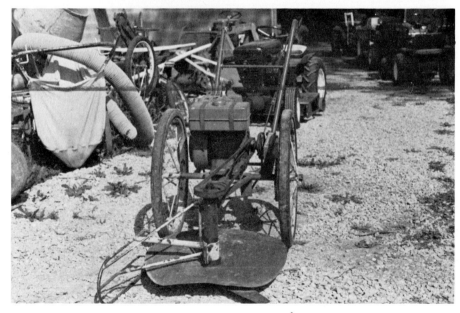

Figure 89.

was on the ground being chopped by the high-speed rotating blade. As a result of this accident, the fellow lost his left hand at the wrist, had a large gouge in the flesh of his hip, as well as the back portion of his left heel.

In an attempt to reconstruct this accident situation, to uncover the particular failure mode in which it occurred, along with the equipment factors which added to the hazardous situation, the investigator selected a simple

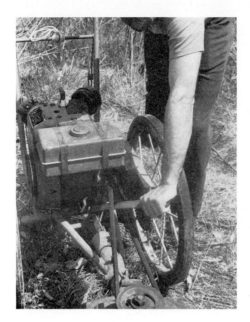

Figure 90.

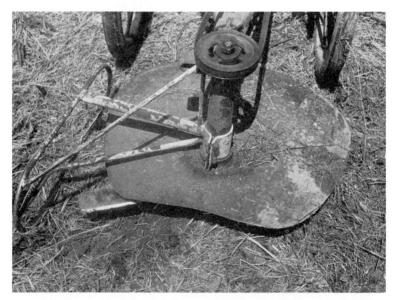

Figure 91.

Failure Mode and Effect analysis as the vehicle to acquire and display information. The analysis matrix in Figure 92 demonstrates the technique and
points up the fact that the power mower possessed several inherent hazards
which contributed to the accident situation. Furthermore, the failure modes
which were most likely associated with the injury situation, were illustrated.
While it is not suggested that this technique is a "cure-all" for all accident
situations, it has, however, proven its value in many circumstances.

Product: All Purpose Mower
H.P.: 7½
Size: 3" x 2⅝"
Blade: 26-inch

Operational Step	Hazardous Element	Hazardous Condition	Trigger	Potential Failure	Effect
1. Start mower	Starting pulley and rope arrangement	Proximity of un-guarded pulley and rope to operator's face	Pulling starting cord to start machine	Rope slipping off pulley, hitting operator in face Pulley binding, causing rope to bruise operator's hand and at the same time pulling operator off balance	Operator slipping and falling Injury to operator's face, hands, back, etc.
2. Activate blade—engage lever	Exposed drive belts Exposed blade (Figure 90 and 91)	Extent of reach required to activate blade lever, forcing operator to bend over side of machine where blade is exposed	Pushing blade activating lever forward	Drive belt snapping—hitting operator in face Operator slipping forward and falling in direct line of exposed blade	Injury to operator from belt Lacerations, contusions, and possible amputation of operator's limbs
3. Activate Drive Lever	Locking linkage on drive lever—(Violation of ANSI B.71.1) "A Dead Man Control will automatically interrupt power to a drive when the operator's actuating force is removed"	Having Dead Man Control made inoperative by having locking linkage activated while machine is in cutting mode	Setting locking linkage after activating drive lever with machine running	Machine running without operator in full control Operator not able to shut machine off without a time lag Operator could be thrown to ground and come in contact with cutting blade which is turning at pre-set revolutions	Injury to operator Injury to others in cutting area Possible runaway machine
4. Cutting Mode	Blade protruding from left side of cowling without adequate guard	Blade striking foreign objects Blade getting caught in rough turf or terrain	Running machine over or into foreign objects or over irregular terrain	Blade throwing objects and dirt back at operator or at others in the area Blade striking substantial object causing machine to yaw—thus creating the torque capable of forcing man to ground or in path of protruding blade Man slipping and falling to side of machine where blade is protruding	Injury to operator Damage to bojects in area
	Heavy machine not equipped with a reverse gear	Undue stress on operator when he changes direction of the machine	Maneuvering the mower	Unnecessary strain on operator	Sprains and Strains

Figure 92. Product hazard analysis.

Figure 92. *Continued.*

Operational Step	Hazardous Element	Hazardous Condition	Trigger	Potential Failure	Effect
5. Disengage Drive Lever	Protruding blade 4½ '' beyond cowling	Rotation of blade after drive lever is disengaged (2-5 secs.)	Momentum of drive shaft Play in actuating lever which doesn't provide full disengagement of blade drive	Operator or others coming in contact with rotating blade	Injury to operator
6. Shutting Machine Off	Exposed belt	Exposed belt in close proximity to shorting mechanism	Shorting-out engine	Operator's hand coming in contact with belt while shorting-out engine	Friction burns and other injury
	Hot Exhaust pipe	Proximity of exhaust pipe to shorting lever	Shorting-out engine	Operator's wrist coming in contact with hot exhaust pipe	Burns

Haddon's Model   Haddon's Model (Figure 93), is another aid that has been developed to help the investigator evaluate all accident contributing factors. Haddon's Model provides an analytical framework that divides the sequence of events leading to the end result—injury and/or property damage—into three phases, preaccident, accident, and postaccident. Factors that determine the accident outcome, human, tool, machine, and environment, can all be operating in each of three phases.

Pre-accident

The pre-accident phases considers all factors that increase the likelihood an accident will occur. Pre-accident countermeasures include, for example: education and training programs, preemployment and periodic medical examinations, tool and machine design, environmental controls, process changes, toxic material substitution, etc.

Accident

The accident phase considers all elements that contribute to its occurrence. During this phase, countermeasures attempt to prevent harmful interaction between the etiologic agent (cause) and the host (worker and/or property). Sample countermeasures involving manipulation of human, tool/machine, and environment factors are machine guards, protective equipment, worker training, removal of hazardous agency, etc.

Factor / Phase	Human	Tool/Machine	Environment
Pre-accident	Lack of: Education/Training, pre-employment medical examination, supervision, maintenance, etc.	Poor: Tool/Machine design, process flow, material selection, etc.	Inadequate: Ventilation, lighting, temperature control, lighting, humidity control, etc.
Accident	Worker unsafe act. Allergic to materials, etc.	Machine improperly guarded, inadequate controls, use of toxic material, etc.	Toxic fumes due to poor ventilation, poor lighting, etc.
Post-accident	Last of first-aid trained personnel, excess delay in obtaining medical treatment	Lack of first-aid equipment, stretcher, gas mask, etc.	Poor lighting, toxic fumes hamper rescue attempts and rendering assistance, etc.

Figure 93. Haddon's model.

Post-accident

During the post-accident phase, methods to prevent death, unwarranted injury, and/or property damage, once the accident has occurred, are considered. Examples are emergency medical care, first aid procedures, safety equipment (eye washes, emergency showers, etc.), emergency shut-offs, firefighting equipment, evacuation plans, sprinkler systems, etc.

By thorough evaluation of the above three phases and all factors affecting each, Haddon's Model can be a valuable aid in the accident investigation process.[3] To better understand the use of Haddon's Model, apply its use to the following accident:

Case Study

A man in the punch press department of a small machine shop has just had a finger amputated. As the punch press department supervisor, you must see to the immediate welfare of your worker. Of primary concern is providing first aid treatment and transporting the injured man to the hospital. You instruct one of your workers to call for an ambulance, and another to get the first aid kit, while you ask the other workers if anyone has been first-aid trained. The worker returns with the first aid kit, and you find it to well-equipped with aspirins and two sizes of band aids. As a stretcher is not provided in the shop, a few co-workers carry the injured worker to the door, anticipating the arrival of the ambulance. Finally, the ambulance arrives, and the employee is taken to the hospital, where he receives medical treatment from trained and prepared personnel, in a well-equipped emergency room.

Now you have the responsibility of completing the accident investigation, while the circumstances surrounding the accident are fresh in everyone's mind.

During the interviews with various workers in the area and a witness you determine the following facts:

- The injured worker had complained of intensive itching of his hands, to fellow workers, during the lunch break.
- The injured worker was placing a part in the die with one hand and actuated the press with the other, when the accident occurred.
- The worker sent to call the ambulance informed you that he was delayed because the telephone number was not available and he did not know whom to call.

After conferring with the injured worker's supervisor, you learn additional facts as follows:

- It has been necessary, on occasion, to remind the injured worker of the hazards concerned with press operation, due to the observation of his committing unsafe acts.
- The press that was being used is not provided with two hand controls or a barrier guard.

As a witness to the post-accident phase of the accident, you know the following facts:

- Adequate first aid equipment was not available.
- First-aid-trained personnel were not available.
- A stretcher was not provided.

After later interviewing the injured worker, you determine the following:

- He had misaligned the part in the die and was in the process of aligning the part with his left hand when the accident occurred.
- The worker believed the area lighting to be inadequate, contributing to the misalignment of the part.
- The worker was not formally trained in press operation, which has become obvious as the investigation is being conducted.
- While at the hospital, the doctor informed the injured man that the itch he had on his hands was dermatitis and believed it to be caused by the lubricant being used on the dies.

The information obtained from these various sources must now be put together, and analysis made if it is to be used, and practical recommendations to prevent a recurrence formulated. This was easily done with the aid of Haddon's Model (Figure 93). Once the information is broken down into the three accident phases and the three factors, many areas in need of improvement can be seen.

To complete the accident investigation process, practical recommendation to prevent a recurrence and minimize delays and injury after the accident must be formulated.

Recommendations

1. Initiate a training program for all new and existing press operators.
2. Find a suitable substitute for the die lubricant that will not cause dermatitis.
3. Conduct a survey of the press department and other areas necessary to determine the need for additional lighting.
4. Provide two hand control devices on all presses.
5. Provide a minimum of two first aid trained employees on each shift.
6. Provide adequate first aid supplies and maintain the supplies.
7. Post emergency telephone numbers at readily accessible telephones, to include the numbers of doctor, ambulance, polices, fire department, and others as necessary.
8. Provide stretchers in appropriate areas of the plant.

Through the process of accident investigation and analysis of the facts, the investigator was able to formulate practical recommendations to prevent a recurrence of of a similar accident and to provide management information that can be used to make informed management decisions.

Coordinating and Evaluating Investigation Findings

After the investigator is satisfied that he has examined all available information, his next task is to analyze this information in the hope of determining the cause or causes of the accident. Again, it is emphasized that the investigator must keep a completely open mind and that he should be looking for reasons both for and against the occurrences of specific events.

In analyzing an accident, it may be helpful to outline a step-by-step sequence of each possible accident mechanism based on the evidence found. If an "evidence gap" is found in one particularly promising mechanism, it may be desirable to reopen the search. If possible, the accident iste should be left undisturbed for a period of time after the investigators leave, to allow for such a possibility. Physical or chemical analyses, detailed equipment disassembly, accident simulation, or other analyses should be performed to verify the final evaluation; . . . "all the screened information must either confirm the final hypotheses, or at the worst, portions of the evidence must neither confirm nor deny it. No reliable circumstantial evidence can be adverse."

Some time should be devoted to evaluating the facility's emergency procedures and their effectiveness during the accident. It is very likely that several useful revisions may be recommended.

Concluding the Investigation

Departure from the Accident Scene   Departure of the investigators is as significant as their arrival. The best time to leave the scene is a matter of judgment. It would not be wise to depart as " . . . thieves in the night.'' An orderly culmination of the on-site effort is required. Many individuals and organizations will desire to know the investigating team's findings. Care should be given in releasing such information, particularly if an important technical analysis remains to be completed.

Preparation of the Final Report   The final report is the product of the investigating team's activities. It should be carefully prepared and adequately justify the conclusions reached. It should be noted that the report preparation phase of the investigation is most significant. A poorly written document will make the most outstanding investigation meaningless.

The timely issuance of the report is equally important. One issued too long after investigative actions are completed will be anticlimatic. If a final report must be delayed pending detailed technical evaluation or analysis, an interim report should be prepared. This document should contain all the results available at its time of issuance. In some cases it may appear unbalanced, since an accident cause at that point might not have been fully accepted. Consequently, the interim report may appear to overemphasize contributing-cause factors rather than the true cause.

In preparation of the final report, the investigator should review the objectives of his investigation, to assure they have been met. The conclusions reached should be supported with the backup data presented in the report. It will not be possible to put all the information gathered in the document, consequently a judicious selection is required.

Additional Important Aspects to be Considered

Public Relations   Man is a social animal and as such has a keen desire to keep abreast of the latest happenings in his environment. An accident in any organization is always of significant interest. The employee's and the public's most common concerns are reflected in the following three questions they so frequently ask: Is there any potential danger to those in the immediate vicinity? What was the cause of the accident? How many people were injured and how badly? With the above in mind, it should not be surprising that a great deal of emphasis, in the early stages of any investigation, will be placed on Public Relations. The significant points to remember in dealing with the public are presented below for guidance. Further points can be obtained from an organization's legal office.

1. Be truthful. Answer questions correctly and be sure of your facts. Don't try to cover up or misrepresent a situation.
2. Know to whom you are talking. If something you say appears in print at a later data, it's nice to know how it got there.
3. Keep a record of all interviews. This might also be significant at a later date.
4. Do not answer questions you do not want to discuss fully.
5. Be certain you are authorized to release information you disclose. Security may be involved in certain accident situations.

Remember, no investigator is under any compulsion to talk. While a cooperative attitude is called for, answers can often be given after due deliberation on the question's import. An investigator should not be rushed into a hasty answer.

The accident report form is the vehicle by which information is recorded for future use in decision-making. A well designed report format will provide sufficient data that can be used for a wide variety of information requirements.

Analysis of Accident Report Forms

Accident report forms are built on the basis of leads, which direct communication flow. They are given or delivered by one person to another and give structure to the communication exchange. Very simply, leads may be thought of as invitations to communicate. There are two broad classifications of leads: open and closed.[5]

Closed leads limit participation by the recipient. They close off the amount of response expected of the recipient. If we picture the basic communication unit, it has two components—the message sender and the message recipient.

The sender uses a lead to frame his wishes for information or participation from the recipient. A closed lead, then, informs the recipient that little response is desired. An example of a closed lead is:

> Did you see this happen?

or:

> I suppose you agree with what the report says.

or:

> How long were you at your work station when you smelled the vapors?

These statements ask for small amounts of information—"Yes," "No," "I don't know," "It fell about 20 feet," etc. People may give more information than they were invited to give by the lead, but the sender cannot or should not expect it. (Note: In court proceedings a witness may be cautioned to restrict his answer to what was asked—yes or no—and not volunteer information. A closed lead preceded that warning.) Closed leads give the sender much control over the information exchange. He conducts the communications according to his particular informational needs. This is not particularly sociable manner of exchange; the sender uses most of the "talk" time, the respondent very little. In the extreme, a closed-lead exchange would sound like a child's game of Twenty Questions. Closed leads, however, are efficient for the sender, he acquires, or may acquire much information quickly.

In a written medium, closed leads appear in polls and survey questionnaires. Computerized information sheets and forms rely exclusively on closed-lead style. Such leads predominate in accident report forms like the OSHA Form 36 (Figure 94).

Open leads invite extended participation from the recipient. Examples of open leads are:

What could be done to make this safe?

or:

How would you compare this situation today with what it was yesterday?

or:

Describe what you saw.

Open leads give senders relatively little control over the information acquiring process. Once the lead has been delivered, the sender is dependent upon the recipient to provide whatever information he has, or is inclines to give. The recipient of the lead also takes whatever direction he wants in answering. The use of a series of open leads may yield much information for the sender, but permits no opportunity for him to pinpoint issues.

In written form, open leads resemble essay-type questions in a classroom test. In accident reporting on report forms usually only one statement is posed in open-lead form—"Describe what happened (in your own words)."

Obviously, a combination of leads produces the most effective information: open leads to produce quantities of information, closed leads to refine and direct information gain.

OSHA—Form 36

Figure 94 illustrates a form which obviously is geared to computerized classification, coding, storage and retrieval of information. The objectives for the form have to be inferred; it becomes clear that the purpose of this form is

Figure 94.

U. S. DEPARTMENT OF LABOR
OCCUPATIONAL SAFETY AND HEALTH ADMINISTRATION
PRELIMINARY FATALITY/CATASTROPHE EVENT REPORT
For Flash Report to National Office, call Items 1-12, 16-17, 19-25, 29-30.

Section I

REPORT IDENTIFICATION

1. Region	2. Area	3. Report Number	4. Date			5. Time	6. Source of Report
			Mo	Day	Yr		1-Employer 5-Hospital 2-Employee 6-Media 3-Police 7-State 4-Medical Examiner 8-Other_____

A B

Section II

EMPLOYER IDENTIFICATION

7. Name of Establishment

8. Address

9. City Code	10. State Code	11. County Code

12. Address at Site of Event if Different than Item 8

13. Name of Person Reporting	14. Job Title	15. Telephone Number

16. Establishment Size

1 - Small (1-19)
2 - Medium (20-499)
3 - Large (500 and over)

17. Type of Business

SIC Code

18. Person to Contact at Site of Event

Section III

FATALITY/CATASTROPHE EVENT DATA

19. Date of Event			20. Time of Event	21. Event Category	Number of Casualties		
Mo	Day	Yr			22. Fatalities	23. Hospitalized Injuries	24. Non-Hospitalized Injuries

AM
PM

1 - Fatality with H/S
2 - Catastrophe with H/S
3 - Fatality w/o Haz Sub
4 - Catastrophe w/o Haz Sub

25. Hazardous Substance (if entry in Item 21 is 1 or 2)

Hazardous
Substance
Code

26. Briefly Describe Fatality/Catastrophe Event

Section IV

DECISION DATA AND ACTION TAKEN

27. History of OSHA Contact	28. History of OSHA Contact Results	29. Is Inspection Planned? (If yes, give date.)
1 - No Previous Contact 2 - Previous Fatality/Catastrophe Event Inspection 3 - Previous Complaint Inspection 4 - Previous OSHA Contact Other Than 2, 3	1 - No Violations Alleged 2 - Nonserious Violation Cited 3 - Serious Violation Cited 4 - Failure to Abate Cited 5 - Willful or Repeated Cited	1-Yes Mo Day Yr 2-No

30. Reason No Inspection Is Planned	31. Date of Flash Report	32. Time	33. CSHO's Assigned
1 - Unresolved Jurisdictional Problem 2 - Inadequate Resources 3 - Excessive Travel Required 4 - Other (Explain in Item 34)	Mo Day Yr		

34. Remarks

35. Signature of Area Director

Date

AREA OFFICE

Form OSHA-36   -36
July 1973

The Process of Accident Investigation   319

Figure 94. *Continued.*

FATALITY/CATASTROPHE EVENT CODE			
1	Fatality With Hazardous Substance	3	Fatality Without Hazardous Substance
2	Catastrophe With Hazardous Substance	4	Catastrophe Without Hazardous Substance

WEATHER AT TIME OF EVENT CODE					
01	Clear	05	Snowing	08	Electrical Storm
02	Overcast	06	Sleet/Ice	09	Smog (Pollution)
03	Raining	07	Windstorm	10	Flooding
04	Fog				

NATURE OF INJURY CODE					
01	Amputation	08	Dermatitis	15	Heat Exhaustion
02	Asphyxia	09	Dislocation	16	Hernia
03	Bruise/Contusion/Abrasion	10	Electric Shock	17	Poisoning (Systemic)
04	Burn (Chemical)	11	Foreign Body in Eye	18	Puncture
05	Burn/Scald (Heat)	12	Fracture	19	Radiation Effects
06	Concussion	13	Freezing/Frost Bite	20	Strain/Sprain
07	Cut/Laceration	14	Hearing Loss	21	Other (Specify)

PART OF BODY CODE					
01	Abdomen	09	Face	17	Lower Arm(s)
02	Arm(s) Multiple	10	Finger(s)	18	Lower Leg(s)
03	Back	11	Foot/Feet/Toe(s)/Ankle(s)	19	Multiple
04	Body System	12	Hand(s)	20	Neck
05	Chest	13	Head	21	Shoulder(s)
06	Ear(s)	14	Hip(s)	22	Upper Arm(s)
07	Elbow(s)	15	Knee(s)	23	Upper Leg(s)
08	Eye(s)	16	Leg(s)	24	Wrist(s)

SOURCE OF INJURY CODE					
01	Aircraft	15	Electrical Apparatus/Wiring	29	Motor Vehicle (Highway)
02	Air Pressure	16	Fire/Smoke	30	Motor Vehicle (Industrial)
03	Animal/Insect/Bird/Reptile/Fish	17	Food	31	Motorcycle
04	Boat	18	Furniture/Furnishings	32	Windstorm/Lightning, Etc.
05	Bodily Motion	19	Gases	33	Firearm
06	Boiler/Pressure Vessel	20	Glass	34	Person
07	Boxes/Barrels, Etc.	21	Hand Tool (Powered)	35	Petroleum Products
08	Buildings/Structures	22	Hand Tool (Manual)	36	Pump/Prime Mover
09	Chemical Liquids/Vapors	23	Heat (Environmental/Mechanical)	37	Radiation
10	Cleaning Compound	24	Hoisting Apparatus	38	Train/Railroad Equipment
11	Cold (Environmental/Mechanical)	25	Ladder	39	Vegetation
12	Dirt/Sand/Stone	26	Machine	40	Waste Products
13	Drugs/Alcohol	27	Materials Handling Equipment	41	Water
14	Dust/Particles/Chips	28	Metal Products	42	Working Surface
				43	Other (Specify)

TYPE OF FATALITY/CATASTROPHE EVENT CODE					
01	Struck By	06	Struck Against	11	Repeated Motion/Pressure
02	Caught In or Between	07	Rubbed/Abraded	12	Cardio-Vascular/Respiratory System Failure
03	Bite/Sting/Scratch	08	Inhalation	13	Shock
04	Fall (Same Level)	09	Ingestion	14	Other (Specify)
05	Fall (From Elevation)	10	Absorption		

CONTRIBUTING ENVIRONMENTAL FACTOR CODE			
01	Pinch Point Action	10	Flammable Liquid/Solid Exposure
02	Catch Point/Puncture Action	11	Temperature Above or Below Tolerance Level
03	Shear Point Action	12	Radiation Condition
04	Squeeze Point Action	13	Working Surface/Facility Layout Condition
05	Flying Object Action	14	Illumination
06	Overhead Moving and/or Falling Object Action	15	Overpressure/Underpressure Condition
07	Gas/Vapor/Mist/Fume/Smoke/Dust Condition	16	Sound Level
08	Materials Handling Equipment/Method	17	Weather/Earthquake, Etc. Condition
09	Chemical Action/Reaction Exposure	18	Other (Specify)

CONTRIBUTING HUMAN FACTOR CODE			
01	Misjudgment of Hazardous Situation	08	Malfunction of Perception System With Respect to Task Environment
02	No Personal Protective Equipment Used	09	Safety Devices Removed or Inoperative
03	No Special Protective Clothing or Appropriate Attire Used	10	Operational Position Not Appropriate for Task
04	Malfunction of Procedure for Securing Operation or Warning of Hazardous Situation	11	Procedure for Handling Materials Not Appropriate for Task
05	Distracting Actions by Others	12	Defective Equipment in Use
06	Equipment in Use Not Appropriate for Operation or Process	13	Malfunction of Procedure for Lock-Out or Tag-Out
07	Malfunction of Neuro-Muscular System	14	Other (Specify)

TASK ASSIGNMENT CODE			
01	Employee Working at Regularly Assigned Task(s)	02	Employee Working at Other Than Regularly Assigned Task(s)

EVENT SITE CODE			
01	Inside a Building or Enclosure	03	Outside but Under Cover
02	Outside in the Open		

much more the recording OSHA-related events than the collection of all relevant data to be used to prevent similar accident situations.

The form is characterized by closed-ended questions. These types of "closed leads" limit the kind of response the witness may give. Only one question, number 26, permits any type of narrative, and by the size of the space provided, there is a strong suggestion that not a great deal of information is required.

It is doubtful that the answer to number 26 can enter data storage for later recall or summarization. This type of form is readily filled out; little thinking is needed, and very straightforward classification of information are requested.

The form leaves the impression that only one entry should be made for any one response group. It is likely that the structure of the form may preclude the detection via any computer analysis of interactions among such factors as weather, injury type and environmental factors.

Because the form is intended for very broad scale use, the classifications are very broad. A refinement of the classification scheme would be needed to assess any particular management failure or action of the individual in relation to the accident. Assessment of multiple events is impossible.

In the type of questioning exhibited in this form, the author must have in mind what he thinks to be the appropriate classifications of information. He has the responsibility for asking them, because he is treating the respondent in a very confining fashion. As in the game "Twenty Questions," he must ask the right questions, lest he get misleading information.

The degree to which an injury or fatality could be reconstructed from a form such as this is questionable.

This form at least has more information in fair detail for detecting or having the potential for detecting interactions than OSHA Form 200 Figure 94a which provides no opportunity for any reconstruction of events. It is a summary statement. However, even though writing is required, these are closed leads—that is the respondent has virtually no chance to expand on an answer. The line of questioning illustrated by Form 200 is very much like the courtroom scene, where the judge reminds the witness only to answer the question as asked and not to elaborate.

In Figure 95, "Supervisor's Accident Investigation Report" we find a total opposite of the OSHA Form 36. To begin with, the questioning style is that of an "open lead," which gives primary control in the communication process to the respondent; whereas, in the OSHA Forms the control rested with the interviewed. This form is much more geared to finding details related to the operations and events associated with the accident, and much less geared to any kind of accounting for OSHA—type purposes. The difficulty with a form like this is that because the type of response and the interpretation of the question rest entirely with the respondent, no classifications of any uniformity exist, to per-

| NOTE: | This form is required by Public Law 91-596 and must be kept in the establishment for *5 years*. Failure to maintain and post can result in the issuance of citations and assessment of penalties. *(See posting requirements on the other side of form.)* | | **RECORDABLE CASES:** You are required to record information about every occupational **death**; every nonfatal occupational **illness**; and those nonfatal occupational **injuries** which involve one or more of the following: loss of consciousness, restriction of work or motion, transfer to another job, or medical treatment (other than first aid). *(See definitions on the other side of form.)* | | |

Case or File Number	Date of Injury or Onset of Illness	Employee's Name	Occupation	Department	Description of Injury or Illness
Enter a nonduplicating number which will facilitate comparisons with supplementary records.	Enter Mo./day.	Enter first name or initial, middle initial, last name.	Enter regular job title, not activity employee was performing when injured or at onset of illness. In the absence of a formal title, enter a brief description of the employee's duties.	Enter department in which the employee is regularly employed or a description of normal workplace to which employee is assigned, even though temporarily working in another department at the time of injury or illness.	Enter a brief description of the injury or illness and indicate the part or parts of body affected.

Typical entries for this column might be: Amputation of 1st joint right forefinger; Strain of lower back; Contact dermatitis on both hands; Electrocution--body. |
(A)	(B)	(C)	(D)	(E)	(F)
					PREVIOUS PAGE TOTALS ⟶
					TOTALS (Instructions on other side of form.) ⟶

OSHA No. 200

FOLD

Figure 94a.

For Calendar Year 19 _____   Page _____ of _____

Company Name	Form Approved
Establishment Name	O.M.B. No. 44R 1453
Establishment Address	

Extent of and Outcome of INJURY						Type, Extent of, and Outcome of ILLNESS													
Fatalities	Nonfatal Injuries					Type of Illness								Fatalities	Nonfatal Illnesses				
Injury Related	Injuries With Lost Workdays				Injuries Without Lost Workdays	CHECK Only One Column for Each Illness *(See other side of form for terminations or parmanent transfers.)*								Illness Related	Illnesses With Lost Workdays				Illnesses Without Lost Workdays
Enter **DATE** of death. Mo./day/yr.	Enter a **CHECK** if injury involves days away from work, or days of restricted work activity or both.	Enter a **CHECK** if injury involves days away from work.	Enter number of **DAYS** *away from work.*	Enter number of **DAYS** of *restricted work activity.*	Enter a **CHECK** if no entry was made in columns 1 or 2 but the injury is recordable as defined above.	Occupational skin diseases or disorders	Dust diseases of the lungs	Respiratory conditions due to toxic agents	Poisoning (systemic effects of toxic materials)	Disorders due to physical agents	Disorders associated with repeated trauma	All other occupational illnesses		Enter **DATE** of death. Mo./day/yr.	Enter a **CHECK** if illness involves days away from work, or days of restricted work activity, or both.	Enter a **CHECK** if illness involves days away from work.	Enter number of **DAYS** *away from work.*	Enter number of **DAYS** of *restricted work activity.*	Enter a **CHECK** if no entry was made in columns 8 or 9.
(1)	(2)	(3)	(4)	(5)	(6)	(a)	(b)	(c)	(d)	(e)	(f)	(g)		(8)	(9)	(10)	(11)	(12)	(13)
										(7)									

Certification of Annual Summary Totals By _____ Title _____ Date _____

OSHA No. 200   **POST ONLY THIS PORTION OF THE LAST PAGE NO LATER THAN FEBRUARY 1.**

SUPERVISOR'S ACCIDENT INVESTIGATION REPORT

CONTRACT NO._____ LOCATION:_____ ACCIDENT REPORT NO._____

Name of Injured or Deceased	Date and Time of Accident	His Craft:

WHAT HAPPENED?

Describe what took place.

WHY DID IT HAPPEN?

Get all the facts by studying the job and situation involved. Question by use of WHY — WHAT — WHERE — WHEN — WHO — HOW

WHAT SHOULD BE DONE TO PREVENT RECURRENCES?

Determine which of the 12 items listed below require additional attention.

Equipment	Material	People
Select	Select	Select
Arrange	Place	Place
Use	Handle	Train
Maintain	Process	Lead

WHAT HAS BEEN DONE THUS FAR?

Take or recommend action, depending upon your authority. Follow up. Was action effective.

HOW WILL THIS IMPROVE OPERATIONS?

Our OBJECTIVE is to PREVENT injuries and ELIMINATE job hindrances.

Accident Investigated by:	Date:	Report Reviewed by:	Date:
Immediate Supervisor of Injured		Job Superintendent	

mit different people to respond in similar ways. It is apparent that the suggestions in the little boxes under the major questions are intended to probe the witnesses' perspective. Nevertheless, because the form is usually handed to the witness to be filled out, considering the work involved, facility to write, etc., the witness is not apt to use the information in the boxes to enhance his responses.

The report format in Figure 96 contains a combination of "open" and "closed" leads and permits one thing which does not appear in the two preceding examples. First, the narrative in the report can be checked against the report's detailed classifications and descriptions. This is a type of reliability estimate. Ideally more forms should have this type of internal check. It is possible with this form to apply interaction analyses among critical conditions of physical surroundings, operations, and equipment. The form, because of its specificity, can be highly detailed in terms of temperature ranges, weather conditions, wind velocities, highly detailed explicit parts of body and types of events related to the actual injury itself.

What is particularly desirable about this form is that the method of data processing, although affecting the format, is not affecting the amount of information and the quality of information to be given. The OSHA Form 36, on the other hand, is virtually the opposite. It seems that computer convenience apparently governed the character of the questions and the amount of information required.

OSHA Form 4, Figure 97 illustrates the use of both open and closed leads although the greatest emphasis is placed on the open lead. In comparing this form with that in Figure 96, it may be observed that no classification system exists making it less possible to obtain any estimate of reliability of the data by analyzing the report form. The report form in Figure 96, on the other hand built into it—a means for coding and classifying the data acquired during the process of investigation. Thus, it is possible for the analyst to go from the narrative part of the report into the classification to find overlaps of discrepancies in the data—thus performing a reliability check.

Accident report forms are exactly that—"report forms." The multitude of various forms in use today are intended to provide the minimum basic information necessary by management for determination of compensation liability, to provide statistical data for accident analyses, etc. Such forms can be used as a guide during the accident investigation, but the investigator must not consider his job as one of simply "filling in the blanks" or as being completed when all questions on the form have been answered.

The Investigation Report

Figure 95. Supervisor's accident investigation report.

```
┌─────────────────────────────────────────────────────────────────────────────┐
│                                                                               │
│                           Dept. Accident File Number_____          │
│   001   Name_____     │
│                    Last              First              Middle                │
│                                                                               │
│   002   Age_____  _____               │
│                    Month            Day           Year                        │
│                                                                               │
│   003   Height_____  004  Weight_____                           │
│                                                                               │
│   005   Social Security Number _____-____-_____ 006  Rank_____   │
│                                                                               │
│   007   Permanently Assigned Unit _____               │
│                                                                               │
│   008   Assigned Unit at Tme of Accident_____ District_____ │
│                                                                               │
│   009   Officer of Company Assigned at                                        │
│         Time of Accident _____             │
│                            Last Name         First        Rank                │
│                                                                               │
│   010   Alarm Number_____ 018  Wind Velocity (Estimate)_____  │
│                                                                               │
│   011   Type of Structure                   0181   Zero-5 mph_____            │
│                                             0182    6-10         _____        │
│         0111   Multiple Dwelling _____     0183   11-15         _____        │
│         0112   One-Family        _____     0184   16-21         _____        │
│         0113   High Rise Office  _____     0185   21-25         _____        │
│         0114   Light Commercial_____       0186   26-30         _____        │
│         0115   Heavy Commercial_____       0187   31-40         _____        │
│         0116   Automobile        _____     0188   41+           _____        │
│         0117   Hotel                                                           │
│         0118   Other (Specify)_____ 019  Temperature Range (Estimate)       │
│                                                                               │
│   012   Fire Building                       0191   Less than Zero°  _____     │
│                                             0192   Zero°-20°        _____     │
│         0121   Occupied          _____     0193   21°- 32°         _____     │
│         0122   Vacant            _____     0194   33°- 45°         _____     │
│                                             0195   46°- 60°         _____     │
│   013   Date of Injury_____          0196   61°- 75°         _____     │
│                  Month   Day   Year         0197   76°- 90°         _____     │
│                                             0198   91°-105°         _____     │
│   014   Time of Day_____ am_____ pm       0199   106°+           _____      │
│                                                                               │
│   015   Light Condition (outside)     020   Activity                          │
│                                                                               │
│         0151   Full Daylight     _____     0201   In quarters                │
│         0152   Twilight          _____                                       │
│         0153   Full Darkness     _____            a. Fire Quarters            │
│                                                       Maintenance   _____     │
│   016   Light Condition (inside)                   b. Office Work   _____     │
│                                                    c. Tending Heating          │
│         0161   Dark              _____               equipment    _____      │
│         0162   Partial Illumination_____          d. Physical Fitness         │
│         0163   Illuminated       _____               Activity     _____      │
│                                                    e. Hose Tower    _____      │
│   017   Weather Conditions                         f. Hose Rack    _____      │
│                                                    g. Hose Drier   _____       │
│         0171   Clear             _____            h. Kitchen      _____        │
│         0172   Rain              _____            i. Sliding Pole _____        │
│         0173   Snow              _____            j. Other (Specify)_____     │
│         0174   Sleet             _____                                        │
│         0175   Fog               _____     0202   Responding to               │
│         0176   Other (Specify)_____                                         │
│                                                    a. En Route to              │
│                                                       False Alarm  _____       │
│                                                    b. Sliding Pole _____        │
│                                                                               │
│   More than one response may be appropriate for any category. Check all those │
│   apply.                                                                       │
│                                                                               │
└─────────────────────────────────────────────────────────────────────────────┘
```

Figure 96.

Figure 96. *Continued.*

0203 Operating at

    a. Apparatus Hook-up _____
    b. Laying Hose Lines _____
    c. Advancing Hose
       Lines   _____
    d. Forcible Entry   _____
    e. Ventilating   _____
    f. Search   _____
    g. Working off
       Aerial Ladder   _____
    h. Raising Ladders _____
    i. Lowering Ladders _____
    j. Boat Activity   _____
    k. Other (Specify)_____

0204 Overhaul_____

0205 Returning from

    02051 False Alarm _____
    02052 Retrieving
            Hose Lines _____
    02053 Directing
            Traffic   _____
    02054 Other_____

0206 Inspection_____

0207 Training (Drills)

    02071 In Quarters _____
    02072 Multi-Unit Drill_____
    02073 Dept. Training
            School   _____
    02074 Other_____

0208 Other (Specify)_____

021 Tools, Equipment, Apparatus Used
    by Injured at Time of Injury

_____

_____

_____

022 Personal Protection Equipment

    Worn at Time of Accident
                 Type Manuf. Age
    0221 Helmet _____ _____ _____
    0222 Bunker _____ _____ _____
            Coat   _____ _____ _____
    0223 Gloves _____ _____ _____
    0224 Boots   _____ _____ _____
    0225 Other
         (Specify)_____ _____ _____

023 Injury Influenced or Caused by

    0231 ☐ using equipment beyond
          specifications
    0232 ☐ using protective equip-
          ment beyond designed
          specifications
    0233 ☐ improper maintenance of
          protective equipment
    0234 ☐ not using protective
          equipment

0235 ☐ inadequate protective
      equipment design
      (Specify)_____

0236 ☐ inadequate equipment
      design
      (Specify)_____

0237 ☐ protective equipment
      failure

0238 ☐ Other (Specify)_____

024 Part of Body Affected

0241 Head
    a. Scalp   _____
    b. Skull   _____
    c. Multiple Injury_____

0242 Eye   _____
0243 Face   _____
0244 Ear   _____
0245 Neck   _____
0246 Shoulder _____
0247 Chest   _____
0248 Lungs   _____
0249 Abdomen _____
0250 Back   _____
0251 Buttocks _____
0252 Groin   _____
0253 Upper Arm _____
0254 Elbow   _____
0255 Forearm   _____
0256 Wrist   _____
0257 Hand   _____
0258 Finger
    (Specify) _____
0259 Leg   _____
0260 Thigh   _____
0261 Lower-Leg _____
0262 Leg, Multiple_____
0263 Ankle   _____
0264 Foot   _____
0265 Toe   _____
0266 Hip   _____

025 Accident Type

0251 Struck Against

    02511 Stationary
            Object   _____
    02512 Moving Object _____
    02513 Cut by
            Tool-Utensil _____
    02514 Stepping on Nails
            Glass, etc. _____
    02515 Other
            (Specify)_____

0252 Struck by

    02521 Falling Object _____
    02522 Flying Object   _____
    02523 Hose Stream   _____
    02524 Vehicle   _____
    02525 Other
            (Specify)_____

Figure 96. *Continued.*

0253 Fall

    02531 From Scaffold,
            Platform, etc. _____
    02532 From Ladder _____
    02533 From Roof _____
    02534 From Vehicle
            or Boat _____
    02535 From or on Stairs _____
    02536 Into Shafts,
            Openings, etc. _____
    02537 Pole Hole
    02538 Fall to Lower
            Level (NEC) _____
    02539 Fall on Same
            Level _____

0254 Caught in, under or between

    02541 Collapsed
            Ceiling _____
    02542 Collapsed Floor _____
    02543 Collapsed Wall _____
    02544 Other
            (Specify)_____

0255 Rubber or Abraded _____

0256 Overexertion

    02561 Lifting Objects _____
    02562 Pulling or
            Pushing _____
    02563 Throwing
            Objects _____
    02564 Making Rescue _____
    02565 Other
            (Specify)_____

0257 Contact with Temperature

    Extremes
    02571 General heat—
            atmosphere _____
    02572 General cold
            atmosphere _____
    02573 Hot objects or
            substances _____
    02574 Cold objects or
            substances _____

0258 Contact with

    02581 Chemicals _____
    02582 Electrical _____
    02583 Embers _____
    02584 Hot tar, etc. _____
    02585 Heat or flame _____
    02586 Hot fluids _____
    02587 Hot metals _____
    02588 Other
            (Specify)_____

0259 Hazardous Conditions

    02591 Lack of
            necessary PPE _____
    02592 Improper or
            inadequate
            clothing _____
    02593 Excessive noise _____
    02594 Excessive heat _____
    02595 Inadequate
            work space _____
    02596 Inadequate
            ventilation _____
    02597 Other
            (Specify)_____

026 Type of Injury

    0261 Sprain _____
    0262 Strain _____
    0263 Abrasion _____
    0264 Contusion _____
    0265 Laceration _____
    0266 Puncture _____
    0267 Burns _____
    0268 Fracture _____
    0269 Respiration _____
    02610 Heat exhaustion _____
    02611 Amputation _____
    02612 Concussion—impact _____
    02613 Electrical shock _____
    02614 Foreign body—eye _____
    02615 Hearing _____
    02616 Cardiac _____
    02617 Systemic poisoning _____
    02618 Multiple Injuries _____
    02619 Other (Specify)_____

027 Vehicle Accident _____

028 Time Lost. ( ) Days _____ No Time Lost ( )

029 Witnesses _____
              Names   Address   Telephone No.

030 First-aid Rendered by _____

031 Attending Physician _____

032 Treatment Center _____

033 Narrative Description of Accident _____

034 What took place? _____

035 Why did accident happen? _____

036 What should be done to prevent recurrence? _____

_____

_____

REPORT IDENTIFICATION

1. Region	2. Area	3. OSHA-1 Identification			4. Fatality/Catastrophe Event Report Number	5. Date of Inspection
		CSHO Nbr	Report Nbr	Fiscal Year		Mo Day Yr

INVESTIGATION FINDINGS

7. Fatality/Catastrophe Event Category	8. Exact Location of Event Site	9. Exact Location of Event at Site	10. Employer Contact

Number Casualties 11. Fatalities	12. Hospitalized Injuries	13. Non-Hospitalized Injuries	14. Estimated Cost of Process Interruption	15. Estimated Cost of Property Destroyed or Damaged	16. Weather at time of event

17a. Name of Injured/Deceased

| BADGE NBR | SEX (M OR F) | AGE | DISP. CODE | NATURE OF INJURY | PART OF BODY |
| SOURCE OF INJURY | EVENT TYPE | CONT. ENVIR. FACTOR | CONT. HUMAN FACTOR | TASK ASSN. | HAZ SUB |

17b. Name of Injured/Deceased

| BADGE NBR | SEX (M OR F) | AGE | DISP. CODE | NATURE OF INJURY | PART OF BODY |
| SOURCE OF INJURY | EVENT TYPE | CONT. ENVIR. FACTOR | CONT. HUMAN FACTOR | TASK ASSN. | HAZ SUB |

17c. Name of Injured/Deceased

| BADGE NBR | SEX (M OR F) | AGE | DISP. CODE | NATURE OF INJURY | PART OF BODY |
| SOURCE OF INJURY | EVENT TYPE | CONT. ENVIR. FACTOR | CONT. HUMAN FACTOR | TASK ASSN. | HAZ SUB |

17d. Name of Injured/Deceased

| BADGE NBR | SEX (M OR F) | AGE | DISP. CODE | NATURE OF INJURY | PART OF BODY |
| SOURCE OF INJURY | EVENT TYPE | CONT. ENVIR. FACTOR | CONT. HUMAN FACTOR | TASK ASSN. | HAZ SUB |

17e. Name of Injured/Deceased

| BADGE NBR | SEX (M OR F) | AGE | DISP. CODE | NATURE OF INJURY | PART OF BODY |
| SOURCE OF INJURY | EVENT TYPE | CONT. ENVIR. FACTOR | CONT. HUMAN FACTOR | TASK ASSN. | HAZ SUB |

18. Equipment, Machines, Materials Involved (be specific about names, size, serial numbers, locations, etc.)

19. Operations Being Performed (include who, what, and where)

20. Describe the Details of the Occurrence of Event (what happened and why)

21. Witness(es) [Eyewitness(es) then Witness(es) to Preceding Circumstances] . List and Attach Statements.

22. Did violation of a standard cause or contribute to occurrence of event? (If yes, list standard(s) cited)
☐ Yes   ☐ No

23. Do you recommend a new or revised standard? (If yes, attach OSHA-9)
☐ Yes   ☐ No

GPO 539-737

1. AREA OFFICE

Signature of CSHO

Form OSHA-4
Rev. July 1973

Figure 97.

It must be remembered that the purpose of accident investigation is to determine facts associated with human situations that can be used by management in the decision-making process, to prevent recurrence of similar accidents. If this purpose is to be realized, complete accident information must be obtained and supplied to management.

The purpose of the investigation report is to convey in concise language the results of the investigation (the facts surrounding the occurrence, the analysis of these facts, and the conclusions). The investigation report constitutes a record of the occurrence by which the investigation is measured as to thoroughness, accuracy, and objectivity, and to which reference may be made at a later data. In addition, any corrective actions directed by the appointing or the reviewing official will be based largely on the contents of the report. The following information would be considered the minimum to be recorded on any accident report.

1. Identification of the persons involved: name, number, shift, age, previous work experience, previous accident record.
2. Time of the accident: hour, day, month, year.
3. Place of the accident: department, specific location in the department. Specific attention should be given here to determine if the injured may have been working at a task not normally associated with his normal work activities.
4. Identification (name and addresses) of all witnesses to the accident. Names of Foremen and Supervisors. Nature and severity of the injury, name of the attending doctor, and record of treatments.
5. Description and cost of property damage or spoilage.
6. An exact description of the accident. Among the items which can be relevant are the following:
   a. A full description of the accident, stating for example, whether the person fell or was struck, and all the factors contributing to the accident.
   b. Identification of the machine, tool, appliance, gas, liguid, or other object which was most closely associated with the accident.
   c. If a machine or vehicle was involved, identification of the specific part which was involved; for instance, the gears, pulley, or motor.
   d. A judgment about the way in which the machine tool, object, or substance was unsafe.
   e. Description of mechanical guards or other safeguards (for example, safety goggles) which were provided.
   f. Statement about whether the injured person or persons used the safeguards which were provided.

g.   Description of the unsafe action of the injured person which resulted in the accident (for example, lifted weight with bent back, removed safety screen from pulley, did not wear goggles, ran down stairs)

h.   The investigator's witnesses', or victim's best guess as to why the person acted unsafely. This is one of the most sensitive areas on an accident report, as it forces the investigator and/or supervisor to make an accusation which could lead to embarrassment, perhaps problems in employer/employee relations. While proofs of human error are very desirable, and many times critical to the investigative process, such determination and subsequent listings on a permanent report must be handled very carefully.

7.   The investigator's witnesses', or victim's opinion about ways of preventing further accidents of this type. (Examples: provide better illumination, provide safety goggles, provide better guards, etc.) are most valuable.

The investigation report shall consist of, but not be limited to, four sections: summary, facts, analysis, and conclusions.

The summary is a brief account of the essential fact of the occurrence, and the investigator's conclusions. The facts section consists of a recitation of the factual information determined in the course of the investigation. It should relate the "who, what, where, and when," of the occurrence. The analysis section of the report is based on the factual information developed and consists of the reasoning of the investigators to support their conclusions. The conclusions section consists of the findings, the probable causes of and contributing factors to the occurrence, and the judgments of deficiencies.

The investigation report shall fully cover and explain the technical elements of the causal sequences of the occurrence and shall also describe the management systems which should have, or could have, prevented the occurrence, e.g., the hazard review system and the quality assurance program from safety, including the monitoring of actual operations.

The investigator(s)' recommendations for corrective actions to prevent a similar occurrence shall not be contained in the report but shall be included in the cover memorandum that transmits the investigation report to the appointing official.

The Investigation Report—Anatomy

1. *Cover.* The cover and title page shall state the subject and date of occurrence, the date of the report, and the security classification. The cover and title page shall not include distribution lists, internal organization nomen-

clature, name or organization participating or preparing the report, or other such information.

2. *Table of Contents.* The table of contents shall identify the sections and subsections of the report, illustrations, charts, and appendixes with their report page number designated.

3. *Scope of Investigation.* This statement shall set forth the issues or objectives to be investigated and any special limitations or instructions to the board.

4. *Summary.* This section shall be written in such a manner that the reader, who may be relatively unfamiliar with the subject matter, can obtain the essential facts, the findings and the probable causes and contributing factors with a minimum of effort and time. The summary shall not contain information that is not discussed elsewhere in the report.

5. *Facts.* This section of the report shall cover the major areas of investigation in a uniform manner and in a reasonable, logical sequence.

    a.   Make this section factual. Do not include any conclusions in this section.

    b.   Give the reader a good account of the accident.

    c.   Stress those areas of the accident investigation bearing on the causal considerations.

    d.   Establish a complete and substantive basis for the analysis and conclusions sections of the report. This assures both accuracy and completeness. It also eliminates the tendency to introduce new facts in the analysis and conclusions sections.

    e.   Stress the areas which form the basis for corrective measures.

    f.   Inform the reader, where appropriate, that additional information on a subject is contained elsewhere in the report. Use a footnote or note of reference naming the section or appendix where such material can be found.

    g.   Do not omit any relevant fact for any reason whatever, i.e., that it might conflict with some preconceived notion of the investigator or interfere with the dissemination of information (bulletins, news releases, etc.). Investigators must, at all times, be critical of their own reasoning, to assure a completely objective and independent account of the occurrence. Examples of information to include are:

        (1)   Pertinent background information, where available, i.e., brief description of facilities, climate, history, etc.

        (2)   Description of injury, exposure, or loss due to occurrences, as well as the property damage or decontamination costs.

        (3)   Physical evidence.

        (4)   Chronological account of events.

        (5)   Physical hazards and review of safety controls.

        (6)   Technical data accumulated.

(7) Related events not in the causal sequence, but revealing deficiencies (to be placed at the end of the section).

6. *The Analysis*

a. This section of the report is intended to present an analysis of the factual material contained in the investigation. Its purpose is to show the reader the interpretation of the facts, conditions, circumstances, and inferences which support the findings, probable causes, and judgments of needs. This section should include a discussion of the causal sequences, and due consideration should be given to charting the relationship of events and causal factors. Speculated events, facts in controversy, denial of allegations, and what could not be determined, should also be discussed in the analysis section.

b. Do not put additional facts in this section. This section is for analysis of the facts.

c. Make the analysis lead up to the findings, probable causes, and judgments of needs. The qualified reader should be able to anticipate the causal factors from the analysis.

d. Make the analysis "accident prevention-oriented" not blame-oriented.

7. *Conclusions*

a. *Findings.* This subsection consists of the significant facts and the analytical conclusions of the investigators.
   (1) Organize findings sequentially, preferably in chronological order or in logical sets of sequences, e.g., hardware, procedures, people, organization.
   (2) State analytical conclusions that are clearly supported by the facts and analysis.
   (3) Keep findings to a minimum. They are a recap of the significant facts and the analytical highlights, a reiteration of the entire sequence of events.
   (4) Keep findings brief, and, as far as possible, put only one highlight in each findings.

b. *Probable causes.* The statement of probable causes shall consist of a series of relatively simple statements which summarize the causes and contributing factors.

c. *Judgments of needs.* This section consists of the investigators' conclusions as to the kinds of managerial controls and safety measures necessary and sufficient to prevent or minimize the probability or severity of a recurrence. These judgments provide the basis for the subsequent recommendations for corrective action. These statements should be clear, concise, direct, and should be based on the weight of the substantive evidence.

8. *Appendix*—Material that is pertinent but need not be made a part of the written report in order to understand or use the report shall be included as exhibits to the report and shall follow the body of the report. These may include written statements, witnesses' remarks, letters, laboratory analyses, memoranda, pictures, death certificates, etc. Medical records and legal opinions shall not be included in the report.

Only material that a reader may want to evaluate, or material that is in controversay should be included in the appendix. All such material should be identified with the same label, e.g., "Exhibit _____," or "Appendix _____." Where more than one such item is used, they shall be numbered in sequence as introduced in the report, i.e., "Exhibit A," "Exhibit B," etc. Every exhibit shall be introduced in the report in appropriate sequence and, at the time introduced, a brief recitation of its contents shall be made. Long, detailed, complex exhibits shall be avoided.

Recommendations

The natural follow-up to the judgments of needs is the recommendations. He who prepares the accident report shall arrive at recommendations intended to prevent similar occurrences. The utmost care should be exerted in forming the recommendations, so that all are clear-cut, feasible, logical, and applicable in the field for which they are intended. These recommendations shall be transmitted to the appointing official in the cover memorandum for the investigation report.

Figures in the Text

Text figures can be a powerful, easy to use aid in reading and understanding.

Maps, schematics, and flow diagrams should be simplified and devoid of unneeded detail. Photographs should have a caption, and also carry labels, measurements or other marks to aid in their interpretation.

In general, the figures can be expected to follow an order similar to the following:

1. General map or aerial photograph.
2. Area of occurrence (use of map or photographs to show location of injured personnel, property damage, witnesses, and equipment).
3. Process flow.
4. The equipment involved (if damages, show; then show a normal counterpart if available).
5. What the operator saw.
6. Closeup photographs or drawings, such as cutaways.
7. Debris (if needed to record magnitude or evidence).
8. Amelioration (fire, rescue, etc.).

All of these are included, if significant. Simple text tables of numbers, if needed to understand findings, can be included; otherwise put over in exhibits.

Exhibits in the Appendixes

1. Exhibits should be relevant, simple, and short. The following are examples of exhibits that should be in the report.
    a. Details needed to assess the accuracy of findings, where such assessment is likely.
        (1) Test methods and results, e.g., in concrete sample test, the results could be relegated to an exhibit.
        (2) Procedures or excerpts to show gaps or deficiencies.
        (3) Written statements.
        (4) Additional maps, schematic, or pictures, if needed.
        (5) Death certificates—(public documents).
    b. Details to help the uninformed understand the report; for example, characteristics of chemicals or explanations of flow or process schematics.
    c. Witness statements. Do not use filler, i.e., witnesses who had few or no observations not covered by the principal witnesses.
    d. "Events and Causal Factors" chart, if it is not included in the analysis section of the report.
    e. Brief description of investigative methods, so silence is not construed as in action; for example, the scene was (was not) secured; the scene was visited and when.
    f. List of participants by name, title, and organization. This is suggested even if names were used in text. Further, the list should show supervision of all relevant units, or an organization chart should be used.
    g. Personal histories, but only matter relevant and nonconfidential and needed to substantiate a finding or conclusion.
    h. Samples of news clippings may help assess public impact.
    i. When classified material is used, include it in a separate classified exhibit if possible.
2. *Do not include in the Report:*
    a. Medical records, even if released. Medical records are exempt from disclosure under the Freedom of Information Act. Let the physician's medical evaluation of event-related matters (either in text or exhibit be self-sufficient.)
    b. Legal opinions consisting of an informed estimate of amounts, probability and validity of possible claims and, where available, information to refute or mitigate the claims of questionable validity.

This information should be prepared by the legal office and transmitted through appropriate channels.

Classifying Accident Report Data

Although accident report forms constitute a critical element in the accident investigation process, they must not be construed as being the last step in the information collection process. Actually, the report form is only the vehicle by which important accident data is transported. Ultimately, the data on each accident report form must be recorded and classified in such a manner that important relationships may be drawn and decisions made, relative to accident reduction.

To aid the accident analyst in his codification and classification activities, ANSI Z16.2, "Methods of Recording Basic Facts Relating to Nature and Occurrence of Work Injuries"—A Standard—has been developed and may be used to identify certain key facts about each injury and the accident that produced it.

Among the key facts about the injury and the accident that produced it which lend themselves to summarization and which tend to indicate general patterns of injury and accident occurrence are the following:

1. Nature of Injury—the type of physical injury incurred.
2. Part of the body—the part of the injured person's body directly affected by the injury.
3. Source of injury—the object, substance, exposure, or bodily motion which directly produced or inflicted the injury.
4. Accident type—the event which directly resulted in the injury
5. Hazardous condition—the physical condition or circumstance which permitted or occasioned the occurrence of the accident type.
6. Agency of accident—the object, substance or part of the premises in which the hazardous condition existed.
7. Agency of accident part—the specific part of the agency of accident that was hazardous.
8. Unsafe act—the violation of a commonly accepted safe procedure which directly permitted or occasioned the occurrence of the accident event.

Supplementary items of information closely related to the key facts, such as age, sex, occupation, and type of work being performed at the time the injury was incurred, are recorded and included in an analysis so that all the facts will be available for taking the proper preventive steps. Contributory factors should be indicated.

The principal source of information for an analysis is the accident report. Complete data regarding all the key facts should be fully and accurately recorded on this form at the time of the accident.

Injury and accident reports, however, commonly consist of a few specific statements relating to the injury plus a narrative account of how and why the accident occurred. The reports vary widely in the amount of detail given and in the clarity and coherence with which the facts are presented. Therefore, the analyst rarely will find the key facts—the items needed for statistical recording—precisely stated. Usually, he must review all the data given in the report, select pertinent items, and fit them into a predetermined recording pattern.

Identifying the Key Facts

Since the reliability of an analysis depends greatly on selection of the correct key facts, the analyst must have a clear understanding of the key facts and of the method for identifying them. The basis on which identification should be made is described and illustrated in the following paragraphs adapted from ANSI Z16.2.

Nature of Injury. The type of physical injury incurred should be designated. If two or more injuries were incurred and one injury obviously was more severe than any of the others, that injury should be selected. For example, an injury involving permanent impairment should be selected in preference to a temporary injury. If there were several injuries of difference natures, such as cuts and sprains, and no one of them was more serious than the others, the term "multiple injuries" should be used.

Part of body. If the injury was localized in one part of the body, that part should be named. If the injury extended to several sections of a major body part, those sections should be named. For example, if a burn affected the fingers, the hand, the wrist, and the forearm, upper extremities multiple should be given as the body part affected. If the injury was internal, the body system should be named. For example, drowning or asphxia would be considered injuries to the respiratory system.

Source of injury. The object, substance, exposure, or bodily motion which directly produced the injury should be identified as the source of injury. In such cases, the source of injury should be determined as follows. When the choice is between two moving objects or between two stationary objects, the one contacted last should be determined as follows. When the choice is between a moving object and a stationary object, the moving object should be selected. When the choice is between two moving objects or between two stationary objects, the contacted last should be selected. For example, if a person fell from an elevation, struck one or more objects in the course of the fall and finally struck the floor, the floor should be named as the source of injury.

If the injury resulted solely from the stress of strain induced by a free movement of the body or its parts for example, in reaching, twisting, or bending, bodily motion should be indicated as the source of injury.

Accident type. The accident type classification is directly related to the source of injury classification and explains how that source produced the injury. If the injury resulted from contact with an object or substance, the action that best describes that contact should be named as the accident type. If exposure, for instance, to extreme heat or cold, produced the injury, contact with temperature extremes would be the accident type. If the source of injury was bodily motion, the personal action or movements during which the bodily motion occurred should be chosen as the accident type.

Hazardous condition. The hazardous physical condition or circumstance which directly caused or permitted the occurrence of the accident should be named. The hazardous condition is related directly to both the accident type and the agency of accident. Generally, therefore, the hazardous condition selected will determine the agency of accident to be named. Since the hazardous condition classification represents the physical or environmental causes of accidents, tabulations of the data in this category properly may be labeled "accident causes."

Bibliography

"Accident/Incident Investigation Manual," U.S. Energy Research and Development Administration, August, 1975.

American National Standards Institute—ANSI 216.2, Methods of Recording Basic Facts Relating to the Nature and Occurrence of Work Injuries.

Baker, Susan P., "Injury Control," Accident Prevention and Other Approaches to Reduction of Injury, Insurance Institute of Highway Safety, 1972.

Chapanis, Alphonse, "Research Techniques in Human Engineering," John Hopkins Press, 1963.

Fine, William T., "A Managment Approach in Accident Prevention," Naval Surface Weapons Center, White Oak Laboratory, 1976.

National Safety Council, "Accident Prevention Manual for Industrial Operations" 7th Edition, 1974.

Wahl, J. E., "Compiling and Comparing Accident Records," National Safety News, December, 1975.

Weintraub, D. J., and Walker, E. L., "Perception" Brooks/Cole Publishing Co., Belmont, California, 1969.

Notes

1. D. Haasl, (From a seminar on Systems Safety) University of Washington, Seattle, Wa., August, 1969.
2. D. J. Dewey, "How We Think." Boston, D. C. Heath & Co., 1910.
3. Susan P. Baker, "Injury Control—Accident Prevention and Other Approaches to Reduction of Injury," Ins. Inst. for Highway Safety, Washington D.C. 20037.
4. D. J. Weintraub, and E. L. Walker, "Perception" Brooks/Cole Publishing Co., Belmont, California, 1969.
5. R. D. Baker, "Communications in Hazard Control," RJF Associates, Inc., 1977.

Monitoring the Workplace for Hazards 9

In Chapter 4, during the discussion of the essential elements of the hazard control process, the role of the monitoring function, an integral part of a viable hazard control system, was discussed. In this Chapter we will continue this discussion, intent on providing the reader with an overall grasp of what this activity is supposed to accomplish, how to make it part of the responsibilities of other members of the organization, and how to use inspection data for informed hazard control decisions.

"Inspection," as discussed in this Chapter is defined as *"That monitoring function conducted in an organization to locate and report hazards emanating from, or existing among components of the workplace that have the capacity to cause accidents."*

Inspection and preventive medicine have something in common. They are concerned with detecting conditions which are known to produce problem situations. The doctor, with his sophisticated equipment, endeavors to prevent the occurrence of disease; the hazard control inspector, equipped with a host of standards and measuring instruments attempts to detect situational, human, and environmental factors that have the potential to cause accidents.

Unlike the doctor, the hazard control inspector's concentration is not limited to the human organism. Instead, he must focus his efforts on physical, mechanical, chemical, and biological elements in the workplace and the interaction between workers, their machines, and the work environment in order to perform a satisfactory job of locating problems and effects of importance.

There are three main motives behind monitoring or inspection activities. First, to provide assurance that controls are functioning as specified. Secondly, to insure that workplace alterations have not nullified the effectiveness of the

The Monitoring Process—An Overview

controls provided. Third, to see that new problems have not entered the workplace, since the last time it was evaluated, and corrections were made.

Those people in the organization who are designated as participants in the monitoring process may be perceived as important "eyes and ears" of the overall hazard control program. These organizational members, are able on a continuous basis, to sense, acquire, and report important information for decision-making purposes. Consequently, if the organization depends so heavily on inspection inputs, then it must make sure that those performing the inspection function receive proper training and education. In addition, and wherever possible, those performing the monitoring function should understand how hazards were ranked according to their importance, as well as the capabilities and limitation of the controls selected to counter the hazard's effects.

Philosophy of Inspection

The philosophy behind the inspection process can be considered from two viewpoints: (1) fault-finding with a view toward criticism; or (2) locating failures that have a profound effect on the operation, in terms of safety, reliability, maintainability, etc.

The second viewpoint is obviously the more desirable. But to be effective, this viewpoint depends—if desired levels of performance are to be reached—upon the following: (1) adequate yardsticks to be applied to a particular situation; (2) comparison made between what is and what ought to be; (3) corrective steps taken to achieve desired performance.

Safety and health standards provide some of these yardsticks.

Unfortunately, because of the nature of workplace operations, even close examination, using the standards as a guide, will not always locate all the problems and conditions responsible for industrial accidents. This is not entirely the fault of the standards. Often, those using them make mistakes.

Mistakes are made mainly because: the standard is not interpreted correctly; the standard is used to evaluate something it was not designed for; those using the standard is not familiar with those interactions in the particular industrial process which can produce accidents; and/or hazards not spelled out in the standard are often overlooked.

Setting Objectives

An inspection program implies the regular systematic and continuing comparison of safety and health standards and other criteria to discrepancies in the industrial environment. The program usually starts by concentrating on those operations of high hazard potential, and it is later extended to other conditions within the plant.

A safety inspection program requires: an understanding of the systematic inspection steps; and a method of reporting, evaluating, and using the data gathered.

When setting objectives for carrying out the inspection function, the following points should be kept in mind: (1) Materials and substances used in operations should be viewed in respect to their capacity to create an injury, occupational illness, fire, or explosion hazard. (2) Machines, materials handling equipment, tools, etc., used during operations should be free from defects and other hazards that could cause injury, death, or property damage. (3) Personal protective and safety equipment must exist, where there is a reasonable probability that any injury can be prevented by such protection, and these devices must be operational. (4) Walking and working surfaces (stairs, ladders, scaffolds, ramps, etc.) must be adequately designed according to standards, and they must be properly maintained. (5) Within the workplace, ventilating, production, fire protection, electrical, heating and cooling equipment, boilers, etc., must be properly installed, used within design limits, and maintained in safe condition. (6) Attention should be given to sanitation, housekeeping, waste disposal, food handling, material storage, etc. (7) Work methods must conform to approved methods and safe practices. (8) Medical services, first aid facilities, and emergency personal protective devices must be available and of adequate quality.

Inspection programs need management's support. In this respect, management should: state the purpose for the inspection program and the goal to which the inspection teams will direct its efforts. The goal, in addition to being concerned with reducing the hazards as listed in OSHA regulations, might also be concerned with cost reduction, reduction of scrap and rework, repair time, elimination of bottlenecks, and other interruptions. In other words, inspection has the triple goal of eliminating hazards responsible for injuries and increasing plant efficiency and effectiveness; conducting a training program to acquaint all production personnel and members of management who will assist in the inspection process with the purposes and techniques of inspection and with safety and health standards; setting up one or more "monitoring teams," with the hazard control specialist as the coordinator, the optimum mix consisting of a production manager, a supervisor, an employee representative, a fire prevention specialist, and an industrial hygienist to perform certain inspectional functions.

Management's Impact

For the most part, inspections can be classified as either one of two types, planned or continuous.

Types of Inspections

Planned Hazard Control Inspections

The planned inspection is what most people think of when they hear the term safety inspection. A planned inspection is deliberate, thorough, and systematic by design.

Planned, inspections range from the daily check of safety equipment or devices by workers as part of a job procedure, to inspection conducted by the hazard control specialist. In many cases, an established procedure or checklist is used in conducting a planned inspection, as specific items or conditions are being looked for and the checklist is a tool that aids in thoroughness.

A disadvantage of planned inspection is that most often it is aimed at, and able to detect, only unsafe conditions. Workers are usually aware of the presence of inspectors, and unsafe acts or practices are rarely discovered under these circumstances.

Continuous Hazard Control Inspections

Continuous inspection is conducted by workers and supervisors alike, incidental to their job, and a part of their job responsibilities. The continuous inspection occurs when a worker notes and reports an unsafe condition or unsafe act, and someone in management then takes corrective action. Likewise, the supervisor must be continuously on the alert for unsafe conditions and unsafe acts and see to their corrections or report them to the individual responsible for correction.

Opponents to continuous inspection say that it usually misses things that require extra effort to note; that it does not get into the out-of-the-way places; that it tends to superficial and erratic; and that when people become engrossed with their work or problems, no "safety" inspection is conducted at all.

It is known that continuous inspection is not fool proof, and that it does not uncover all unsafe conditions and unsafe acts, but neither does planned inspection. The truth is—both are necessary and, if all concerned are made aware of and accept their roles and responsibilities relating to safety inspection, most unsafe acts and unsafe conditions can be detected and eliminated prior to their causing accidents

Preparation for Hazard Control Inspections

If inspections are to be conducted according to a systematic process, it is necessary to plan and prepare for the inspections beforehand. It is necessary to determine what areas are to be inspected, what is to be inspected in each area, at what frequency the inspections can be conducted, what conditions are to be inspected for, and who should inspect.

The best method, of determining what various factors will affect the inspection, is to conduct an inspection inventory.

Hazard Control Inspection Inventory

A hazard control inspection inventory is the result of a thorough analysis of the various factors and problems associated with conducting the actual inspection of an area. It is the foundation upon which a program of planned inspection is based and can be compared to and in fact related to a planned preventive maintenance system, and can be expected to yield many of the same benefits.

Defining Inspection Areas

The entire facility should be divided into areas of: responsibility, including yards; building; equipment and machinery; vehicles; and others, as is fitting.

Once the areas of responsibility have been determined, they should be listed in an orderly fashion, and possibly a color-coded map of the facility or floor plan developed. In large areas or departments it may be desirable to further subdivide each area or department into the specific area of responsibility for each first line supervisor and/or the hazard control department's inspector.

Determine What to Inspect

Once specific areas of responsibility have been determined, it will be necessary to determine what specific items within each area require inspection, such as: tools; machines supplies; systems, e.g., ventilation, sprinkler, etc.; equipment—e.g., safety, fire protection, etc.; specific operations; etc.

The list of specific items should preferably be developed by the hazard control specialist for each area and verified with the department head, to assure that it is complete and accurate. Perhaps, it may be more beneficial to subdivide the list into specific items to be inspected to facilitate the overall process. Such specific items may be: parts subject to rapid deterioration; machine guards; safety controls; safety devices, e.g., safety valves, etc.; and system parts, e.g., sprinkler control valves, exhaust system filers, etc.

The items requiring separate inspection can be determined from many sources such as: operating experience; instruction manuals; accident reports; maintenance records; and specific standards and codes, e.g., vehicle, elevator, boiler and pressure vessel, crane, fire extinguishers, etc.

Determine what Conditions to Inspect for

After having determined what areas and items are to be inspected, it is necessary to determine what conditions to inspect for. Many times, the inspector will have a general knowledge of adverse conditions that will affect the safety of a particular item, but guidelines should be developed to remind and assist him. The conditions requiring inspection can be determined from the same sources listed under "Determining What to Inspect," and can be used to develop forms, checklists, or other inspection aids.

Determine Inspection Frequency

As previously described, an inspection program can be compared to a preventive maintenance system. The frequency of performing inspections of specific items, pieces of equipment, areas, etc., will vary just as the frequency of performing preventive maintenance on a specific piece of equipment, and the frequency will be determined by many of the same factors, such as: potential severity; potential cost; potential delay; history of past failures; manufacturer's recommendations; or specific standards and code requirements.

The frequency of inspections can vary from hourly to annually. Most workers, supervisors, and managers consider hourly, once a shift, or daily inspections of equipment, machinery, log keeping, etc., as a required part of proper operation and protection of the equipment, itself. While this is many times true, inspection is also required for the safety and protection of personnel and other equipment in the area. Inspections that are made less frequently—e.g., monthly, quarterly, semi-annually, etc.—are often taken less seriously and at times overlooked, yet they are often more important. The required frequency of inspections must be determined as indicated above, and followed if the program is to be successful in accomplishing its objectives.

Determine Who Should Inspect

In many cases, the individual who should complete the inspection will be the one most familiar with the items of concern. In the case of continuous inspection and planned inspections to be conducted at frequent intervals, this is especially true.

Inspections of a specific nature or concerning specific equipment should be conducted by qualified individuals from within the organization, whenever possible. At times, it may be required that licensed inspectors complete routine inspections of certain equipment, e.g., cranes, elevators, boilers, pressure vessels, etc. When such inspections are necessary, arrangements must be made with the authority having jurisdiction.

Inspections of a general nature that are to be conducted on a planned basis should be conducted by various personnel within the organization. A suggested guide for general safety inspections is as follows: daily—area supervisor; weekly—department head; monthly—a committee or group consisting of worker, supervisor and department head, and specialists, as required. The hazard control department may also be actively involved in monthly, quarterly, semi-annual and annual inspections.

At this point, it should be noted that higher management officials should make planned inspections of the facility periodically, to indicate and emphasize their interest in the overall hazard control effort. It is recommended that such inspections can be conducted at least quarterly.

Using Data Acquired During Inspection

What is done with the information derived from an inspection program is as important as the inspection process itself. It is to be hoped that the inspection team will bring faults to management's attention, accompanied by recommendations for corrective action.

Fault-finding, in itself, does nothing significantly to alter existing inadequacies within the organization. The information provided by the inspection team should, in one way or another, pinpoint a weakness in the management control system. The theory behind this statement is that the discrepancies uncovered during the inspection didn't just "fall out of the sky." Instead, they were the results of factors or combination of factors (situational, human, environmental) that were allowed in the workplace.

For instance, if the purchasing department ordered equipment for the plant from a supplier without having the necessary safety devices installed, it contributed to the accident problem by bringing additional hazards into the plant. The same holds true for the maintenance department which, by ineffective repair work, by poor maintenance, by makeshift repairs, etc., also contributes to the overall problem. Other members of the management team (e.g., production control, process engineering, personnel, etc.) may be at fault in causing inconsistencies that inadvertently create potential accident situations.

In order for the inspection team to do its job properly, it should concentrate on providing inputs into the operations of each of the management systems involved, making certain that the information is credible and accurate.

Some of the more general recommendations that might be made by inspection teams are to:

- Set up a better process. The data from inspections may be used as inputs for Process Engineering to modify existing processes or to construct new ones.
- Suggest that the present process be relocated in such a way as to make it less hazardous, while at the same time providing better results. For instance, the hazard may emanate from a fault in the operational sequence, routing methods, etc.
- Suggest redesign of a tool or fixture, or a change in the operator's work pattern that may reduce the hazard potential and be of significant value to the production control department.
- Recommend methods of cost reduction and increased plant efficiency.
- Suggest more adequate training of personnel engaged in a particular operation. This information would be used advantageously in modifying existing training methods.

Based on the problems uncovered and recommendations made by the inspection team, management must decide what course of action it will take.

Usually these actions will be based on the cost-effectiveness of the recommendations. As an example, it may be more feasible and practical, from a cost standpoint, for a plant manager to substitute a highly toxic material with one that will work just as effectively and be less toxic. On the other hand, a particular hazardous machine may be too costly to replace. In this case, the less expensive approach of installing a guarding device might correct the problem.

Information from inspections should never be used for punitive action. It must be viewed as an additional input into the overall control process—one that will reduce accident-injury experience, improve maintainability in the plant, and increase overall productivity.

Inspection Scheduling

The hazard control specialist will have to develop a schedule for inspection, in addition to drawing up checklists. The object of inspection scheduling is to inspect often enough so that the establishment is hazard-controlled at all times. The schedule should state when each item should be inspected, and in what degree of detail. Safety and health inspections should be an integral part of the supervisor's regular production, and quality inspections and tests and should be scheduled to coincide with the other inspections of facilities where possible. Other factors also influence scheduling. Equipment such as two-hand controls, machine guards, fire extinguishers, and activities or work practices which must be constantly relied on for safety and health require frequent and thorough inspection.

New equipment should be inspected thoroughly before use. During the shakedown period, new equipment merits more frequent attention than older, dependable machinery. Once a new machine is found to be dependable, the inspection schedule may be changed. Machines and equipment with poor safety and health or reliability records, rate frequent inspection. Accident records are a guide to those items. Such records also can point out the processes and equipment that are costly and damaging to production, because of their repeated failure. The amount of time a machine is in use also influences scheduling. For example, a machine operating 24 hours a day will likely merit more frequent inspection than one in use only 4 hours a day.

The degree of detail required also affects the frequency of inspection. For example, the line supervisor could be expected to inspect all his machinery on a daily basis to see that machine and equipment guards and machine adjustment tools are in place, personal protective equipment is used, and employees are working according to acceptable hazard control practices. On a weekly basis, the line supervisor would inspect such items as the security of safety guard mountings, functioning of retractable guards, condition or adjustment and other tools, and the need for lubrication or servicing. On a monthly or less frequent basis, he would cover still other items. He would inspect holding-down bolts, see that travel-stop on moving machines are securely bolted in place, and test the operation of limit switches and all other safety devices which do not need more frequent attention. Thus, a general check of vital safety and health features should be made continuously, and more detailed inspections regularly, on a weekly, monthly or other basis, as needed.

The main question to ask in deciding how often to inspect an item is, "How fast can something to wrong with it?" The answer depends on the nature of the device or condition, its history of reliability, and the supervisor's experience with it. However, equipment whose constant functioning is necessary to life and limb should be checked daily, regardless of its past reliability.

Inspection Checklists

Many different types of checklists are available and in use today, which vary in form and length from thousands of items to only a few. Each type has its place and can be of benefit to all kinds of operations and organizations, if properly applied. Generally, the longer form of checklist is known as a General Industry Inspection Checklist, which usually references numerous OSHA Standards and can be used to complete an initial survey of an organization, to determine which standards apply to a particular operation and to check for compliance with standards. The General checklist is a very valuable tool in conducting initial or annual inspections of an organization, but should not be used as, for example, a monthly inspection checklist form.

The best form of checklist, however, is one that has been developed by an individual organization to suit its own needs. The development of individualized checklists should not be a difficult task if the inspection inventory, as previously described, has been completed.

A good checklist clarifies inspection responsibilities, provides a basis for reporting inspection activities and findings, and controls inspection activities.

Regardless of how complete the inspection checklist is, the results of the inspection will be no better than the individual performing the inspection. Inspectors must be realistic and use common sense—a hazard observed during an inspection must be commented on and reported, even though not required by the checklist, if the inspection is to be complete. The inspection checklist must be used to augment continuous safety inspections, and not relied on to cover all possible conditions and situations.

A checklist which is of exceptional value for making thorough safety and health inspections is that published by the National Safety Council under the title "Self-Evaluation Checklists." Figure 98.

The self-evaluation checklists, when properly utilized, will aid the inspector in revealing apparent violations of the OSHA Standards. They will also reveal conditions which may not be already known.

SUBPART P SEC. 1910.243 TITLE		GUARDING OF PORTABLE POWERED TOOLS

AREA INSPECTED

INSPECTED BY		DATE

REQUIREMENT	EVAL	COMMENT

(A) PORTABLE POWERED WOODWORKING TOOLS
 	
(1) **Portable Circular Saws (blade diameter greater than 2 in.)**
 	
   (i)   Are portable circular saws equipped with guards above and below the base plate?
 	
       ✓ Does the upper guard cover the saw to the depth of the teeth, except for minimum arc needed to tilt base for bevel cuts?
 	
       ✓ Does the lower guard cover the saw to the depth of the teeth, except for minimum arc required for proper "backing up," and contact with the work?
 	
       ✓ When the saw is withdrawn, does the lower guard automatically and instantly return to covering position?
 	
   (ii) The above subdivision does not apply to circular saws used in the meat industry for meat-cutting purposes. [38 F.R. 14373 (June 1, 1973)]
 	
               ***
 	
Note. The following two questions recommended by NSC are not specifically spelled out in OSHA Standards.
 	
And are the guard pivots lubricated?
 	
Is the trigger switch free from binding or sticking?
 	
(more)		

These checklists present OSHA standards in such a manner as to enable employers to determine apparent compliance with them. Notes have been inserted to explain, illustrate or amplify the regulations.	EVALUATION KEY	YES—Apparently meets requirement NO—Apparently does not meet requirement NA—Not applicable U—Undetermined If NO, specify location, equipment, facility, other details under COMMENT

© 1972 National Safety Council   Stock No. 115.27-0243   Rev., July 31, 1973

Figure 98. (Reproduced with permission of the National Safety Council.)

The 15 subparts of 29 CFR part 1910 and 21 subparts of CFR part 1926, form the organization of the OSHA regulations and each subpart covers a special subject. The subparts address the topics of:

Part 1910	*Part 1926*
Walking and working surfaces	General safety and health provisions
Means of egress	Occupational health and environmental controls
Platforms and manlifts	
Health and environment	Personal protective and life saving equipment
Hazardous materials	Fire protection and prevention
Personal protective equipment	Signs, signals and barricades
General environment	Materials handling, storage, use, and disposal
Medical and First aid	
Fire protection	Tools—Hand and power
Compressed gas and air	Welding and cutting
Materials handling and storage	Electrical
Machinery and machine guarding	Ladders and scaffolds
Hand and portable power tools	Floor and wall openings and stairways
Welding and cutting and brazing	Cranes, derricks, hoists, elevators, and conveyors
Electrical	Motor vehicles, mechanized equipment and marine operations
Special industries	Excavations, trenching, and shoring
	Concrete, concrete forms, and sharing
	Steel erection
	Tunnels and shafts, caissons, cofferdams, and compressed air
	Demolition
	Blasting and use of explosives
	Power transmission and distribution
	Rollover protective structures; overhead protection.

The Hazard Control audit checklists which appears on page 356 is an example of a format designed to facilitate the inspection process on construction job sites.

Hazard Analysis Data—An Inspection Aid

In Chapter 6 hazard analytical techniques were examined for their potential utility as methods to extract and facilitate the evaluation of hazard information. The data on page 196 to page 200 also serves other valuable purpose. Such data provides the basis for conducting thorough inspections. With such hazard information in hand, the inspector is in a more enlightened position when it comes to understanding the problem for which specific controls have been provided for. In addition, such information will allow the inspector to more readily determine how alterations in the workplace reduce the effectiveness of existing controls.

Assessing Health Hazards in the Workplace

As previously stated, a thorough inspection requires that emphasis be given to both safety as well as health hazards.

In order to be able to recognize health hazards during an inspection process, the inspector requires the knowledge and understanding of the environmental factors in his workplace, which have the capacity to impair the health of workers.

An evaluation of health hazards requires that the inspector consider:

- The nature of the product being produced;
- The raw materials being used;
- The materials and substances being added in the process;
- By-products produced;
- The equipment involved;
- The cycle of operations;
- Operational procedures being used;
- Health and safety controls utilized; and
- Number or workers and level of worker exposure to harmful chemical, biological, and physical agents.

To aid the inspector in accomplishing the environmental health aspects of the inspection process the following guidelines are offered:

1. List all hazardous chemical, physical, and biological agents. Figure 99: Hazardous Materials Information sheet will serve as an aid in identifying the specific characteristics and harmful effects of hazardous materials.
2. Determine what state the hazardous agents will assume in the workplace environment—particulate matter (dust), mists, fumes, vapors, smokes, gases.
3. Determine the threshold—limit values for all chemical, physical, and

HAZARDOUS MATERIALS INFORMATION SHEET

(Please complete all applicable sections.)

1. Product Name, Number, Synonym _____ Chemical Formula _____
2. Manufacturer's Name _____
3. Manufacturer's Address _____
4. Chemical and Physical Properties: a. Molecular Wt. _____ b. Boiling Point _____ °C

    c. Melting Point _____ °C d. Specific Gravity (water = 1) or Bulk Density _____

    @ _____ °C e. Vapor Density (air = 1) _____ f. Vapor Pressure (mm Hg) _____

    @ _____ °C; _____ @ _____ °C; _____ @ _____ °C;

    g. Solubility _____

    h. pH/conc. _____ i. Index of Refraction _____ @ _____ °C

    j. Corrosive action on materials (e.g. aluminum, carbon steel, copper, rubber, plastics, etc.) _____

    _____

    k. Does the material decompose when exposed to air? water? heat? strong oxidizers? possible

    products? _____

    l. Does the material generate heat through polymerization or condensation? _____

    m. Composition *(give chemical names of components; information will be treated as confidential)*

COMPOUND	PERCENT	COMPOUND	PERCENT

NOTE: *Please be specific. For example, it is important to know whether an alcohol is methanol; an aromatic hydrocarbon is benzene; a chlorinated material is carbon tetrachloride.*

5. Flammability and Explosive Properties: a. Flash Point, F, Closed Cup _____

    Open Cup _____ If flash point changes during evaporation give data _____

    b. Explosive limits (% by vol. in air): LOWER _____ UPPER _____

    c. Susceptibility to spontaneous heating: YES _____ NO _____

    d. Fire point, F _____ Auto-ignition temp., F _____

    e. What products might be formed in the event of fire or abnormal temperatures? _____

    f. Suitable extinguishing agents _____

6. Procedures in Case of Container Breakage or Leakage _____
7. Transportation and Storage Requirements _____
8. Physiological Properties *(give animal tested, observation time, dosage value and range, dilution medium, etc.):*

    a. Acute oral toxicity _____

    b. Acute local effects on eyes _____

    c. Acute local effects on skin. Primary irritant? _____

    Sensitizer? _____

    d. Acute inhalation toxicity *(vapor, mist, fume, dust. Indicate effects of concentration and time.)*
    _____

    e. Chronic effects _____

    f. Warning properties *(odor; irritation of eyes, nose, throat)* _____

    g. Threshold limit value *(estimate, if not on current list of ACGIH)* _____

9. First Aid Treatment:

    a. Skin contact _____

    b. Eye contact _____

    c. Inhalation _____

    d. Antidote and treatment in case of swallowing _____

10. Recommended Pre-placement or Periodic Medical Examination *(health standards, clinical tests, frequency, etc.)* _____
11. Precautions for Normal Conditions of Use _____
12. Recommended Personal Protective Equipment _____
13. Suggested Method for Air Analysis _____
14. Pertinent Literature References _____
15. Information Furnished By: NAME _____ DATE _____

    TITLE _____

    COMPANY _____

    ADDRESS _____

(If more space is needed for comment, please attach an additional sheet. Please attach product information data sheets or other publications related to the safe handling and use of this material.)

Figure 99. Hazardous materials information sheet. (Reproduced with the permission of the National Safety Council.)

Monitoring the Workplace For Hazards   **351**

biological agents and compare against actual conditions in the workplace.

4. Consider the synergistic effects which could be produced, via the reactions of raw materials used in the production process.

5. Determine which processes and pieces of equipment are capable of producing hazardous levels of either chemical, physical or biological agents during normal operation.

The charts in Figure 100 and 101 will be of value in illustrating the types of health hazards associated with various processes and operations.

Managing the Inspection Program

As discussed previously, management should define and assign inspection areas, supervise formulation of inspection inventories, and develop well-tailored checklists. Such activities are no different than other management activities: they require planning, setting objectives, expected completion dates, etc., and then, close supervision and follow-up to insure completion.

When the inspection program has been prepared and readied for implementation, it is essential that everyone completely understands its purpose and the desired results.

Completed hazard control checklists and inspection reports submitted to management are important records which should be reviewed and acted upon with promptness. Such documents are comparable to quality control and production records and deserve the same attention and concern. In addition, management personnel should personally conduct periodic safety inspections and become involved in corrective action, to indicate management's concern for hazard control and to provide a stimulus for participation at all organizational levels.

Summarizing Inspection Data

Upon completing the inspection process, the inspector must be able to convert his findings into a format which will allow for proper communication and management actions.

In addition, consideration must be given to sorting out the most important problems from those of less importance, so that management may be guided toward correcting hazards on a worst-first basis.

Although there are almost as many systems for judging hazard importance as there are hazards, nevertheless, a single system, understood by organizational members must be instituted. From the suggested alternatives in Figure 20, page 81, a hazard classification scheme can be tailored to fit individual needs.

Figure 102 illustrates an Inspection Summary Report. Such a system proves very beneficial in displaying hazard data for decision-making purposes. A more detailed version of this report is found on page 87.

It is critical to the inspection process that inspection results be displayed, so that important information is communicated properly. The easier it is for

PROCESS OR OPERATION	NATURE AND DESCRIPTION OF HAZARDS
Abrasive blasting	Abrasive blasting equipment may be automatic or manually operated. Either type may use sand, steel shot, or artificial abrasives. The dust levels of work-room air should be examined to make certain that the operators are not over-exposed.
Assembly operations	Improper positioning of equipment and handling of work parts may present ergonomic hazards due to repeated awkward motion resulting in excessive stresses.
Bagging and handling of dry materials	Conveying, sifting, sieving, screening, packaging, or bagging of any dry material may present a dust hazard. The transfer of dry, finely divided powder may result in the formation of considerable quantities of air-borne dust. Inhalation and skin contact hazards may be present.
Ceramic coating	Ceramic coating may present the hazard of air-borne dispersion of toxic pigments plus hazards of heat stress from the furnaces and hot ware.
Dry grinding	Dry grinding operations should be examined for air-borne dust, noise, and ergonomic hazards.
Dry mixing	Mixing of dry material may present a dust hazard and should take place in completely enclosed mixers whenever air sampling indicates excessive amounts of air-borne dust are present.
Electron beam welding	Any process involving an electric discharge in vacuum may be a source of ionizing radiation. Such processes include electron beam equipment and similar devices.
Fabric and paper coating	The coating and impregnating of fabric and paper with plastic or rubber solutions may involve evaporation into the workroom air of large quantities of solvents.
Forming and forging	Hot bending, forming, or cutting of metals or non-metals may have the hazards of lubricant mist, decomposition products of the lubricant, skin contact with the lubricant, heat stress (including radiant heat), noise, and dust.
Gas furnace or oven heating operations (annealing, baking, drying, etc.)	Any gas or oil fired combustion process should be examined to determine the level of by-products of combustion that may be released into the work-room atmosphere. Noise measurements should also be made to determine the level of burner noise.
Grinding operations	Grinding, crushing, or comminuting of any material may present the hazard of contamination of work-room air due to the dust of the material being processed or of the grinding wheel.
High temperatures from hot castings, unlagged steam pipes, process equipment, etc.	Any process or operation involving high ambient temperatures (dry-bulb temperature), radiant heat load (globe temperature), or excessive humidity (wet-bulb temperature) should be examined to determine the magnitude of the physical stresses that may be present.

Figure 100. (Reproduced with the permission of the National Safety Council.)

PROCESS OR OPERATION	NATURE AND DESCRIPTION OF HAZARDS
Materials handling, warehousing	Work areas should be checked for levels of carbon monoxide and oxides of nitrogen arising from internal combustion engine forklift operations.
Metalizing	Uncontrolled coating of parts with molten metals present hazards of dust and fumes of metals and fluxes in addition to heat and non-ionizing radiation.
Microwave and radio frequency heating operations	Any process or operation involving microwaves or induction heating should be examined to determine the magnitude of heating effects and in some cases noise exposure on the employees.
Molten metals	Any process involving the melting and pouring of molten metals should be examined to determine the level of air contaminants of any toxic gas, metal fume, or dust produced in the operation.
Paint spraying	Spray painting operations should be examined for the possibility of hazards from inhalation and skin contact with toxic and irritating solvents and inhalation of toxic pigments. The solvent vapor evaporating from the sprayed surface may also be a source of hazard, because ventilation may be provided only for the paint spray booth.
Plating	Electroplating processes involve risk of skin contact with strong chemicals and in addition may present a respiratory hazard if mist or gases from the plating solutions are dispersed into the work-room air.
Punch press, press brake, drawing operations, etc.	Cold bending, forming, or cutting of metals or non-metals should be examined for hazards of contact with lubricant, inhalation of lubricant mist, and excessive noise.
Vapor degreasing	The removal of oil and grease from metal products may present hazards. This operation should be examined to determine that excessive amounts of vapor are not being released into the work-room atmosphere.
Welding, gas or electric-arc	Any process involving the melting and joining of metals parts should be examined for toxic fumes and the possibility of production of ozone and oxides of nitrogen. If there is an arc or spark discharge, the effects of radiation and the products of destruction of the electrodes should be investigated. These operations also commonly involve hazards of high potential electrical circuits of low internal resistance.
Wet grinding	Wet grinding of any material may produce possible hazards of mist, dust, and noise.
Wet mixing	Mixing of wet materials may present possible hazards of solvent vapors, mists, and possibly dust. The noise levels produced by the associated equpment should be checked.

Figure 101. (Reproduced with the permission of the National Safety Council.)

354   The Process of Hazard Control

Prepared by:_____
Dept.:_____

Violation Number	Description of Hazard	Specific Location	Standard Violated	Hazard Cl.	No. People Exposed	Remarks Action
1	Lack of personal protective equipment or ventilation to minimize respiraton of aluminum oxide from grinding wheel	Tool grinding area	OSHA Subpart I Section 1910.132 and 1910.34	III	3	Short Term: Respirators should be required for grinding operation Long Term: An adequate local exhaust system should be installed to control airborne particulate matter

management to read and understand the logic behind the recommended improvements along with available alternatives, and the cost for improvements, the better the chance that what needs to be done will be one in a timely and efficient manner.

Figure 102. Inspection summary report.

Summary

Effective inspection is a necessary part of the total hazard control effort. A good inspection requires that:

1. A determination be made of:
   a. What should be inspected and for what;
   b. When to inspect;
   c. Where to inspect;
   d. How to inspect; what special knowledge, training, etc., is required; and
   e. Who should inspect; what special knowledge, training, etc., is required.
2. The inspection be carried out thoroughly and effectively.
3. The facts and information obtained during inspection are carefully assessed as to their risk potential.
4. Facts and information noted during inspection, be forwarded to management along with alternatives for both short and long term corrective action.

Inspection programs are similar to other programs in that, to be effective and provide the desired results, they must be well-designed, implemented, and supported at all levels of the organization. Positive results can and should be expected from such a program in the form of reduced accidents and their resultant losses.

Hazard Control Audit

To: _____   Date: _____

From: _____   Subject: _____

                                  Area: _____

                                  Location: _____

Date(s) of Audit: _____

Persons Contacted: _____

_____

_ _

Purpose of Audit: To provide management with assistance in the evaluation of the organization's safety program, compliance to specific administrative requirements, and the condition of the job relative to safe working conditions.

Foreword: The following is a checklist of records, reports, posted materials, equipment condition, personnel conduct and job conditions which are either required by safety laws, codes or organizational policy. This list does not encompass *all* necessary items but a portion of each activity is examined.

Notes: A notation of N.A. indicated that the item is not applicable to the site being audited.

__This notation indicates that corrective action is required.

Section I—General—Determination of Requirements

1.0 Has a survey been made to determine what laws, regulations, codes apply to the specific location? (Y) (N). The following jurisdictions exercise regulatory authority: Federal O.S.H.A.? (Y) (N), agency? (Y) (N), activity of organization? (Y) (N), other _____
Are copies of the (Y)'s requirements on file at the site? (Y) (N)
Comments: _____
_____
_____.

2.0 What is the nature of organization's involvement in job?
   1. Direct hire
   2. All work subcontracted
   3. Combination of 1 & 2
   4. Advisory only
   5. Subcontractor

Courtesy—The Rust Engineering Company.

Have agreements with others being reached concerning various Safety, First Aid, Communications, Transportation and Inspection Obligation?
Comments _____
_____
_____
_____

3.0 Based upon an interpretation of the most restrictive of the law(s), regulation(s), or code(s) it was determined that the following safety, first aid, facilities and equipment was required to service a force of _____ employees.
　1. Is a safety coordinator required? (Y) (N).
　2. Are first aid attendants required? (Y) (N); number _____.
　3. Communications (Y) (N). Type_____; Proximity to work area
　　_____.
　4. First aid room? (Y) (N).
　5. First aid room equipment? (Y) (N); Examining table? (Y) (N); Others
　　_____.
　6. Is there a specified list of medical supplies? (Y) (N).
　7. Is there a requirement for stretchers and for baskets? (Y) (N); Quantity(s)
　　_____
　8. Is there a transportation requirement? (Y) (N); If (Y), Specify ____
　　_____.
　9. Is there a requirement for fire trucks, major fire fighting equipment or water supply? (Y) (N). If (Y), Specify _____
　　_____.

4.0 Has a written summary being made of this major safety and health requirements for the workplace? (Y) (N). Does this Safety and Health Summary include a list of the required reports, records, notifications, and communications? (Y) (N). To Whom? (Y) (N). When? (Y) (N). If the necessary information is provided by reference to existing documents, was the document provided? (Y) (N). Is the reference specific, article, page, or paragraph? (Y) (N).
Comments: _____
_____

Note: The following sections of this Audit are based upon the Occupational Safety and Health Act of 1970 and Executive Order 11807. The interpretations are in keeping with the understood intent of the law. The person conducting the audit must consider O.S.H.A. and the addition of other regulations which may be more restrictive. In any case, the *most* *restrictive requirement will determine acceptable conduct* of safety and health operations in the workplace under inspection.

Section II—Posting and Recordkeeping

5.0 Has the Department of Labor *"Safety and Health Protection on the Job"* poster been displayed in a prominent place on the site to which the employees report? (Y) (N). Where office employees report? (Y) (N). See Appendix B.

6.0 Are copies of the organization's General Safety Rules (employees) posted where employees report? (Y) (N). Have the Safety Rules been explained to all supervisors and employees, does evidence in writing exist? (Y) (N). Are emergency phone numbers posted prominently? (Y) (N). Are fire department, police, emergency medical service and first aid telephone numbers posted near field office phones? (Y) (N); at the guard post(s)? (Y) (N), on office boards? (Y) (N).

7.0 Have there been any citations, temporary variance or regulations requiring posting? (Y) (N). Are these posted as required? (Y) (N). Comments: _____

_____.

8.0 Are the following records satisfactory? First aid log? (Y) (N); medical log? (Y) (N); accident investigation report file? (Y) (N); daily safety inspection report file? (Y) (N); monthly safety report file? (Y) (N); work permit file? (Y) (N).

9.0 Are the following records required by OSHA being kept? OSHA No. 100. Log of Occupational Injuries and Illnesses? (Y) (N); OSHA No. 101 or its equivalent? Is OSHA 102 posted? (Y) (N). Note, not required except each February for preceding year. Additional records, reports etc. which are required by other Regulations:

_____

_____

_____.

Section III—General Health and Safety Conditions

10.0 Has a workplace Safety Plan been established? (Y) (N). Has budget been established? (Y) (N). Does budget include—employee charges for safety inspections and meeting? (Y) (N). Cost of; training materials? (Y) (N), signs? (Y) (N), protective equipment? (Y) (N), others _____

_____.

11.0 Have Safety Program goals been established? (Y) (N). Does the supervisor conduct Monthly Safety Meetings during which the Safety

Record is compared to the goals? (Y) (N). Corrective action planned? (Y) (N). Is each employee informed of the Safety Rules upon employment, (a signed acknowledgement of instruction is a part of personnel file)? (Y) (N). This training is evidenced by the supervisor giving the instruction attached to the employees file? (Y) (N).

Comments: _____

_____

_____ .

12.0 Are there any harmful materials, substances, plants, or natural conditions which present potential hazard to employees? (Y) (N). Have warnings been posted? (Y) (N). Have instructions relative to potential danger been given? (Y) (N). Have preventive actions been taken as applicable? (Y) (N). Comments: _____

_____

_____

_____ .

13.0 Are there any employees who are required to handle or use poisons, caustics, and other harmful substances? (Y) (N). If (Y), have appropriate instructions been given? (Y) (N).

14.0 Are there any employees who are required to enter confined areas with limited routes of escape? (Y) (N). If (Y) have appropriate instructions been given? (Y) (N). Did the evaluation of such conditions determine if supplementary ventilation is required? (Y) (N).

Section IV—Occupational Health and Environmental Controls

15.0 Are medical personnel available for advice and consultation on matters of Occupational Health? (Y) (N). Name: _____ .
Location: _____ .
Have provisions been made for prompt medical service in case of serious injury(s)? (Y) (N). Name of Facility _____ ,
Person contacted _____ ,
Distance _____. Has a suitable enclosed area been provided for first aid? (Y) (N). Is there a first aid kit or minimum required first aid supplies available? (Y) (N). Are medical attendents at site? (Y) (N). Are copies of certificates or evidence of qualification at site? (Y) (N). Have provisions been made for emergency medical communication? (Y) (N), transportation? (Y) (N).

16.0 Sanitation

16.1 Is portable water available in adequate quantity? (Y) (N). Are portable containers in use capable of being tightly closed? (Y) (N); equipped with spigot (dipping prohibited)? (Y) (N). Is nonportable water identified with signs stating approved use? (Y) (N). Have systems been checked to assure no cross connections? (Y) (N).

Comments: _____

_____

_____.

16.2 Are toilets and urinals provided according to the standard? (Y) (N). Have local codes been checked to assure that disposal system is compliance? (Y) (N).

16.3 Are sleeping quarters available? (Y) (N). Comments: _____

_____.

16.4 Have washing facilities been provided for employees engaged in the application of paints, coating, herbicides, insecticides, etc.? (Y) (N). Are such facilities in near proximity to work site and so equipped so that employees can adequately remove such harmful substances? (Y) (N).

17.0 Occupational noise exposure survey of the site was last made on / / . Were areas found which required protection? (Y) (N).

Comments: _____

_____

_____.

18.0 A hazardous gas, fume, dust or mist survey of the site was performed / / . Were any hazards found which are not provided for in Installations Safety Regulations? (Y) (N). Comments: _____

_____.

Was ventilation provided if applicable? (Y) (N). Has protective equipment been provided? (Y) (N). Have enforcement steps been taken? (Y) (N).

19.0 An illumination survey during work hours was last conducted / / . Were values according to standard? (Y) (N).

Section V—Personnel Protective and Life Saving Equipment

20.0 Have (ANSI Z-89-2-1971) hard hats been provided for all employees entering head impact areas? (Y) (N). Have enforcement steps been taken? (Y) (N).

Comments: _____

_____.

21.0 An eye and face protection survey was last conducted / / . Were any hazards found which are not provided for in the organizations Safety Regulations? (Y) (N). Comments: _____

_____.

Has adequate protection been provided? (Y) (N). Have enforcement measures been taken? (Y) (N). Comments: _____

_____.

22.0 Are safety belts, life lines, and lanyards or nets provided in all areas not protected by adequate guard rails (where a 10 ′ or more fall hazard exists)? (Y) (N). Is the use of this equipment enforced? (Y) (N). Comments: _____

_____.

23.0 Are U.S.C.G. approved life vests provided for employees working on or above water? (Y) (N). Are ring buoys with 90 ′ of line readily available? (Y) (N). Is a life saving skiff available? (Y) (N). Comments: _____

_____.

Section VI—Fire Protection and Prevention

24.0 Has a fire protection and prevention plan been prepared? (Y) (N). Does plan include fire prevention inspection? (Y) (N). Does a record of inspections exist? (Y) (N). Do inspections show inspection of equipment? (Y) (N); of area for hazards? (Y) (N). Has corrective action been effective to eliminate inspection deficiencies? (Y) (N). Have fire drills or tests of fire fighting plans been accomplished? (Y) (N). Have these forces made trial runs to the jobsite? (Y) (N). Have appraisalls of drills or tests been made? (Y) (N). Were communication plans adequately tested? (Y) (N). Comments: _____

_____

_____.

25.0 Fire protection equipment checks have been made to assure: Equipment is immediately available? (Y) (N). Access to equipment is open at all times? (Y) (N). Fire roads for equipment are adequate to permit passage at all times? (Y) (N). Fire fighting equipment is conspicuously located? (Y) (N). Fire fighting equipment is periodically inspected, defective equipment is replaced? (Y) (N). Has a water supply been provided? (Y) (N). Have provisions for adapting fire fighting equipment to water supply been made? (Y) (N). Have water supplies been protected from freezing? (Y) (N).

    25.1 Fire extinguishers or other suitable fire fighting equipment or facilities have been provided near accumulations of combustible materials storage areas? (Y) (N). In or near areas where combustible materials are present? (Y) (N). In offices? (Y) (N). In all warehouses? (Y) (N).

    25.1 All fire extinguishers and/or water barrels are clearly identified as to type of fires for which they are to be used? (Y) (N). Comments: _____

_____.

26.0 If workplace is near existing plants, refineries, buildings, storage facilities, pipelines or flammable natural growth, has the fire hazard external to the site been evaluated? (Y) (N). Does the external condition present a hazard to the site? (Y) (N). Is there liquid or gaseous materials that could pass in or out which constitute a fire hazard? (Y) (N). Is there grass or other vegetation which could be a fire hazard? (Y) (N). Can or have steps been taken to eliminate or minimize these hazards (fire walls, fire breaks, flame screens, sparks arrests etc.)?

Comments: _____

_____

_____.

27.0 Are daily fire prevention inspections conducted? (Y) (N). Does inspection include: Housekeeping? (Y) (N), fire extinguishers? (Y) (N); no smoking and enforcement? (Y) (N); electrical installations? (Y) (N); access and road checks? (Y) (N); material storage conditions? (Y) (N); fuel storage? (Y) (N); paint storage? (Y) (N); heaters? (Y) (N); appliances? (Y) (N); hazards in welding and cutting areas? (Y) (N); oil or gas leaks? (Y) (N); explosive storage? (Y) (N); distance of explosives, fuels, and paint storage facilities from other facilities? (Y) (N); review of material receiving report? (Y) (N).

Section VII—Signs, Signals and Barricades

28.0 Are accident prevention signs used as applicable for: danger signs where immediate hazard exists? (Y) (N); caution signs, potential hazards? (Y) (N); exit signs? (Y) (N); directional signs? (Y) (N); traffic signs? (Y) (N); accident prevention tags? (Y) (N). Does the color and shape of signs comply with standards? (Y) (N).

29.0 Are barricades used to control vehicular and or pedestrial traffic hazard areas? (Y) (N). Are barricades erected around open excavations? (Y) (N); holes in floors? (Y) (N); around moving or revolving equipment? (Y) (N); under overhead operations? (Y) (N)?

Section VIII—Material Handling Storage, Use and Disposal

30.0 Are materials stored so that material will not fall? (Y) (N); so as not to exceed the load supporting ability of the ground or structure where stored? (Y) (N). Is clearance provided for passage of vehicles plus personnel? (Y) (N); at least 6′ is open adjacent to floor openings or hoistways? (Y) (N), or 10′ from wall that does not extend above the top of the material? (Y) (N); noncompatible materials are segregated? (Y) (N).

31.0 Is there a periodic inspection of slings, clamps, shackles, hooks, chains, links and cables used to handle materials? (Y) (N). Are the items used examined before use? (Y) (N). Are items found to be defective removed from service? (Y) (N). Is each item above marked with rated capacity? (Y) (N).

32.0 Is the disposal of waste materials, rubbish and scrap from the work areas accomplished without allowing accumulations? (Y) (N). Are oily rags, solvent waste and flammable liquids kept in fire resistant covered containers until removed from work site? (Y) (N).

Section IX—Tools—Hand and Power

33.0 General—Are all tools, whether furnished by employee or employer, maintained in good condition? (Y) (N). Are power tools that are designed to accomodate guards operated with the guards in place? (Y) (N). Are all belts, gears, shafts, pulleys, sprockets, spindles, drums, flywheels, chains, or other reciprocating, rotating or moving parts of tools or equipment guarded if such parts can come in contact with employees or other cause of hazard? (Y) (N). Are all hand held powered tools, except those specifically exempted, equipped with constant pressure switches or operating valve that automatically release when pressure is released? (Y) (N).

34.0 Is the use of unsafe hand tools permitted whether personal or issued? (Y) (N). Are sprung wrenches or sockets being used? (Y) (N). Are impact tools and chisels kept free of mushroomed heads? (Y) (N). Are handles kept tight, and free of splinters or cracks? (Y) (N). Note: excessively painted or otherwise covered handle may hide hazardous defects.

35.0 Are electrical power tools of the double insulated type on a grounding circuit? (Y) (N); or in conformance with standards on ground fault circuit interrupters? (Y) (N). Are pneumatic power tools secured to the hose by some positive means to prevent accidental disconnection? (Y) (N). Are impact tools provided with a retainer to prevent chisel or tool from being accidentally expelled? (Y) (N). Are power stapler, nailers and similar equipment which operate at more than 100psi equipped with safety muzzles to prevent the accidental ejection of nail or staple? (Y) (N). Are precautions taken to prevent operation of tools, valves, fittings, and pipe at pressures higher than specified by the manufacturer? (Y) (N). Is the use of compressed air over 30psi allowed for cleaning only when a protective equipment is used? (Y) (N). Are hoses larger than 1/″ I.D. provided with a safety device at the source or branch to reduce pressure in case of hose failure? (Y) (N). Are airless spray guns (high pressure 1,000psi or more) equipped with double safety switches or valves? (Y) (N).

36.0 Are fuel powered tools, stopped for fueling, servicing, and maintenance? (Y) (N). Is the tool and fuel handled, stored and transported as provided for fuels and internal combustion engine equipment? (Y) (N). Are hydraulic tools operated with fire resistant fluids? (Y) (N). Are personnel and special safety precautions enforced for powder-activated tools? (Y) (N). Are the rules for jacks, being followed? (Y) (N).

37.0 Are abrasive wheels and tools examined to assure sufficient power to maintain safe spindle speed? (Y) (N); proper guarding? (Y) (N); proper alignment of wheel? (Y) (N); proper fit of wheel to shaft or spindle? (Y) (N); that wheel is not cracked or broken by visual examination or ring testing? (Y) (N). Are operators prohibited from using abrasive tools in a manner not recommended by the manufacturer? (Y) (N); without tool rests properly adjusted? (Y) (N); without protective equipment? (Y) (N).

Section X—Welding and Cutting

38.0 Are protection caps kept secured on compressed gas cylinders when transported, moved and stored? (Y) (N). When cylinders are hoisted are they secured on a cradle, slingboard or pallet, not by means of the magnets, choker slings or protective cap? (Y) (N); when moved individually rolled on their bottom edge, and not intentionally dropped, struck or permitted to strike each other violently? (Y) (N); when transported by powered vehicles secured in a vertical position? (Y) (N). Are cylinders with regulators attached being moved other than in a carrier designed for the purpose? (Y) (N). Are cylinders secured to prevent falling, using securing chain or other steadying device? (Y) (N); when empty or not in use is the valve of cylinder closed? (Y) (N). Are cylinders stored vertical, away from heat, electrical circuits, slag, sparks and being struck by arc welding electrodes (in cases where not possible protected by resistant shield)? (Y) (N). Have employees being instructed to momentarily open and close valve before attaching regulator, open valves slowly, use gases only for specified use, never use without regulator or suitable-device to reduce pressure, keeping wrench available if required for valve, to place aside and return damaged or leaky cylinders, to ventilate hoses before storage and not use hose, fittings, regulators, torches valves or other components for gas welding or cutting that are suspected of being defective or damaged? (Y) (N). Have instructions been given regarding the hazards involved in the use of grease or oil on oxygen cylinders, fittings, valves, or parts? (Y) (N). Are manifolds marked with at least 1″ letters to identify the gas, and fitting such to prevent accidental connection to the wrong line? (Y) (N). Are torches, manifolds, valve fittings examined daily before use? (Y) (N). Are torches lighted only by friction lighter or other approved lighter, not by match or by hot work? (Y) (N).

39.0 Are arc welding and cutting electrode holders, cables, connectors or any current-carrying parts of a capacity capable of safety handling the maximum rated capacity considering duty cycle and insulated against the maximum voltage encountered to ground? (Y) (N). Are welding machines equipped with machine grounds? (Y) (N). Are the frames of arc welding machines grounded through a third wire or a separate wire at the source of current and of sufficient capacity to assure that a fuse or circuit will interrupt the power? (Y) (N). When electrode holders are left unattended, are electrodes removed and the holder placed in a safe position? (Y) (N). Is the dipping of hot electrode holders in water prohibited? (Y) (N). Are welding machines turned off when the welder leaves his work? (Y) (N). Are welding and cutting operation shielded when practicable by the use of noncombustible or flameproof screens? (Y) (N). Are fire prevention techniques being followed such as: Moving to safe area when possible? (Y) (N); using spark and slag confining methods? (Y) (N); forbidding welding or cutting in the presence of flammable or explosive compounds such as point, gas, dust in concentrations when creates a hazard? (Y) (N); suitable fire extinguishing equipment and a plan for use when fire hazard exists? (Y) (N). Are pipes, tanks or barrels that contained toxic or flammable substances filled with water or thoroughly cleaned, vented, and tested before cutting and welding? (Y) (N).

40.0 Ventilation and protection in welding, cutting and heating—Is welding and cutting in enclosed, unventilated or poorly ventilated areas prohibited? (Y) (N). Are adequate precautions being taken when cutting or welding toxic substances such as metals containing or coated with zinc, lead, cadmium, chromium berryllium or mercury? (Y) (N). Are other employees working near welders protected from fumes and ultra-violet radiation? (Y) (N).

Section XI—Electrical

41.0 Have the pertinent provisions of the National Electrical Code, NFPA 70–1975, ANSI C1—1975 (Rev. of 1968), and the National Electrical Safety Code, National Bureau of Standards, Part 4 (ANST C2.4) for all electrical work, installations and wire capacities both for temporary and permanent installations? (Y) (N). Are circuits de-energized before work is performed, or protective precautions taken? (Y) (N). Are areas of electrical hazard posted, provided with barriers and insulated if possible? (Y) (N). Are the working spaces around electrical equipment sufficient to allow the safe, operation? (Y) (N); opening of hinged doors or panels 90°? (Y) (N); clearance of 6-1/4 ' high and 3 ' wide? (Y) (N). Are circuits or installations which have been de-energized in the course of work locked out and tagged to prevent accidental energizing? (Y) (N). Do all electrical personnel who may have cause to de-energize circuits carry tags and locks for this purpose at all times? (Y) (N).

42.0 Grounding and bonding—Are the noncurrent—carrying parts of portable fixed and/or plug—connected equipment grounded? (Y) (N). Has grounding been checked to assure that resistance to ground does not exceed 25 ohms for driven rod electrods? (Y) (N); (2 or more electrodes connected in parallel may be required). Are all extension cords in good repair? (Y) (N); of the 3 wire type? (Y) (N); of sufficient capacity to carry the electrical load? (Y) (N). Are all portable lighting cords used in vessels, tanks, and towers or other hazards locations at a maximum of 12 volts? (Y) (N). Are all portable lights protected with an adequate protective cover to prevent accidental contact with bulb? (Y) (N). Are temporary lights equipped with heavy duty cords and connectors? (Y) (N).

43.0 Equipment installation and maintenance—Are flexible cable and cords of an approved type with concealed contacts with provision for extending ground? (Y) (N); designed so that plug can be disconnected without leaving live parts exposed? (Y) (N); equipped with different types of fittings for different voltages, frequencies, or types of current (a.c. or d.c.) to avoid accidental hazardous connections? (Y) (N), equipped with skirts for supplying equipment over 300 volts or otherwise designed to confine arc? (Y) (N); equipped so the attaching end and connecting end is protected to avoid the effect of mechanical strain from affecting the mechanical or dielectric integrity of the cable or cord? (Y) (N). When passing through work areas are they elevated or covered to protect from damage or hazard to employees? (Y) (N); not used if frayed or worn? (Y) (N).

44.0 Are overcurrent protectors provided for all circuits? (Y) (N). In the placing of overcurrent devices prohibited except where the device opens all conductors of the circuit or for motor running protection? (Y) (N). Are special insulated fuse removal tools used for removal and installation of fuses? (Y) (N). Are switches, circuit breaker and disconnectors marked legibly to indicate use unless the arrangement is self-evident? (Y) (N). Are boxes for disconnects securely fastened to the surface where mounted, shielded and located to avoid employee injury? (Y) (N). Are water-proof boxes and disconnects used in wet or damp locations? (Y) (N). Are all energized transformers, except these mounted on poles 12 ' or more from the ground, or over 150amps to ground protected from personnel by covering housing, fence secured by lock or other fastening requiring the use of tools to open? (Y) (N). Are signs prohibiting unauthorized access to these displayed on cover or other type enclosure? (Y) (N).

45.0 Is the battery room and battery charging facilities for nonseal types located in an enclosure with outside vents or in well ventilated rooms? (Y) (N); so as to ensure diffusion of gases and prevent accumulation and explosive mixtures? (Y) (N). Are workmen provided face shields, aprons and rubber gloves for handling acids and batteries? (Y) (N). Are quick drench facilities provided within 25 ' of work area? (Y) (N).

Section XII—Ladders and Scaffolding

46.0 Are the following rules relative to ladders being adhered to? Are ladders with defects, broken rungs, broken or split side rails prohibited and when found immediately removed from service? (Y) (N). The local manufacturer of ladders is controlled so as to comply with ANSI A 14.1—1975? (Y) (N); metal ladders comply to A 14.2—1972? (Y) (N); portable ladders are used at a pitch so that the base is placed out approximately 1/4 the working height? (Y) (N); ladders are not placed in doors, drives, aisles, or other locations where accidental displacement is possible? (Y) (N).

47.0 The top of portable ladders are blocked and or tied off to prevent movement? (Y) (N). The side rails extend at least 36 ″ above the landing or grab rails are provided? (Y) (N). Portable metal ladders are not used for electrical work or where contact is possible? (Y) (N). For ladders exceeding 30 ' is the ladder offset at a landing with a platform between each ladder and guard rails and toe boards are erected on exposed sides? (Y) (N).

48.0 Scaffolding

Guard rails and toe boards are provided on all open sides of scaffolds over 10 ' high? (Y) (N). Guard rails are 2 × 4 material or equivalent, approximately 42 ″ high with supports at least each 8 ' and with toeboards a minimum of 4″ high? (Y) (N). Note: Midrails are required when a hazard exists that a midrail prevents or mitigates. In areas where persons are required to pass under the scaffold, 1/″ mesh screen is attached between the toeboard and handrail? (Y) (N). Scaffolds are designed to support at least 4 times the maximum intended load? (Y) (N). No damaged scaffold parts are used? (Y) (N). Are scafolds constructed of woods which have a minimum 1,500 fiber strength? (Y) (N). The maximum span for 2 × 10 or wider full thickness planking is: workload/span 25 lbs/10 ', 50/8 ', 75/6 '; Nominal thickness: 25/8 ', 50/6 '? (Y) (N). All planking is overlapped 12 ″ or secured from movement? (Y) (N); planks extend at least 6 ″ and not more than 12 ″ over the end support? (Y) (N); legs, poles or uprights are plumb? (Y) (N). Are all scaffolds provided with ladders or stairs or equivalent safe access? (Y) (N). Welding, burning or riveting is not performed on staging suspended by fiber or synthetic rope? (Y) (N). Wire, synthetic or fiber rope used for scaffold support has a rated capacity of 6 times the expected load? (Y) (N). Shore pump jack, or lean to scaffolds are not used? (Y) (N). The specific rules for scaffolds as shown in 1926.451 are being followed? (Y) (N). Note: All scaffolds over 125' must be designed by a registered engineer and have drawings and specifications.

49.0 If tube and coupler scaffolds are used, has an examination of the tubing, clamps and other materials been made? (Y) (N). Are the pole spacings and height criteria according to Table L. 10, 1926.451? (Y) (N). Have runners been interlocked to the inside and outside posts at even heights and not more than 6'-6" on centers with the bottom runners as close to the base as possible? (Y) (N). Are bearers at least 4" longer but not more than 12" longer than the post spacing? (Y) (N). Has cross bracing been installed across the width of the scaffold at least every third set of posts and every fourth runner? (Y) (N). Has diagonal longitudinal bracing on the inner and outer rows of poles been installed at approximately a 45° angle from the bottom of the scaffold to the top at least each fifth post? (Y) (N). Is the entire scaffold tied to and braced securely to the building at least each 30' horizontally and 26' vertically? (Y) (N).

50.0 Are tubular welded frame scaffolds being used as intended by the manufacturer's design? (Y) (N). Are the cross and diagonal braces being used on all sections? (Y) (N). Are scaffolds attached to the building or structure at intervals not exceeding 30' horizontally or 26' vertically. When used as manually propelled mobile scaffolds does the height exceed 4 times the minimum base dimension? (Y) (N). Are the casters designed to support-4 times the intended load and equipped with wheel locking devices? (Y) (N).

Section XIII—Cranes, Derricks and Hoists

51.0 Are copies of the manufacturers operating specifications available at the jobsite for all cranes and derricks? (Y) (N). Are rated capacities, operating speeds, special hazard warnings conspicuously posted on the equipment? (Y) (N). Is all equipment being inspected by a competent employee prior to each use to assure safe operating condition? (Y) (N). Are thorough annual inspections of hoisting machinery made by a competent person or governmental, or private agency recognized by the U.S. Department of Labor? (Y) (N). Is a record of the dates and results of these inspections maintained? (Y) (N). Is wire rope replaced for the following conditions: In running ropes, 6 randomly distributed broken wires in one lay or 3 in 1 stand of lay? (Y) (N). Wear of 1/3 the original diameter of outside individual wires? (Y) (N). Crushing or bird caging which results in distortion of rope? (Y) (N). Evidence of heat damage? (Y) (N); reduction of 1/64" in diameter of rope up to 5/16", 1/32" for 3/8" to 1/2", 3/64" for 9/16" to and including 3/4", 1/16" for 7/8' to 1-1/8" and 3/32" for 1-1/4" to 1-1/2"? (Y) (N). In standing lines is rope replaced when more than 2 broken wires in 1 lay? (Y) (N). Have reciprocating, rotating and other moving parts which are exposed to employees been guarded? (Y) (N). Are precautions being taken, such as barricades, to prevent striking or crushing injuries in the swing area of the crane? (Y) (N). Are all exhaust pipe guarded if located where they might be touched by employees during normal duties? (Y) (N). Are all windows safety glass or equal? (Y) (N). Are adequate ladders, steps, guard rails provided for access work areas of machine? (Y) (N). Does each crane have an accessible fire extinguisher of 5 BC rating? (Y) (N). Are the required clearances from powerlines being observed 10' to 50 KV' + 0.4"/1KV up to and including 345 KV' and 16' for voltages up to and including 740 KV? (Y) (N). Is a person designated to observe and give timely warning when work is being performed in electrical hazard areas? (Y) (N). Have the safety requirement of special cranes or elevators been investigated and a separate checklist provided? (Y) (N). Attach copy of list if required.

Section XIV—Summary of Audit

The following is a summary of the observations giving (1) checklist, page and description of observed condition, and (2) recommended corrective action.

Item 1 Page _____ Description _____
_____
Recommendation _____
_____

Item 2 Page _____ Description _____
_____
Recommendation _____
_____

Item 3 Page _____ Description _____
_____
Recommendation _____
_____

Item 4 Page _____ Description _____
_____
Recommendation _____
_____

Item 5 Page _____ Description _____
_____
Recomendation_____
_____

Item 6 Page _____ Description _____
_____
Recommendation _____
_____

Item 7   Page _____ Description _____
_____

Recommendation _____

Item 8   Page _____ Description _____
_____

Recommendation _____

Item 9   Page _____ Description _____
_____

Recommendation _____

Item 10   Page _____ Description _____
_____

Recommendation _____

Item 11   Page _____ Description _____
_____

Recommendation _____

Item 12   Page _____ Description _____
_____

Recommendation _____

Item 13   Page _____ Description _____
_____

Recommendation _____

Item 14   Page _____ Description _____
_____

Recommendation _____

Item 15   Page _____ Description _____
_____

Recommendation _____

Item 16   Page _____ Description _____
_____

Recommendation _____

Item 17   Page _____ Description _____
_____

Recommendation _____

_____

Item 18   Page _____ Description _____

_____

Recommendation _____

_____

Item 19   Page _____ Description _____

_____

Recommendation _____

_____

Item 20   Page _____ Description _____

_____

Recommendation _____

_____

"Accident Prevention Manual for Industrial Operations," 7th edition, National Safety Council, Chicago, Illinois, 1974.

Binford, Charles M., Fleming, Cecil S., and Prust, Z. A. "Loss Control in the OSHA Era," New York, 1975.

Brown, Thomas, C., "Compliance and Enforcement," Occupational Safety and Health, A Transcript of a MAPI Seminar, Machinery and Allied Products Institute and Council for Technological Advancement. Washington, D.C., (Feb. 1973).

Browning, R. L., "Calculating Loss Exposures," Chemical Engineering, November 1969.

Concklin, Bert., "National Emphasis Program: View from the Top," Job Safety and Health, Vol. 4, no. 2 (April 1976).

Foster, James F., "OSHA Launches Voluntary Compliance Course," Job Safety and Health, Vol. 1, no. 2 (January, 1973).

Gilmore, Charles L., "Accident Prevention and Loss Control," American Management Association' 1970.

"Guidebook to Occupational Safety and Health," Commerce Clearing House, Inc., New York, 1973.

"Guide for Compliance with General Industry Standards," Job Safety and Health, Vol 2, no. 9 (September 1974).

"Hazardous Working Conditions in Seven Federal Agencies," Report to the Congress by the Comptroller General of the United States, HRD-76-144, Washington, D.C.: Government Printing Office, 1976.

Kerns, Bernard A., "Safety and Health in the Engineering and Manufacturing Functions," Occupational Safety and Health, A Transcript of a MAPI Seminar, Machinery and Allied Products Institute and Council for Technological Advancement, Washington, D.C., 1973.

LeClaire, Charles H., "A Safety and Health Audit," Occupational Safety and Health, A Transcript of a MAPI Seminar, Machinery and Allied Products Institute and the Council for Technological Advancement Washington, D. C., 1973.

Martin, W. A., "Inspection, Surveys and Audit," National Safety News, Vol. 104, no. 5 (November 1971), pp. 50-53.

McMannis, Donald, "At Ball State, We Chose Compliance" Job Safety and Health, Vol. 4, no. 1 (January 1976).

Moore, Robert L., "How to Inspect for Accident Prevention—Physical Condition of Buildings," National Safety Congress Transactions, Vol. 12, 1963.

Olishifski, Julian B., "How to Evaluate On-the-Job Health Hazards," National Safety News, March 1973.

Polling, Vincent, "Safety Sampling," Journal of the American Society of Safety Engineers, August 1962.

Tarrants, William E., "Research" (Critical Incident Technique), National Safety Congress Transactions, Vol. 12, 1966.

Wirfs, Ralph, "An Industrial Hygenist Inspects a Plant," Job Safety and Health, Vol. 1, no. 4 (March 1973).

Product Safety 10

Introduction

Product safety is definitely here to stay. Looking at the stipulations with which insurance companies are providing their risks, the rising costs of product liability insurance, and the fact that consumers are becoming more and more aware of a manufacturer's obligation to provide safe products, as well as their right to claim damages against a manufacturer or seller who fails to do so, has stimulated manufacturers to take a very hard and long look at how and with what resources within their companies a program could be put together to assure, at the very least, that they can stay in business while producing the safest product possible.

The National Commission on Product Safety estimates that 20 million injury-producing accidents occur each year in and about the household. Individuals, products, and their environments are all involved in these accidents, and the contributing factors are varied and complex.

The Problem

While precise statistics are not available, a consensus of opinion by the Federal Interagency Task Force on Product Liability is that over 500,000 product liability suits are experienced by industry each year. The increasing number of suits has driven the cost of insurance up from approximately $25 million a year in premiums back in 1950 to approximately $125 million a year by the early 1970s.[1] The reason for the increase is clear. The awards are averaging better than $100,000 per case. Since the insurance company doesn't want to get stuck with the tab, the manufacturer finds that the problem comes to rest in his lap. A close analysis of the situation however, reveals that after all is said and done it is the consumer—you and I—who eventually end up absorbing the cost.

Product liability, as it exists today, can be traced back to 1916, New York State, and the case of MacPherson vs. Buick Motor Company. This landmark case made significant inroads emasculating the rule of privity of contract. In this case the defendant, the Buick Motor Company sold a car to a retailer who in turn resold it to MacPherson, who was injured as the direct result of a defective wheel. Evidence demonstrated that the defect could have been discovered by a prudent person performing a reasonable inspection, and that in the opinion of the Court, an inspection had not been made. Buick argued that MacPherson bought the car directly from a dealer and not from Buick and therefore its obligation did not extend to the ultimate buyer—consequently, no privity. The Court, in a controversial ruling, ruled that Buick made a car with a defective component which left the car a dangerous instrument capable of inflicting injury and damage, and thus the manufacturer could not escape liability. Before this decision, privity had always been considered an integral part of breech of warranty claims.[2]

Another significant case, Escola vs. Coca-Cola Bottling Company of Fresno, California, 24 2d 453, in 1944, involved the doctrine of Res Ipsa loquitur—"The Thing Speaks for Itself." Simply stated, the accident, on the basis that it occurred, proved negligence. Under this doctrine, the manufacturer of a product doesn't have to be proved negligent. All that needs to be established is that he manufactured a product which caused an injury. Presiding Judge Traynor stated, "In my opinion it should now be recognized that a manufacturer incurs an *absolute liability* when an article that he has placed on the market, knowing that it is to be used without inspection, proves to have a defect that causes injuries to human beings . . . The cost of injury and loss of time or health may be an overwhelming misfortune to a person injured, or a needless one, for the risk of injury can be insured by the manufacturer and distributed among the public as a cost of doing business."

As time passed product liability cases became directed more in terms of breach of contract, and by the early 1960's, the theory of strict liability in tort had won broad acceptance by the courts. In the case Greenman vs. Yuba Power Products, Inc., et al.—59 Cal. 2d 57 (1963) the Court said, "A manufacturer is strictly liable in tort (personal injury), when the article he places on the market, knowing that it will be used without inspection, proves to have a defect that causes injury to a human being." This case brought out the significant fact that strict liability has two meanings—one legal, the other socio-economic. From a legal standpoint, it frees the buyer of the burden of proving fault against a manufacturer. The socio-economic meaning is best spelled out by the following quote taken from the Greenman case: "The purpose of such liability is to insure that the costs of injuries resulting from defective products are borne by the manufacturers that put such products on the market rather than by the injured persons who are powerless to protect themselves.'' Cases involving strict liability in tort have been increasing since early 1970. As a result of the shift in the orientation of liability cases, manufacturers must prepare themselves to withstand many more claims than even before and take necessary precautions to meet the potentially heavy costs of the judgments which can be placed on them.[3]

The shifts that have taken place in product liability law are having significant impact on industrial accident situations, where the workers compensation laws have had jurisdiction for years. Today, an injured worker can collect worker's compensation, and he then may have the option to sue the manufacturer of the product that injured him for damages. The product liability problem coupled with meeting the OSHA standards has placed, and will continue to place increasingly more strain on the manufacturer to establish a system which will insure that his products have been carefully assessed for the purpose of identifying and controlling hazards which are capable of causing injuries.

Occupational Safety and Product Liability

The experience of Marsh and McLennan[4] indicates that rising costs and limited availability of products liability insurance is a severe problem for certain small businesses and an increasingly difficult problem for others. Those firms currently experiencing most difficulty can be categorized as follows:

Insurance Ramifications to the Manufacturer

1. Manufacturers or distributors of products which have a catastrophic loss potential (e.g., aircraft parts).
2. Manufacturers or distributors of products with "batch exposure" (e.g., flu vaccine).
3. Manufacturers or distributors of products with sophisticated medical applications.
4. Manufacturers or distributors of products used in hazardous occupations.
5. Manufacturers or distributors of products which have a history of loss frequency (e.g., power lawn mowers).
6. Manufacturers and distributors of capital equipment and other long-life products.
7. Distributors of a wide range of products imported from other countries.

The difficulty in obtaining coverage for manufacturers and distributors in categories four and six is compounded by the exposure that their products have to industrial accidents. As was already pointed out in this chapter, this exposure results in a high incidence of suits from injured workers and from insurance companies seeking recovery of Workers' Compensation payments.

Negligence

Negligence may be summarized as lack of due care under the circumstances. Insofar as manufacturer negligence is concerned, it is generally said to be the failure to exercise reasonable care in the design, construction, and assembly of products, to keep them free from latent or hidden defects. Manufacturers have been charged with negligence in cases of defective design, defective construction, defective assembly, failure to warn, inadequate warning and failure to use adequate "Safety Features."[5]

The Concept of Unreasonable Risk

In Chapter two risk was defined as the product of the amount to be lost times the probability of losing it. Risk is associated with almost every facet of life and, as some of the theorists expound, life wouldn't be much without it. However, when we are speaking about safety, risk takes on an important meaning. Deciding what is reasonable risk versus what is unreasonable risk has been a very perplexing question to today's manufacturers. Many liability suits have been won primarily on the basis that the manufacturer had not taken measures to eliminate or safeguard a hazardous product to the extent that a prudent individual, in the use of the product would not be injured. Edwards,[6] explains the phenomenon of reasonable risk as follows: "Risks of bodily harm to users are not unreasonable when consumers can: understand that risks exist; appraise their probability and severity; know how to cope with them; and voluntarily accept them to get benefits that could not be obtained in less risky ways." Implicit in this statement is the fact that the consumer must be acquainted with the risk via instructions, warnings, etc., understand the pros and cons of taking the risk and for all practical purposes understand the full ramifications of what he could lose versus what he can gain from taking the risk in the first place. Edwards[7] goes on to state that "when there is a risk of this character, consumers have reasonable opportunity to protect themselves, and public authorities should hesitate to substitute their value judgments about the desirability of the risk for those of the consumers who choose to incur it. On the other hand, preventable risk is not reasonable, (a) when consumers do not know that it exists; or (b) when, though aware of it, consumers are unable to estimate its frequency and severity; or (c) when consumers do not know how to cope with it, and hence are likely to incur harm unnecessarily; or (d) when risk is unnecessary in . . . that it could be reduced or eliminated at a cost in money or in the performance of the product that consumers would willingly incur if they know the facts and were given the choice." As it turns out, design choices are made by manufacturers or regulated by government agencies on the basis of their perception of the reasonableness of the risk placed on the consumer, given the fact that the consumer will use the product within its design parameters.

A case of unreasonable risk is illustrated by the following example: A large consumer manufacturer of electrical appliances produced a hair drier, which, on the basis of all design review, quality checks, and so forth, was considered to be a safe product. As the story goes, while a female consumer was drying her long hair, her hair was caught into the rotating parts of the drier. In the process of trying to free her hair from the drier, she decided to cut it with a knife. In so doing, she stuck the point of the knife in her eye, and as a result became blinded in one eye. When this case reached the Courts, the plaintiff pleaded her case on the grounds that the manufacturer should have known that hair could get caught in the drier and thus, the manufacturer should have provided an adequate safeguard to prevent such a situation from occurring. In this case, the court ruled in favor of the plaintiff. There was ample information and techniques available for the manufacturer to have countered the hazard during the design and manufacture phases of the products life cycle. Unfortunately, the product went all the way through the system without anybody asking the right question, learning about the deficiency, and thus doing something about it.

In order to counter the rising trend in losses resulting from product defects and cope with the tasks of providing product safety assurances, the manufacturer must establish a well-integrated cooperative system, within his organization, capable of assuring the highest degree of safety for his manufactured products.

The large firm should consider the impact of its product safety program on a corporate-wide scale. Common to large companies are organizational structures consisting of a single corporate headquarters with numerous divisions, subsidiaries and subordinate corporations, each nearly autonomous and each responsible for its own management and direction. In situations like this, it is imperative that the corporate product safety policy emanate from the parent corporation, with firm directions provided to guide the operation of subsidiary programs. Although the safety requirements may vary for each subsidiary, the policy established by the central headquarters should have impact on every aspect of the subsidiaries organization.

The small firm should place the same emphasis on the safety of its products as the larger one. There is, however, one important difference: product liability loss can mean the end of a small firm which lacks the financial resources to absorb the tremendous losses possible today. Although the small company looks toward the insurance company for liability insurance, that in itself is not the total answer. Many of the same product safety program elements employed by the large companies—and discussed in this chapter—must be incorporated into the small company's total operations, if it is going to enjoy the benefits of producing products which are safe. Actually, the small firm, unlike

The Manufacturer's Defense

the large firm, usually finds it easier to develop a close working relationship between management and employees to foster product safety consciousness. With communication problems lessened, the owner of a small firm is able to transmit and reinforce his decisions on a daily basis—seeing to it that everybody knows what is going on and what his roles are in meeting specific objectives.

Elements of a Product Safety Program

A well-rounded program for product safety should include the following elements:

Issuance of Policy Statement

Under the signature of the Chief company executive, a policy statement must be established which will establish specific responsibilities, procedures, and operations relating to the Company's products. The policy statement should delegate appropriate authority to the key people relied on to carry out the product safety mission. Additional information to be conveyed in the policy statement include: specific company objectives for product safety, guidelines for safe product design, product safety test procedures, quality control procedures, final audit procedures, need for product identification systems, and the designation of a coordinator of the product safety program.

The policy statement should be revised periodically to reflect any new changes in the overall systems operation.

Assigning a Coordinator of Product Safety Activities

Critical to the development of any program designed to cope with the issue of product liability is the designation of a person in top management as the overall product safety coordinator. This individual should preferably be an engineer or someone with knowledge of the concept of system safety and hazard control and, of product safety laws and standards. Someone capable of devising a program which will insure the cooperation of all key organizational members. This individual must be capable of evaluating the company's products from the standpoint of how they can cause harm to the consumer and of perceiving how consumer carelessness and error, combined with the characteristics of the product, could lead to a death or injury situation.

Develop a System for Identifying and Evaluating Hazards in Products

A typical system for the identification and evaluation of product hazards is shown in Figure 103. The systems approach illustrated in Figure 104 demonstrates the Royal Glove Insurance Company's Plan for a coordinated effort among all the organization's management systems—each obliged to contributing a specific expertise to the overall product safety goal.

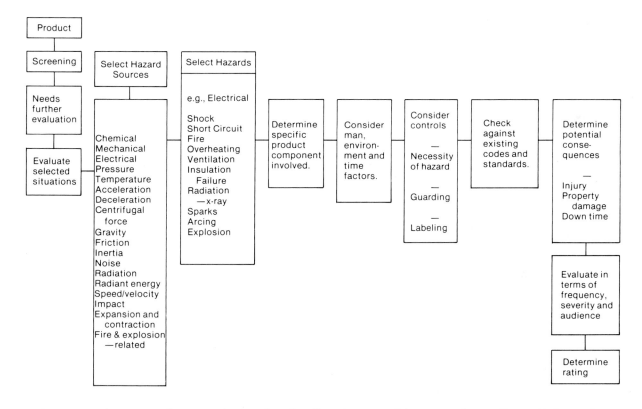

Figure 103. System for identifying and evaluating product hazards. (Reprinted from ASM Report System paper C70-29.3, originally presented at the 1970 ASM Materials Engineering Congress.)

A systematic approach to product safety implies that provision must be made to include a thorough analysis of the product during its entire life cycle—namely its conceptual, engineering development, manufacturing and distribution phases. As a result of the evaluation, inherent product hazards will be identified, and necessary safeguards provided prior to the time the product reaches the consumer.

During the conceptual phase of a product's development, consideration should be given to: the adequacy of design concepts to meet the safety demands of the consumer; comparison of the design against standards established for the product; evaluation of design criteria, proposed hardware materials, etc. The utilization of many systems safety analysis techniques may prove valuable. During the *engineering development phase* of the products' life cycle, consideration is given to the: identification and evaluation of critical production techniques; review of fabrication and assembly procedures; identification and evaluation of testing and inspection requirements; prescription of packaging and warning instructions; establishment of quality control and final audit tests. During the product's *manufacturing phase,* all those involved in the total product safety program must pool their resources and observations toward the objective of locating product hazards and making necessary corrections before the product reaches the hands of the consumer. In this phase, worker involvement in the product safety program is critically important.

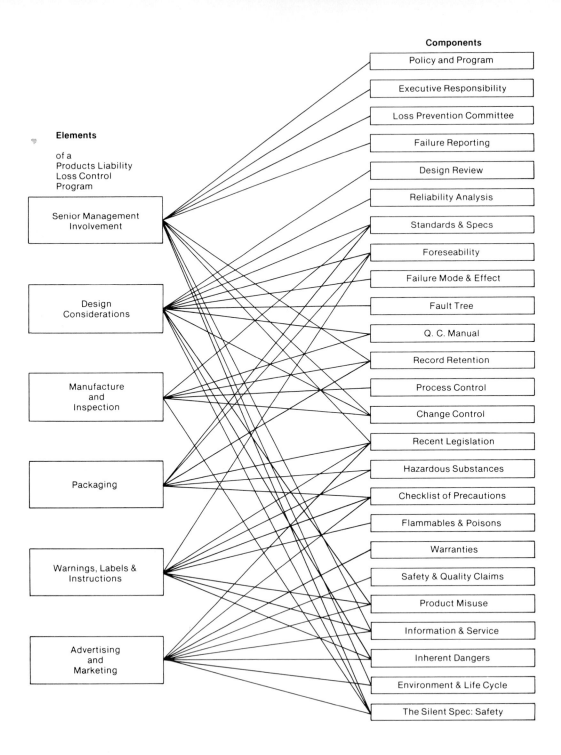

Components

Policy and Program

Executive Responsibility

Loss Prevention Committee

Failure Reporting

Design Review

Reliability Analysis

Standards & Specs

Foreseability

Failure Mode & Effect

Fault Tree

Q. C. Manual

Record Retention

Process Control

Change Control

Recent Legislation

Hazardous Substances

Checklist of Precautions

Flammables & Poisons

Warranties

Safety & Quality Claims

Product Misuse

Information & Service

Inherent Dangers

Environment & Life Cycle

The Silent Spec: Safety

Elements

of a
Products Liability
Loss Control
Program

Senior Management
Involvement

Design
Considerations

Manufacture
and
Inspection

Packaging

Warnings, Labels &
Instructions

Advertising
and
Marketing

When workers are encouraged to detect and report their observations of deviations in product manufacture, materials, techniques, etc. a greater likelihood exists that additional—and often extremely important information—will reach the hands of management in time for corrections to be made, prior to being shipped to the consumer. Prior to the distribution phase of a product's life cycle the product should receive a final test. A real-life simulation of the products' use will often reveal problems which can be countered.

The Product Hazard Analysis technique illustrated on page 313 has been successfully used to record hazard data during the time when a product is being put through tests prior to its delivery to the marketplace. Although the technique was introduced as an aid in investigating a product-related accident (after-the-fact), it is nonetheless a valuable tool to acquire essential hazard data, before the fact. During the *distribution phase,* shipping and packaging plans are adopted and procedures enacted to prevent the product from being harmed en route to the consumer. The proper handling, storage, and transportation of a finished product is a science in its own right. The design of a container in which a product will be stored and shipped is often not an easy task. Awareness must be had of materials which may adversely affect the product under handling, transporting, and shipping conditions, to avoiding the use of materials which might themselves be a safety or health hazard after the product is unpacked. During this phase of a products' life cycle, additional consideration is given to the potential deterioration of materials in the product of its package from exposure to extremes of temperature, humidity, shock, and vibration.

Establishing a Standard of Competence for Product Design Before a Products' Life Cycle Begins

This includes a close evaluation of a products' critical parts and their ability to last beyond a products' expected life; packaging which will help in reducing product damage; provision for adequate warnings, labels, and instructions consistent with hazard awareness and safety; specification of procedures for preparing and recording design reviews; surety that there is minimum risk associated with the use of new materials, and production techniques.

Testing Design Against Standards

Once the product has successfully passed the conceptual and design phases, a prototype should be constructed. The purpose behind this activity is twofold: First, to determine specific requirements for materials, processes, inspection,

Figure 104. Products liability loss prevention plan. (With permission of Royal Globe Insurance Company, N.Y.)

etc., and second, to evaluate the products' performance when subject to the types of failure modes that it will be subjected to by the consumer.

Manufacture and Inspection

At this stage of a product's life cycle a great reliance is placed on quality control, as this function is one of the most critical functions to insure that a product is not being produced with observable flaws, faulty design configurations, or other factors which have the capacity to cause injuries or damage. In addition to the inspection function, Quality Control evaluates all raw materials and sub-contractors or vendors components and parts, as well as maintaining a complete set of records of the product's life cycle including inspections, rejected products and/or materials and test data.

The manufacturer should note that all written communications pertaining to the product, no matter if it be only a—handwritten note, are subject to *"discovery"*—the right of a plaintiff's attorney to request and receive from the manufacturer's files, reports or similar information concerning any aspect of design, testing, manufacturing, or manufacturing control including inspection records, hazard and failure data, control charts, quality and reliability reports, etc.

During the quality control aspects of the program, written instructions for the production of the product are essential. Manufacturing process instructions, quality control inspection and in-process instructions, quality assurance test methods, quality audit test instructions, and any other applicable procedures need to be documented.

Packaging

Before the product is ready to be shipped to its ultimate destination, an analysis of those hazards which may be encountered en route, which have impact on the product's integrity and capacity to harm, must be conducted, and as a result of such analysis, appropriate shipping and packaging plans established.

Warnings and Instructions

This very critical aspect of the overall product safety venture requires that the manufacturer, once the specific danger of the product is determined, sees to it that adequate warnings, and other instructions are provided, to place the consumer in an enlightened position to understand the product's inherent hazardous shortcomings while at the same time explaining what evasive actions are required to avert injuries and other damage. Instructions must be explicit enough to preclude the possibility of misinterpretation. The manufacturer is responsible for warning the consumer of all hazards which cannot be engineered out of the product and which cannot be adequately guarded against.

"The Courts have often ruled that a manufacturer must give appropriate warning of known dangers which the user would not ordinarily discover. The likelihood of an accident taking place and the seriousness of the consequences are always to be considered, with respect to the duty to provide sufficient warning. It must be adequate, since insufficient warning is, in legal effect, no warning. Whether sufficient warning is given depends on the "language used, and the impression which it is calculated to make upon the mind of an average user of the product." Reference should be made to the Federal Hazardous Substances Labeling Act and subsequent regulations published in the Federal Register.[8]

Preparing Advertising

In the preparation of advertisements for the media, messages must be carefully scrutinized to avoid inferences or statements which suggest that misuse of the product is acceptable. Safe product performance must not be countered by attempts to demonstrate the products durability and performance capabilities.

Review of Advertising Literature

In addition to the previously mentioned protections against product liability claims a manufacturer has at his disposal, there are other protections which encompass aspects of advertising and marketing. At that time in the product's life cycle when the manufacturer is prepared to turn it loose on the consumer population, considerable thought needs to be given to the plan and methods by which the product will be marketed and advertised. Primary among the considerations is that those in a selling capacity be attuned to the product's capabilities and limitations to such a degree that they will not purport that the product exceeds the capabilities intended by its designers, nor will they infer that the product's inherent hazards are safeguarded when they are not. A thorough review of all manufacturer specifications and other printed sales documents should be reviewed, to ascertain that no claims are made which cannot be supported, or even worse, that no claims are made for things which cannot be substantiated.

Legal Counsel Review of Warranties and Guarantees

Provisions should be made for a very careful review of warrantees, guarantees, disclaimers, exculpatory clauses, etc. by the legal staff to ascertain their accuracy, validity, and that the consumer is not being mislead into believing that the product is safe when there is reason to want him to understand otherwise.

Establishing Product Identification Systems and Maintaining Records of Product Distribution

In the event a product or one of its components or parts, through an oversight in manufacturing or because of a lack of sufficient experience data, proves to be defective, and hazardous, such components or parts must be located and recalled for upgrading or replacement. To counter this problem, the manufacturer must devise a system to readily identify the product system and its parts, so they can be readily located. In recalling products after sale, the manufacturer has three options: (1) he can contact the consumer directly—providing he has their names and addresses (reason for establishing and maintaining a buyer identification system); (2) he can contact them through their distributors, providing the distributors have maintained a record of product sale; (3) in lieu of no other alternative, he can attempt to contact the consumer through the public news media.

The Role of the Hazard Control Specialist in Product Safety

The job of hazard and risk reduction, whether it pertains to the industrial process in general, or specifically to those products generated by it, must rely on a coordinated effort of the entire organization to carry the burden. Although each member of the management and worker teams is tasked with certain involvement in the overall product safety mission, one member of the management team, who can add significant contribution to the program, is the company's hazard control specialist. The work activity involved in plant safety is in many instances very compatible to product safety itself. A question that often arises concerns the issue of where industrial hazard control stops and product safety begins. In reality, such a split in program missions is not clearly made, although it can be agreed that certain designated functions are fairly much in one camp or another. The fact remains that the two missions have a lot in common. A case in point may help to illustrate this compatibility between functions. Several years ago a toy company manufactured a plastic rifle which was capable of producing a cloud of white smoke. After the toy was unleashed on the public, it was determined after many complaints, that the "smoke" contained silica—a health hazard. While the problem of the toy's potential to cause harm to children confronted the manufacturer from the liability standpoint, another question entered the picture. What affect had the silica had on the workers during the manufacturing process? If there had been a hazard control specialist working for the company, and if he had determined that silica dust was a health hazard to workers and should be either eliminated or controlled, he might have, at the same time, been able to point out to management the likelihood of problems they might encounter down the road, when the product fell into the hands of the consumer. The hazard control specialist, by virtue of his knowledge of locating failure modes, extracting and evaluating hazard data, choosing solution alternatives for hazard reduction or elimination, and utilizing standards and monitoring methods to insure acceptable system performance, is in a position to add a significant contribution to the overall product safety effort. With some modification to the in-plant hazard control objectives, the hazard control specialist can utilize his staff most effectively, to aid those other management groups which have responsibility for the safety of company products. Staying on top of changes in the product liability laws and the current proven methods to acquire hazard information from products, along with aiding the company with product hazard analyses, the hazard control specialist can and will be of significant benefit towards the overall company goal of—producing safe products.

Guide for Assessing Product Safety Needs[9]

1. What are the in-house product design capabilities?
2. What standards or codes apply to the product?
3. Are those standards or codes used as a minimum?
4. Does the company maintain a current reference library concerning those standards or codes which apply to their products?
5. Does the company belong to any organizations or societies which contribute to the development of standards or codes?
6. Are new product designs analyzed from a safety standpoint?
7. Is foreseeable/reasonable product abuse or misuse considered in the safety analysis?
8. How is the analysis documented?
9. Are prototypes or models produced and tested?
10. What problems exist in communications between design and production?
11. Are outside testing agencies used?
12. When design and development work is contracted out, how are such consultants selected?
13. Are their specific insurance requirements specified for outside consultants?
14. If manufacturing to a customer's specifications, is the final use of the product determined?
15. Is a key engineer trained in proper handling of litigation and in how to function as an expert witness?
16. Determine the extent of the quality control program's involvement as it pertains to:
    a. purchased materials or components.
    b. materials in-process.
    c. finished goods.
17. Review quality control records in relation to each of the above and determine what major shortcomings have been uncovered through quality control.

18. When was the quality control program last updated and by whom?
19. Is there a formalized action plan to deal with nonconforming materials, components or products?
20. Who determines when variations from given standards will be allowed?
21. Is company capable of performing all quality control tests inhouse?
22. If outside laboratories are used, how are delays in test results handled?
23. Is there a system to provide for regular, documented calibration of testing instruments, gauges, and equipment in accordance with recognized standards?
24. Is quality control responsible for final sign off or approval to ship the product?
25. What happens when products are shipped before quality control tests are complete?
26. What training has been given to quality control personnel as regards product safety?
27. How are conflicts between production or product design departments handled?
28. Determine ability to trace defective products back to individual inspectors.

Useful Legal Terms and Their Meanings

actionable   The breach of any legal duty that will form the basis of a remedy by action.

Ad damnum clause   A clause in a declaration or complaint of the plaintiff that makes the demand for damages and sets out the amount.

Ad Hoc   Latin words meaning, "for this." An ad hoc refers to a limited or particular situation. An ad hoc decision means, for this purpose only. An ad hoc committee is one limited to a special purpose. An ad hoc attorney is one appointed to do a special task in a particular case.

Adjudicate   The exercise of judicial power by hearing, trying, and determining the claims of litigants before the court.

Affidavit   A voluntary statement of facts formally reduced to writing, sworn to, or affirmed before, some officer authorized to administer oaths. Such officer is usually a notary public.

A fortiori   Latin words meaning "by a stronger reason." The phrase is often used in judicial opinions to say that, since specific proven facts lead to a certain conclusion, there are for this reason other facts that logically follow which make stronger the argument for the conclusion.

Agent   An agent is a person authorized to act for another (a principal). The term may apply to a person in the service of another, but in the strict sense an agent is one who stands in place of his principal. A works for B as a gardener and is thus a servant; but he may be an agent. If A sells goods for B, he becomes more than a servant. He acts in the place of B.

A priori   A generalization resting on presuppositions and not proven facts.

Authority   The power of government as evidenced by an executive order, by legislation, or by the decision of a court.

Bad faith   The term means "actual intent" to mislead or deceive another. It does not mean misleading by an honest, inadvertent, or careless misstatement.

Carelessness   A word sometimes used synonymously with "negligence." It means lack of ordinary care, i.e., lack of such care as a man of diligence and care would exercise under the particular circumstances.

Case   The term used to name a cause of action in a court of law or equity. Any issue which is to be heard, tried, and decided by a judicial tribunal may be called a case.

Case (action on)   The term distinguishes between a common-law action used as a remedy for damages resulting from the indirect consequences of a tort and a cause of action used to collect damages resulting from the direct result of a tort. Damages caused by a patent infringement would be a basis for "action on the case." The immediate damages caused by A striking B's car would give rise to a remedy in trespass, not case.

Case law   The law as found in cased decided by the courts. Through what is called "common law judicial process," the courts, by deciding cases, evolve legal principles that become law. This law is called "unwritten law," as distinguished from laws passed by Congress, state legislatures, and city councils.

Cause of action   When one's legal rights have been invaded either by breach of a contract or by a breach of a legal duty toward one's person or property, a cause of action has been created.

Caveat   A warning enjoining from certain acts or practices; an explanation to prevent misinterpretation; a legal warning to a judicial officer to suspend a proceeding until ths opposition has a hearing.

Caveat emptor   These words express an old idea at common law—"let the buyer beware"—and mean that when goods are sold without an express warranty by the vendor as to their quality and capacity for a particular use and purpose, the buyer must take the risk of loss as to all defects in the goods. The rule of caveat emptor applies at judicial sales. The buyer takes no better title than that held by the debtor or defendant.

Caveat venditor   These words mean "let the seller beware" (in contradistinction to caveat emptor "let the buyer beware"). Caveat venditor means that unless the seller by express language disclaims any responsibility, he shall be liable to the buyer if the goods delivered are different in kind, quality, use, and purpose from those described in the contract of sale.

Chattel   The word "chattel" is derived from the word "cattle." It is a very broad term and includes every kind of property that is not real property. Movable properties, such as horses, automobiles, choses in action, stock certificates, bills of lading, and all "goods, wares, and merchandise," are chattels personal. Chattels real concern real property, such as a lease for years—in which case the lessee owns a chattel real. A building placed on real property by a lessee is a chattel real.

Circumstantial evidence   If from certain facts and circumstances, according to the experience of mankind, an ordinary, intelligent person may infer that other connected facts and circumstances must necessarily exist, the latter facts and circumstances are considered proven by circumstantial evidence. Proof of fact A from which fact B may be inferred is proof of fact B by circumstantial evidence.

Civil Action   A proceeding in a law court or a suit in equity by one person against another for the enforcement or protection of a private right or the prevention of a wrong. It includes actions on contract, ex delicto, and all suits in equity. Civil action is in contradistinction to criminal action in which the state prosecutes a person for breach of a duty.

Claim   A claim in a legal sense is a request by one person against another for the recovery of money or property. Such request must arise out of a right one person has against another, to do, or forbear to do, some act or thing as a matter of duty. A debt is a claim for money. A true owner claims the right to title and possessions of property. 'A' claims damages because of an injury to his person by B.

Claimant   One who makes a claim. One who files a claim against a deceased person's estate. A creditor who files a claim against an insolvent debtor's estate. A material man who files a claim under the mechanics' lien law is a claimant.

Code   A collection or compilation of the statutes passed by the legislative body of a state. Such codes are often annotated with citations of cases decided by the State Supreme Courts. These decisions construe the statutes. Examples—Oregon Compiled Laws Annotated, United States Code Annotated.

Damages   A sum of money the court imposed upon a defendant as compensation for the plaintiff because the defendant has injured the plaintiff by breach of a legal duty.

Dealer   One who makes a business of dealing; a merchant, broker, factor. One who buys and sells "goods, wares, and merchandise."

Deceit   A term to define that conduct in a business transaction by which one man, through fraudulant representations, misleads another who has a right to rely on such representations as the truth, or, who by reason of an unequal station in life, has no means of detecting such fraud.

Decision (judicial)   The word "decision" may mean a final judgment of a court of last resort, a conclusion of law or facts, the opinion of the court, or the report of the court. Generally speaking, a decision means the judgment of the court as to the disposition of the case—for the plaintiff, for the defendant, or for neither. Decision must be distinguished from opinion. An opinion of the court constitutes the reasons given for its decision or judgment. The report of the case is a printing of the opinion and decision.

Declaration   At common law, a word used to name the plaintiff's first pleading in which are set out the facts upon which the cause of action is based. The word "complaint" is used synonymously with declaration.

Defendant   A person who has been sued in a court of law; the person who answers the plaintiff's complaint. The word is applied to the defending party in civil actions. In criminal actions, the defending party is referred to as the accused.

Defense The word "defense" applies to all methods of procedure used by the defendant and to all facts alleged by way of denial by the defendant in his response to the plaintiff's complaint. Demurrers, set-offs, pleas in abatement, answers, denial, confession, and avoidance are procedural means of defense.

Dictum An expression of an idea, argument, or rule in the written opinion of a judge that has no bearing on the issues involved and that is not essential for their determination. It lacks the force of a decision in a judgment.

Directed verdict If it is apparent to reasonable men and the court that the plaintiff by his evidence has not made out his case, the court may instruct the jury to bring in a verdict for defendant or himself direct a verdict for the defendant. If, however, different inferences may be drawn from the evidence by reasonable men, then the court cannot direct a verdict.

Discretion A privilege of a judge, in absense of a definite rule of law, to decide a case upon its merits in light of what is fair, right, just, and equitable under the circumstances of the particular case.

Due Care The words express that standard of conduct which is exercised by an ordinary, reasonable, prudent person. See 'Negligence.'

Equity Because the law courts in early English law did not always give an adequate remedy, an aggrieved party sought redress from the king. Since this appeal was to the king's conscience, he referred the case to his spiritual adviser, the chancellor. The chancellor decided the case according to rules of fairness, honesty, right, and natural justice. From this there developed the rules in equity. The laws of trusts, divorce, rescission of contracts for fraud, injunction, and specific performance are enforced in courts of equity.

Error A mistake in fact or law committed by the court in the trial of a case that may be the basis of an appeal to a higher court. The admitting of improper evidence is "error of law occurring at the trial." Assumption that a fact exists when it does not is error of fact.

Exception An objection taken by an attorney at a trial because of some ruling made by the court upon a matter of law. It forms the basis of an appeal to a higher court.

Exemplary Damages   A sum assessed by the jury in a tort action (over and above the compensatory damages) as punishment in order to make an example of the wrongdoer and to deter like conduct by others. Injuries caused by willful, malicious, wanton, and reckless conduct will subject the wrongdoers to exemplary damages.

Express warranty   When a seller makes some positive representation concerning the nature, quality, character, use, and purpose of goods, which induces the buyer to buy, and the seller intends the buyer to rely thereon, the seller has made an express warranty.

Facts in Issue   Those facts in the particular case upon which the party, either plaintiff or defendant, rests his legal right to remedy or defense.

Fraud   An intentional misrepresentation of the truth for the purpose of deceiving another person. The elements of fraud are: (1) false representation of fact, not opinion, intentionally made; (2) intent that the deceived person act thereon; (3) knowledge that such statements would naturally deceive; and (4) that the deceived person acted to his injury.

Gross negligence   The lack of even slight or ordinary care.

Inference   A deduction or conclusion from known facts.

Injunction   A writ of judicial process issued by a court of equity by which a party is required to do a particular thing or to refrain from doing a particular thing.

Interlocutory decree   A decree of a court of equity that does not settle the complete issue, but settles only some intervening part, awaiting a final decree.

Joint-tort-feasors   When two persons commit an injury with a common intent, they are joint tort-feasors.

Label   The term is broader than "trademark" in that it particularly includes a general description of the goods and indicates the source of the chattel.

Latent defect   A defect in materials not discernible by examination. Used in contradistinction to patent defect which is discernible.

Liability   In its broadest legal sense, the word means any obligation one may be under by reason of some rule of law. It includes debt, duty, and responsibility.

Misrepresentation   The affirmative statement or affirmation of a fact that is not true: the term does not include concealment of true facts or non-disclosure or the mere expression of opinion.

Mistake of law   An erroneous conclusion of the legal effect of known facts.

Negligence   The failure to do that which an ordinary, reasonable, prudent man would do, or the doing of some act which an ordinary, prudent man would not do. Reference must always be made to the situation, the circumstances, and the knowledge of the parties.

Nonsuit   A judgment given against the plaintiff when he is unable to prove his case or fails to proceed with the trial after the case is at issue.

Opinion   An opinion is a conviction founded upon probable evidence. In a strict legal sense, the opinion of a court is the reason the court gives for its decision. See 'Decision.'

Ordinary care   That care that a prudent man would take under the circumstances of the particular case.

Patent ambiguity   An uncertainty in a written instrument that is obvious upon reading.

Pendente lite   A Latin phrase which means ''pending during the progress of a suit at law.''

Per curiam   A decision by the full court in which no opinion is given.

Plaintiff   In an action at law, the complaining party or the one who commences the action is called the plaintiff. He is the person who seeks a remedy in court.

Precedent   A previously-decided case that can serve as an authority to help decide a present controversy. The use of such case is called the doctrine of "stare decisis," which means to adhere to decided cases and settled principles. Literally, "to stand as decided."

Preponderance   Preponderance of the evidence means that evidence which in the judgement of the jurors in entitled to the greatest weight, which appears to be more credible, has greater force, and overcomes not only the opposing presumptions, but also the opposing evidence.

Privity   Mutual and successive relationship to the same interest. Offeror and offeree, assignor and assignee, grantor and grantee are in privity. Privity of estate means that one takes title from another. In contract law, privity denotes parties in mutual legal relationship to each other by virtue of being promisees and primisors. At early common law, third party beneficiaries and assignees were said to be not in "privity."

Proximate cause   The cause that sets other causes in operation. The responsible cause of an injury.

Punitive damages   Damages by way of punishment allowed for an injury caused by a wrong that is willful and malicious.

Ratify   To ratify means to confirm or approve.

Reasonable care   The care that prudent persons would exercise under the same circumstances.

Re-insurance   A contract of re-insurance is where one insurance company agrees to indemnify another insurance company in whole or in part against risks which the first company has assumed. The original contract of insurance and the re-insurance contract are distinct contracts. There is no privity between the original insured and the re-insurer.

Remand   To send back a cause from the appellate court to the lower court in order that the lower court may comply with the instructions of the appellate court. Also to return a prisoner to jail.

Remedy   The word is used to signify the judicial means or court procedures by which legal and equitable rights are enforced.

Remise   The word means discharge or release. It is also synonymous with "quit claim."

Special verdict   A special verdict is one in which the jury finds the facts only, leaving it to the court to apply the law and draw the conclusion as to the proper disposition of the case.

Stare decisis   Translated, the term means "stand by the decision." The law should adhere to decided cases. See 'Precedent.'

Statute   A law passed by the legislative body of a state is a statute.

Suit   The term refers to any type of legal proceeding for the purpose of obtaining a legal remedy; the term "suit" generally applies to "suit in equity," whereas, at law, the term is "action at law."

Tort   A wrongful act committed by one person against another person or his property. It is the breach of a legal duty imposed by law other than by contract. The word tort means "twisted" or "wrong." 'A' assaults 'B,' thus committing a tort.

Trial   A proceeding by the properly authorized officials into the examination of the facts and for the purpose of determining an issue presented according to proper rules of law.

Verdict   The decision of a jury, reported to the court, on matters properly submitted to it for its consideration.

Warranty   An undertaking, either expressed or implied, that a certain fact regarding the subject matter of a contract is presently true or will be true. The word has particular application in the law of sales of chattels. The word relates to title and quality. The word should be distinguished from "guaranty" which means a contract or promise by one person to answer for the performance of another.

Bibliography   Anderson, R. T., "Product Safety: Analysis and Control," Technical Note PS + R – 100 ITT Research Institute, November 1971.

Bruce, R., "The Consumer's Guide to Product Safety," Award Books, New York, 1971.

Byington, S. J., "Prospectives in Product Safety," *Professional Safety,* May 1977.

"A Capsule History of Product Liability," Occupational Hazards, Executive Report-ER 11, 1976.

Clements, R., "Product Liability," Viewpoint, Marsh and McLennan Companies Quarterly, 1977.

"Consumer Sounding Boards," *Professional Safety,* May 1977.

Firenze, R. J., "Tomorrow's Product Safety Specialist," National Safety News, January 1974.

Hammer, W., "Handbook of System and Product Safety," Prentice-Hall, 1972.

Leight, W. G., "Product Safety, In What Direction Should We Be Going?" Professional Safety, May 1977.

Manuele, F. A., "The Elements of a Product Loss Control Plan," Viewpoint, Marsh and McLennan Companies Quarterly, 1977.

O'Sullivan, J. F., "Problems of Small Businesses in Obtaining Products Liability Insurance," Viewpoint, Marsh and McLennan Companies Quarterly, 1977.

Peters, G. A., "Product Liability and Safety," Coiner Publications, LTD., Washington, D.C., 1971.

"Product Liability," Executive Action Series, #143, Bureau of Business Practice, Waterford, Conn. 06385.

"Safety in the Marketplace," National Business Council for Consumer Affairs, April 1973.

Notes

1. A Capsule History of Product Liability," Occupational Hazards, Executive Report-ER 11, 1976.
2. Product Liability, Executive Action Series, Bureau of Business Practices, Waterford, Conn. 1971.
3. "Product Liability," Executive Action Series, #143, Bureau of Business Practice, Waterford, Conn. 1971.
4. Viewpoint, Marsh and McLennan Companies Quarterly, 1977. "Problems of Small Businesses in Obtaining Product Liability" Insurance by John F. O. O'Sullivan.
5. J. E. DuBois, and T. R. White, "Product Liability—The Pendulum Swings," ASSE Journal, Mar. 1968.
6. R. Bruce, "The Consumer's Guide to Product Safety" Award Book, N.Y., 1971 from Corwin D. Edwards—University of Oregon.
7. R. Bruce, "The Consumer's Guide to Product Safety" Award Book, N.Y., 1971 from Corwin D. Edwards—University of Oregon.
8. L. Faulkner, "Safety Professionals' Role in Product Safety," ASSE Journal, March 1968.
9. With permission of Marsh and MacLennan, Inc.

Labor-Management Relations in Hazard Control 11

Throughout this book a theme has been reinforced many times. It deals with the need for a cooperative effort which must be developed between the hazard control specialist and the other members of his or her organization. Through this cooperative spirit, prejudices are reduced, respect for individual contribution is increased, and important, necessary things get done.

While cooperation between the hazard control specialist and the management systems in his or her organization is critical to the success of any hazard control program, there is another dimension of cooperation that is equally critical, namely the cooperation between labor and management.

The controversial passage of the OSHA Act, enacted into the law of the land in 1970, provoked many stresses between labor and management. In retrospect, each side established a very rigid position from the onset: Labor on the offensive—management on the defensive. Both groups did all they could to protect their own interests within the limits of the law. Many confrontations occurred. Each group argued its positions informally, legislatively, and through litigation. Over all, a vast amount of energy, dollars, and time was spent, in an attempt to reach compromises on what had to be done, how it would be done, and who would do it. During this period of ironing issues out, one thing became very clear, workers were still injured, diseased, and dying, as a result of exposure to hazards in the workplace. It was also clear to labor and management that neither side was going to solve the problem of controlling hazards in the workplace by themselves. The job was an extensive one. They realized that only through a joint effort would full benefits of death, injury and illness reduction become a reality.

This Chapter deals with several important issues pertaining to labor/management relationships in hazard control. Among these issues are: joint procedures for inspecting the workplace; education and training of representatives of labor and management to mutually form knowledgeable and functional teams who can perform adequately in their roles of hazard identification, evaluation and control; specific contract language in collective bargaining agreements where they exist; and labor and management consultations on standards adoption, modification, and deletion.

Cooperation in Enforcing the Law

With the passage of the OSH Act and its subsequent regulations came the concommitant obligation of both labor and management to put forth effort in reducing or eliminating hazards in the workplace. The Company was ordered to make reasonable provisions for the safety and health of its employees during the hours of their employment. At the same time, the Union and workers were obliged to recognize their responsibilities as well as their rights under the law.

An examination of employer and employee responsibilities under the Act points up just how critical a joint-effort is, in transforming a list of requirements into a viable program for accomplishing needed results.

Employer's Obligations

To fulfill their duty of furnishing a safe and healthy workplace, all employers covered by the Act, in addition to providing a workplace free from recognizable hazards, must provide certain information to their employees. This information includes: *Protections and obligations of employees under the OSH Act.* (With the worker knowing his or her role in the program and how much he or she will be relied on to make the hazard control program work, communication and cooperation between the employees and the employer will be established. Such a cooperative spirit will form the basis for a viable joint effort). This will develop providing the opportunity is given for employees to equally participate in monitoring, measuring and evaluating their exposure to toxic chemicals and harmful physical agents. In so doing, the employer accomplishes three things. First, he draws the employees closer into the hazard control program by involving them in the hazard assessment process. Second, with the employees or their representatives involved as observers of the monitoring and measuring process, it is more likely that, should the data be agreeable, the employees or their representatives will support management in the adoption of new procedures to correct the hazardous situation. Third, the more often employees or their representatives participate in monitoring and measuring procedures, the more knowledgeable they become of the details concerning the capabilities and limitations of monitoring and measuring worker exposure. As their knowledge increases, the more viable their recommendations and inputs to the total hazard control program becomes. *Notification must be given to any worker who has been or is exposed to excessive toxic materials or harmful physical agents, and notification to that employee of the corrective action being taken must be followed up.* (It is here that the system of cooperation is tested to its fullest. The potential for hazards occurring in the workplace is reasonably high. New materials, new processes, new knowledge of the hazards of materials which have been used for many years, etc., are problems which the employer must solve on a continuous basis. Given that hazardous materials must often be used in the workplace, the employer, by making all information known to each of his workers, accomplishes three objectives. First, he provides the worker with information which can be used in diagnosis by the worker's physician.

Second, the employer demonstrates intent to correct hazards as they arise. Third, the employer establishes the logic behind the necessity for new controls and the participation necessary by the employees to make the controls work. Management should post labels or other types of warning to ensure that employees are informed of all hazards to which they are exposed. This includes relevant symptoms and when appropriate, the recommended medical treatment, and proper precautions. This requirement, even when met, does not always solve the problem at hand. There may be instances where the very nature of the work sets-up hazards which cannot be adequately corrected using conventional methods. The employer and employees may not be able to produce a workable answer. The employees may not accept a less than adequate solution. A perfect case for example, involves a suitable means of protecting Ironworkers during the phase of construction requiring the connecting of structural steel. Conventional life lines and safety belts do not readily lend themselves to this type of work mode. In fact, they can actually precipitate accident situations. In a case like this, and there are many others, a compromise must be made. Here, cooperation is critical. Each side may have to take less than they would like to have—from the standpoint of production—in order to get the job done.

Since there is less protection, the work pace or rate must be modified accordingly to compensate for the employees inability to reach the original production standard. In cases like this one, management must be willing to accept lower production in order to assure the safety of its employees. It is important that management, in addition to accepting lower production, communicate their understanding and acceptance of the problem to the employees.

If the employees and management both know and understand that production is secondary to safety in a high hazard endeavor, then the mental strain of equal production is reduced. It is crucial that both sides evaluate the issue together, decide on the benefits vs. the costs associated with the control of the hazard, and reach a conclusion satisfactory to both sides. An important factor emerging from this situation is that labor and management—together—establish their own standard to satisfy their needs at hand. In doing so they are able to confront the lawmakers with a rationale for a better regulation which would address their hazard more effectively, or the need for a variance to govern their particular situation; *providing employees with the results of any medical examination or tests made at employer's expense in connection with occupational health and/or safety.* Here a great amount of discretion must be placed. From both a moral as well as a legal standpoint, the employer must appraise his or her workers about all medical tests and diagnostic results. Such data, once in the hands of the employee, can be a highly valuable aid to his physician in assessing and drawing conclusions about his health. On the other hand, the communication of an employee's health information is not a one-way deal—only traveling from employee to his or her physician. Maximum utilization of the data is realized only when the employer learns about the general consequences of employee exposures and uses this information to upgrade his workplace. This open distribution of information between management and worker is another critical link in the total program of joint-efforts toward improving the safety and health of workers. However, one important issue needs to be discussed: the problem associated with maintaining the confidentiality of information between the employer and the employees. In many instances, for reasons private to the worker, they do not want their medical data openly disclosed to anyone but their physicians. Not only do the employees want their medical data associated with a job-related health problem kept confidential from anyone but their employers, they want assurances that their employer be privileged to only information which is pertinent to a job-related problem. They want their general medical information to remain a confidential, private matter between themselves and their physicians regardless of who pays the physician's bills. A recent U.S. District Court decision upheld the right of government investigators to gain access to medical records and work histories of past and present employees at DuPont's West Virginia plant under authority of the Occupational Safety and Health Act. While collecting and using medical data for the benefit of employees is mandatory if occupational illness reduction will ever be realized, the issue of protecting employee's right of confidentiality must be continuously considered. Many compromises will have to be made on all sides, in order to produce the data for needed improvements.

Worker's Obligations

The OSH Act charges employees with certain responsibilities for their own and their fellow workers safety and health. Among these responsibilities are that a worker must:

1. Not deface or remove posted notices which prohibit use of unsafe machinery or equipment or entry to an unsafe area.
2. Obey approved safety and health notices prohibiting the use of unsafe equipment or entry to unsafe areas which are posted by the federal government, the state OSHA agency, or the employer. In this regard, it must be understood that these areas must be mutually agreed on by labor and management. Employers cannot arbitrarily make unilateral

safety rules and regulations that may differ from state or federal OSHA.

3. Not remove, displace, damage, destroy or carry off any approved safety device, safeguard, notice or warning furnished for use in any place of employment.
4. Must not interfere with the use of any safety device or safeguards mutually agreed to. This applies to methods, processes, and employer orders. Unilateral employer orders are unacceptable!!!
5. Must not interfere with the use of any method or process adopted for the protection of any employee, including himself or herself.
6. Must not fail or neglect to do everything reasonably necessary to protect the life, safety, and health of fellow employees.
7. Must comply with all occupational safety and health standards, rules, regulations, which are applicable to actions and conduct on the job.

In each of the listed employee obligations under the OSH Law, it is evident that unless the employee is willing to cooperate with approved and acceptable rules and procedures for hazard control (unless of course, circumstances demonstrate a rational reason not to) then there is a very real limit to how many deaths, injuries, and illnesses will be reduced in the workplace.

Cooperation and the Filing of Complaints

Under the Act, the worker has the right to lodge a complaint with the government for a suspected safety or health hazard. Such legitimate complaints, should lead to an inspection of the employer's workplace.

If there was a single factor which has hindered cooperation between labor and management, worker safety and health complaints would head the list. While this provision in the law has a definite use, and may be the only recourse a worker has to obtain necessary action, indiscriminate use of the complaint provision can prove to be counterproductive. When an employee files a complaint without attempting corrective action first through the normal chain of command, a situation is created not conducive to a cooperative effort. Second, filing complaints indiscriminately has proven counterproductive by preventing the Federal OSH Compliance Inspectors from devoting their time to workplaces that have high risk and hazard situations. This has happened in several regions of the United States. In the past five years, many employers, in generally good compliance with OSH regulations, were being inspected more often than most of their counterparts who had more hazardous workplaces and never saw a federal inspector.

Organized labor has taken a giant step forward in attempting to maintain an employee's right to file safety and health complaints while at the same time doing everything possible to reduce the strains and maintain a cooperative effort between labor and management. The Building and Construction Trades Department—AFL-CIO, has established a model formula to guide its seventeen affiliated unions in filing worker complaints. Below is a summary of the Building and Construction Trades Department's recommended procedures for rectifying safety and health hazards.

Model Procedures for Rectifying Hazards in the Workplace

Steps to follow when a hazard is observed

1. If the hazard is within the authority of the craftsman, he or she should take steps to personally solve the problem. This may include talking to the craft foreman if appropriate.

If the situation is not corrected

2. The craftsman should bring the hazard to the attention of the craft steward. The steward should try to correct the problem by working with job supervisors.

If the situation is not corrected

3. The craft steward should inform the Business Agent (BA). The Business Aqent should try to resolve the issue with the Project Management, Failing this, the BA, depending on local union policy, should inform the Business Manager.

If the situation is not corrected

4. The Business Manager, depending on the nature and immenency of the hazard, should bring the matter to the Local Building Trades Council. The Council should meet with the Project Management to resolve the situation.

If the situation is not corrected

5. With the recommendation of the Building and Construction Trades Council and Local Unions, a formal OSHA complaint should be filed with OSHA.

If OSHA fails to correct the situation

6. The Building and Construction Trades Department and International Unions should be asked to bring the matter before the Secretary of Labor through the appropriate area, regional or national office.

What the Building and Construction Trades Department has done, through the issuance of its complaint procedures, is to place greater emphasis on solving safety and health problems within the construction industry by the people—both labor and management—who have the most experience and expertise in construction along with the knowledge of coping with the hazards associated with it.

The inspection process holds one of the keys to the establishment and maintenance of a true cooperative spirit between labor and management.

Over the past few years, some unions have carefully bargained, into their agreements with management, special clauses which call for the establishment of joint safety and health committees. As a result of negotiations for safety and health, union leaders have had significant impact on stimulating management to develop new safety and health programs and/or foster their existing ones.

Cooperation in Inspections

A joint labor/management safety and health committee should serve an important role in the total hazard control program. Organized properly, given adequate direction and support, the joint committee will return high dividends for the resources committed.

Joint Safety and Health Committees

The joint committee concept is cooperative in nature. From the viewpoint of the employer and the employees, the committee concept provides the opportunity for employees to become personally involved in and make positive contribution to the company's hazard control program. In addition, the joint committee concept serves as the forum for the discusssion of suggested changes in programs or rules and potential new hazards. Most important is the cooperative effort created by the committee which encourages workers to communicate problems to management without fear of reprisals.

Generally, the committee serves in an advisory capacity and to a practical extent, observes the following guidelines:

1. Advise both management and labor concerning issues of safety and health matters other than complaints or grievances.
2. Schedule meetings monthly or other agreed time intervals for the sole purpose of discussing issues relevant to safety and health hazards in the workplace. It is mandatory that minutes be recorded for each meeting and copies provided for the committee members as soon after the meeting as possible. Segments of each meeting should be devoted to: reviewing and evaluating the activities of the preceding month, keeping aware of accomplishments, new problems encountered, and new issues which have impact on collective activities, etc. Prior to meetings, the chairperson or designee shall coordinate an inspection to be made of mutually selected areas of the workplace. At the conclusion of the inspection, a written report should be prepared by the inspector setting forth the findings to the committee. A copy of the report should be furnished to the Union representative and the Company's hazard control specialist.
3. The joint committee should provide advice and recommended alternatives for the solution of hazardous situations along with sup-

porting ideas for their implementation. These should be submitted to the appropriate management authority for consideration and follow-up action as necessary. The Committee should record each of its recommendations by type, date, and persons *provided with recommendation.*

4. Review safety and health matters raised by members of the Bargaining Unit.

5. Review published company safety and health reports and develop other data which would be useful in identifying accident sources and injury trends. In addition, the Committee should consider and offer ways of improving the workability of company safety and health rules and regulations on the job.

6. Committees can assist, under the direction of the hazard control specialist (if one exists), in conducting accident investigations.

7. Monitor the workplace and serve or assist in the role of safety and health inspectors, directing their efforts towards detecting hazardous physical conditions and unsafe work methods.

8. Encourage workers to abide by procedures established jointly by the committee for their safety and health.

9. From an educational and training standpoint, promote and evaluate in-house training and education programs in hazard recognition and control and first-aid training for workers and their supervisors.

10. Be available for consultation when the company proposes to introduce new items of personal protective and safety equipment and for the purpose of establishing agreement on the selection of the particular item and strategy. They should support the employers and employees joint endeavors by gaining the cooperation of the workers involved.

11. Recommend ideas to modify or delete the use of safety devices and protective equipment in the workplace in order to arrive at a more effectively hazard-controlled situation.

12. From the standpoint of maintaining a perspective on the success or failure of the Company's attempts at hazard control, the Company should keep the Committee informed of accident, injury, illness, and loss data. Such data, and data trends can be compared with the data acquired by the Committee and will form the basis for further inquiry.

13. The Committee, through their combined experiences and knowledge of their crafts, including their knowledge of how hazards are caused in their workplace, are in an exceptional position to offer suggestions pertaining to the use and enforcement of certain standards, justification for requesting variances from others, and setting and adopting additional standards of their own which will guarantee the existence of a workplace where hazards are controlled to an acceptable level.

Although the usefulness of the joint-committee cannot be emphasized enough, there are two points which need to be underscored.

First, even though management has the prime responsibility of conducting and owning up to the results of safety and health inspections, the existence of joint labor/management inspection teams suggests equal responsibility for recommendations made and actions taken. For the protection of both sides, before any final agreements are reached, it is mandatory that the committee's analyses and recommendations be reviewed and confirmed by those with sufficient expertise in the specialty areas involved e.g., industrial hygiene, electrical safety, etc.

Second, and crucial to the organization, members of the joint-committee must be adequately educated on the purposes and methods of the inspection process and be trained in the use of survey and inspection instruments. At this step, the hazard control specialist plays a key role, being in a position to instruct and counsel the joint-committee. An active role in the committee's daily duties is discouraged. However, the hazard control specialist should establish a relationship with the committee whereby open communication exists. More often than not, hazardous situations and other problems uncovered by the joint-committee can be solved with the cooperation of the hazard control specialist, without having the problems ever reach top management.

Recent studies demonstrate the traits of joint-committees which function adequately, as compared to those which do not. This research revealed some interesting data. Those joint-committees which make measurable contribution in controlling hazards in the workplace have the following common characteristics: (1) They use a locally negotiated Collective Bargaining agreement covering one specific plant, as compared to corporate-wide agreements unilaterally applied to all plants throughout the Corporate-wide system; (2) the company employs a staff officer, (a full-time hazard control specialist), who is given necessary authority to make decisions concerning hazard and loss control; (3) layers of supervision are minimized between the hazard control specialist and the chief decision maker; (4) representatives of the company's line management consistently attend and contribute to joint-committee meetings; (5) management demonstrates commitment in the hazard control program by conscientious encouragement of labor and management cooperation and also provides resources to allow the program to function adequately; (6) the union is represented on the joint-committee; (7) "safety" stewards are appointed for each work shift providing continuous worker representation in matters of "safety" and "health"; (8) management and labor exchange a monthly report of issues, problems, etc., which relate to safety and health; (9) a high level of joint problem solving is evidenced by joint-committee decisions and actions; (10) the committee meets every month, and each meeting is preceded by a workplace tour and in-

Characteristics of Committees Which Are Effective

spection; (11) union and management act to translate external safety and health pressures imposed on them into concrete plans of action that become well integrated into the firm's overall policies for safety and health; (12) management conscientiously works at buffering the committee members from the collective bargaining process; (13) management and the union promotes the recruitment and selection of committee members who exhibit a genuine interest in safety and health and who are interested in spending some of their time acquiring the skills necessary to function as committee members.

Characteristics of Committees Which Are Not Effective

In contrast, those joint-committees which are not able to demonstrate favorable impact possess some or all of the following characteristics: (1) the company employs a safety director who operates from a corporate base removed geographically from the local plant; (2) at the local level safety and health matters are handled by a "coordinator" of employer relations who is given little authority for decisions relating to safety and health; (3) many layers of supervision exist between the coordinator of employer relations and the chief decision maker; (4) the "safety director" is directed to preside over the joint-committee; (5) line department heads do not regularly attend joint-meetings; (6) monthly committee meetings are often postponed; (7) committee meetings are perfunctory and do not accomplish a fraction of their capabilities; (8) management gives lip-service to its hazard control program's mission instead of demonstrating an active and assertive role; (9) although there is a strong contract clause for safety and health, the union does not provide a chairperson to preside over its company department safety representatives; (10) poor two-way communication exists between department safety representatives and the rank and file.

Voluntary Self-Inspection Programs

A practical idea, introduced by the State of California and organized labor/management, for establishing cooperation between labor and management in hazard control, is voluntary self-inspection programs aimed at monitoring the workplace.

The California OSHA program (CAL/OSHA) concluded that the governmental inspection/enforcement program alone is not effective in reducing job-related deaths and injuries on construction job-sites because very many deaths and injuries are the result of momentary hazards or behavioral problems. CAL/OSHA also concluded that voluntary employer/employee group programs aimed at locating and eliminating or reducing hazards not normally controlled under the inspection format would make a significant contribution in upgrading job safety and health for workers. CAL/OSHA determined after an extensive study that several classes of construction accidents, not directly related to safety standards, have been relatively unaffected by its compliance activities. Thus, inspection and enforcement efforts alone do not constitute a viable prevention program for the construction industry. CAL/OSHA found further accurate evidence that standards cannot be written to cover every possible hazard in construction. An inspection force cannot monitor all hazards. Compliance inspections in themselves may not motivate employers and workers to police their own workplaces. However, daily and hourly vigilance at the worksite by workers and supervisors is a key factor in controlling hazards. Concluding, CAL/OSHA, attempting to be more effective, realized that it would have to broaden its existing program. Employers and employee groups needed to be encouraged and stimulated to develop jobsite voluntary self-inspection safety and health programs involving employees and supervisors.

The State of California's Department of Finance Study of the concept of "voluntary self-inspection," indicated that injury rates in places of employment vary widely, even in hazardous industries. The difference in rates within an industry group, as a rule, corresponded with the individual plant or jobsite safety program. Programs which seriously involved workers and supervisors in safety committees and special training activities tended to have low injury rates. Those without serious worker and management involvement usually experienced higher rates. A study of safety program practices in high accident versus low accident rate companies by NIOSH[1] described some of the practices which are associated with an effective hazard control program. NIOSH concluded that in general, the low rate companies demonstrated the following characteristics: (1) greater stature and staff commitment given to the director of the company safety effort; (2) greater utilization of outside influences in instilling safety consciousness in workers (this includes involvement of union representatives in the development of safety programs and in accident investigations). (3) multiple use of variety of safety promotional incentive techniques; (4) greater opportunities for general and specialized training with supplemental modes of instruction for all production personnel, e.g., group discussion, lectures by safety specialists; (5) more humanistic approach in disciplining risk takers and violaters of "safety" rules; (6) more frequent though less formal inspections of the workplace as a supplement to or instead of formal inspections at relatively infrequent intervals; (7) a "safety" program emphasizing better balance between engineering and nonengineering approaches toward accident prevention and control; (8) more stable qualities in the make-up of the workforce, i.e., more older married workers with longer time on the job.

California Building Trades/National Constructors Association (NCA) contends that it should be able to adopt a method to promote—on an experimental basis, a pilot program of jobsite self-inspection between companies within the National Constructor Association (NCA), and members of the California Building and Construction Trades Council. Such a program would be designed to cope with the mandatory hazards and the behavioral problems that constitute the basis for a large fraction of job-induced injuries. California, like many other states, legislated their Occupational Safety and Health Act understanding the need for voluntary joint-programs for accident and injury control. Of course, these states have stipulated that mandatory compliance investigations are required only when a complaint is received from an employee, a representative of an employee, an employer of an employee, or when there has been a fatality or catastrophe.

The Issue of Union Liability

In working out the details of this program a question arose, whether this program could create union or employee liability for construction site injuries. After an extensive legal review of this question, it was determined that "although a risk of liability does exist, that risk is not substantial."[2] Thus, it was determined that the California building trades unions can participate in jobsite safety committees without incurring any substantial risk of being held liable for jobsite injuries. Following is the background information which supported this position.

Studies show that 82 percent of all collective bargaining agreements and 79 percent of all agreements in the construction industry contain safety and health provisions. Yet, only 39 percent of the collective bargaining agreements in all industries and only 4 percent of the agreements in the construction industry establish safety committees, and less than one-half of these call for periodic inspections of the worksite by the committees.[3] Although relatively few contracts establish safety committees, a large percentage of the suits against unions for on-site injuries involve contracts creating such committees. The existence of a safety committee in which union members participate encourages suits against unions and union members.

Traditionally the employer has been the only party responsible for maintaining a safe workplace. Nevertheless, several suits seeking to hold unions liable for work-related injuries have been filed during recent years. A union or union member may be brought into a suit by the injured plaintiff employee or by the defendant employer. State worker's compensation laws often preclude an injured employee from suing his employer. These laws generally do not provide complete relief to an injured disabled employee. Consequently, such an employee may sue his union seeking additional relief. On the other hand, an injured employee may decide to sue an employer. Should this happen, the employer will often file a third-party complaint against a union, alleging that the union is also responsible for the employee's injuries.

Suits against labor unions involving safety and health issues have rarely succeeded. Generally, in these suits the union is charged with negligence or with breaching its duty of fair representation. Those lawsuits in which negligence is charged are based on the theory that the union has a common-law obligation to exercise reasonable care in enforcing the safety provisions of its contract and in performing those functions, such as safety inspections, which it is contractually obligated to perform. History illustrates that most courts have dismissed suits based on this theory. Federal law controls the obligation of a union to its members and completely preempts state law; the only obligations which a union has to its members are those imposed by federal law. Federal law imposes a duty of fair representation on unions, but not a general duty of care. Consequently, a union cannot be sued for common-law negligence.[4] Nevertheless, in one case, *Helton v. Hake,* a plaintiff did succeed in holding a local union liable for an allegedly negligent failure to enforce contractual safety provisions. The plaintiff recovered a $150,000 judgement from an Ironworkers local union in Missouri state court. That decision was recently affirmed by a Missouri court of appeals and will be appealed to the Missouri Supreme Court. The attorneys in that case, however, do not expect to prevail in Missouri Supreme Court and anticipate filing a petition for certiorari with the Supreme Court. Moreover, courts have rejected the contention that by agreeing to include safety provisions in its collective bargaining agreement, a union assumes a duty to its members to provide a safe workplace. A Washington state court, for example, states:

> The Defendant Union by attempting to improve the working and safety conditions of its members (including the Plaintiff) through the introduction into its collective bargaining agreement with Plaintiff's employer of provisions dealing with safety, did not thereby assume a duty or liability to its members (including Plaintiff) to provide them with a safe place to work and is not chargeable with the duty with reasonable care in making the safety inspection.

Higley v. Disston, Inc., 92 LRRM 2443, 2444 (Wash. Super. Ct. 1976); *see Bryant v. Mine Workers,* 467 F.2d. 1, 81 LRRM 2401 (6th Cir. 1972), *cert. denied,* 410 U.S. 930, (1973); *House v. Mine Safety Appliances Co.,* 47 F. Supp. 939, 92 LRRM 3638 (D. Idaho 1976).

The lawsuits alleging a breach of the duty of fair representation have also been generally successful. A union has a federal statutory duty to represent all members of its bargaining unit fairly and without discrimination. A union breaches its duty of fair representation when "its conduct toward a member of the collective bargaining unit is arbitrary, discriminatory or in bad faith." *Vaca v. Sipes,* 386 U.S. 171 (1967). Those suits in which a breach of the duty of fair representation is alleged are usually based on what is in effect alleged negligent conduct by the union. Courts have rejected these claims because the duty of fair representation does not encompass a general duty of care; a union does not breach its duty of fair representation by acting negligently. *Bryant v. Mine Workers; Brough v. Steel Workers,* 437 F.2d. 748, 76 LRRM 2430 (1st Cir. 1971); *House v. Mine Safety Appliance Co.* The only case based on a duty of fair representation theory, which the court refused to summarily depose of, is *Wentz v. IBEW,* No. CV76-L-60 (D. Neb.). In *Wentz,* however, the plaintiff alleged that the union *willfully* refused to negotiate safe working conditions or enforce the existing contractual safety provisions. It remains to be seen whether the plaintiff can actually show such willful conduct by the union.

In dismissing suits against unions, courts have also relied on public policy. They recognize that to impose liability for employee injuries on labor unions which have negotiated safety provisions in their contracts would discourage unions from attempting to make the workplace safer. *Bryant v. Mine Workers; House v. Mine Safety Appliances Co.; Higley v. Disston, Inc.* Accordingly courts have been reluctant to hold unions liable under any theory for employees' injuries.

Significantly, one of the theories advanced by the plaintiffs in *Wentz* was that the union was liable for the plaintiff's injuries because it failed to negotiate adequate contract safety provisions. Thus, even if a union did not become actively involved in a safety and health program, there is no guarantee that it would not be sued for worksite injuries.

It was concluded that a means does exist by which unions can reduce the likelihood of being held liable. If the collective bargaining agreements between management and the union states that the responsibility of maintaining a safe worksite is the employers' and the employers' only, a court would be less likely to find that the unions had assumed a duty to maintain a safe workplace for their members. Also, if the agreement describing the duties of a workplace safety committee describes those duties in permissive rather than mandatory terms (the committee "may" inspect rather than the committee "shall" inspect) union liability would be less likely. In addition, an agreement by management to identify employee members of the safety committee for any liability resulting from their service on the committee, would provide added protection.

An issue somewhat related to whether unions can be held liable for work-related injuries, is whether employees can refuse to work under dangerous conditions and whether employers can hold unions liable for such refusals. Section 502 of the National Labor Relations Act (NLRA) states that "the quitting of labor by an employee or employees in good faith because of abnormally dangerous conditions for work at the place of employment of such employee or employees (shall not) be deemed a strike under this Act." In 1974, the Supreme Court held that this section authorized work stoppages called to protect employees from immediate danger, but only if "ascertainably objective evidence supporting (the) conclusion that an abnormally dangerous condition for work exists." *Gateway Coal Co. v. Mine Workers,* 414 U.S. 368 (1974). If such evidence exists, a work stoppage cannot be enjoined and cannot be the basis of a suit for damages against the union.

In a recent case the United Staes Court of Appeals for the Fifth Circuit invalidated a Department of Labor regulation which interpreted OSHA to permit employees to refuse to work under conditions threatening serious injury or death. *Marshall v. Daniel Construction Co.,* No. 76–1465 (5th Cir. November 21, 1977). The National Labor Relations Board (NLRD), however, treats such safety related protests and work stoppages as protected activity under the NLRA. The Board has held that the NLRA does not permit an employer to discharge or discipline an employee who refuses to perform dangerous work. *Roadway Express, Inc.,* 217 NLRB No. 49, 88 LRRM 1503 (1975), enforced 532 F.2d. 751 (4th Cir. 1976). In one case the Board held that when an "abnormally dangerous" condition exists, employees may refuse to work even if the contract contains a no-strike clause. *Combustion Engineering, Inc.,* 224 NLRB No. 76, 93 LRRM 1049 (1976).

Thus, it was concluded that the California building trades unions can participate in jobsite safety committees without incurring any substantial risk of being held liable for jobsite injuries. Moreover, if abnormally dangerous work conditions actually exist, their members can refuse to work without being disciplined or discharged, and that work stoppage cannot be enjoined or be the basis of a suit for damages against a union.

To induce employers and employee groups to organize and support such voluntary programs, CAL/OSHA decided to provide a meaningful incentive. The employer will be removed from routine scheduled inspections by State/OSHA compliance personnel so long as the voluntary program is effective. However, employee rights will be protected by assuring that any formal complaints coming from employees to CAL/OSHA will be summarily investigated by the Division, without regard for the voluntary program. In other words, once a voluntary self-inspection safety program is in force at a place of employment, the employer's name will be removed from the routine of self-initiated inspection program of CAL/OSHA. Further, that place of employment will not be visited by CAL/OSHA personnel except to review and monitor the program or for consultative purposes or to investigate a formal complaint or a fatality/catastrophe/serious accident. Such a program, in addition to being highly attractive to employers and employee groups, would free CAL/OSHA compliance personnel to concentrate their efforts on places of employment with high injury rates.

As this proposed program was still being developed at the time this book was going to press, comments on its successes and/or failures cannot be made. However, the author finds the whole idea of voluntary compliance programs very commendable. They have a potential for high pay-off, if they are organized and administered properly. If this experimental voluntary program succeeds in this pilot attempt at bringing labor and management together for the purpose of improving overall hazard control on the construction jobsite, then perhaps those in other industries may embark on similar programs.

Cooperation at the Bargaining Table

When all is said and done, one of the most important advances that can be made toward increasing cooperation between labor and management, is that of formulating and carrying out safety and health provisions in contract agreements. The existence of the OSHA law and its promulgated standards, has actually, in an indirect way, called for a closer attention to Labor relations—as the cooperation of the union is essential in dealing with the important safety and health issues and in achieving compliance with the standards.

Over the past five years higher priority has been assigned to the safety and health aspects of union contracts than during any time before. The union's stance, for the most part, has reflected increasing membership pressures for safety and health. On the other hand, progressive company negotiators are beginning to emphasize the need for worker involvement in the safety and health program. Employers recognize that such worker involvement will add credibility to management's overall hazard control program effort, and thus improve the safety and health climate while increasing labor/management cooperation. Furthermore, management has demonstrated that it can better protect its own authority and its need for flexibility of safety and health policy by taking the initiative in bargaining.

As a result of collective bargaining, many agreements have been signed which specify the establishment of programs designed to study safety and health problems and to arrive at more favorable solution alternatives. The AFL-CIO United Rubber Workers contract signed in 1970 is a classic case in point. In the URW case, 0.5 cent per hour per worker was agreed to be used for long-range occupational health research program to be conducted at a recognized school of Public Health. The five-year comprehensive program involved epidemiology, industrial hygiene, industrial medical, and toxicological studies for the purpose of recognizing, evaluating, and controlling health situations and conditions which confront the URW membership.

Since 1970, other labor/management agreements have produced similar joint programs in both research, education, and training. More of these programs will emerge as safety and health becomes more and more of an issue at the bargaining table, and as labor and management begin to see the total benefits derived from understanding and coping with safety and health hazards associated with their operations.

Safety and Health Contract Provisions

As was stated several times in this chapter, the thrust of a viable joint safety and health program lies with clearly defined safety and health provisions in collective bargaining agreements. The following serves to highlight some of the agreement's major issues of concern.

1. Compliance required with recognized safety and health standards.
2. Information to employees concerning harmful contaminants in the environment (including noise and radiation).
3. Formation of, and increased functions for, joint safety and health committees at department, plant and corporate levels.
4. Opportunity for union representatives to make plant safety inspections.
5. Union participation in investigations of lost-time and fatal accidents.
6. Information to the union concerning reports of surveys by state and federal safety and health inspectors—and the right to accompany such inspectors on their tours.
7. Measurement of contaminants at the work place on union request.
8. Provision by the company at its expense of needed personal protective wear (safety shoes, safety glasses, hard hats, metatarsal protection, heat protective clothing, chemical protection aprons, shields, etc.)
9. Consultation with union prior to changes in safety rules, regulations, and programs.
10. Right of the employee to be relieved of a job he considers to be unsafe, other work at no financial or seniority loss.
11. Information on company plans and expenditures for the solution of remaining safety and health problems.
12. Joint committees to propose company-financed research on occupational safety and health programs and joint monitoring of such research.
13. Specific measures of protection against known hazards—i.e., radiation, noise, carbon monoxide.
14. Cooperation in the handling of health problems which are not basically occupational, such as alcoholism, mental health, drug addiction, etc.
15. Special procedures for the settlement of disputes concerning safety and health.
16. Inspection of new equipment and processes prior to their being put into use.
17. Transfer or discipline unsafe workers by joint decision.
18. No loss of pay for union representatives on joint safety committees for time spent on safety inspections and other safety and health activities.
19. Heating and ventilating improvements in the workplace.
20. Invalidation of disciplinary warnings for violations of safety rules after a given period, in case of subsequent discipline.
21. Special status of injured employees with respect to transfer, promotion, and other aspects of seniority.
22. Union involvement in company programs pertaining to air and water pollution outside of the plant.[5]

The following contract language, although it represents an ideal situation, nevertheless does serve as indicators of what may be possible to accomplish.

Suggestions for Contract Safety and Health Clauses
Place of Employment

- Management will provide places of employment where recognized hazards are eliminated or at least effectively controlled, by safeguards or other such protective devices.
- Job methods and procedures shall be in conformance with safe work practices.
- Management will repair and maintain all workplace facilities and tools and equipment therein.
- Management will, at no cost to the employees, provide, maintain, and train employees in the use of personal protective devices and safety equipment and will monitor the workplace for safety and environmental hazards and make this information available to the worker and/or his representative.

Joint Labor-Management Safety Committee

- A joint Labor-Management safety and health committee will be established which will consist of members selected by management and representatives chosen by the Local Union. This committee will establish and adopt safety and health rules, regulations, and procedures as well as making recommendations for corrective action.
- The joint-committee will hold regular monthly meetings and when necessary special meetings to review and evaluate safety and health conditions on the job as well as making recommendations to upgrade the safety and health program.
- Committee members shall be permitted to distribute to other workers all information regarding health and safety conditions in the workplace results of medical tests and workplace inspections, and other relevant information.
- Safety committee members shall be paid by the company at their standard rate for all the time spent on committee business, including time spent at meetings, inspecting and handling safety and health information, and accompanying government inspectors.
- Safety committee members shall, under the direction of the Company's hazard control specialist, have access to Company testing equipment. They shall also have the right to use other testing equipment and to bring in outside experts to inspect the workplace.

Safety and Health Inspections

- Either labor or management can request for an inspection by government or state inspectors, private organizations, or agents of the union. All data evolving from such inspections shall be made available to the entire safety and health committee.

Safety and Health Training, Education and Research

- Management will provide a continuous training and education program to insure that all workers are capable of recognizing, assessing, and taking proper action against hazards located in their workplaces.
- No worker will be required to operate equipment on which he has not received appropriate safety and health training.

Education and Research

Note: Where labor and management have negotiated for the establishment of a program for worker safety and health research and/or training the following clause might apply.

- Management will contribute a negotiated sum for each man-hour worked to a special health and safety research trust fund, to be administered jointly by the company and the union, for studying health hazards peculiar to the industry and for the training and education of workers in safety and health matters.

Labeling Toxic Materials

- Management will make available to the joint-committee the toxicity rating of all substances used in the workplaces—emphasizing those which may be unhealthful or dangerous to employees.
- Management will inform workers of the hazards associated with the toxic materials they are using and take all precautions necessary to prevent employee exposure to the hazards.
- All hazardous materials shall be labeled in a prominent manmer with standard hazard information to acquaint and instruct employees with the hazards involved, safe use, handling, and emergency procedures.

Medical Services

- Management will make available, at no cost to the workers, competent medical services of the employees choice and facilities for the proper diagnosis and treatment of cases resulting from injuries, physical impairments, etc., incurred during employment.

- Copies of all employer generated medical reports shall be furnished to the employee or employees physician.
- First-Aid facilities will be provided for worker injuries on the job.
- Employees will be compensated with full pay for the entire shift they were working when injured.

Safe Work Practices

- Employees shall not be required to work on a job or machine until its safety can be determined by the joint-committee. During such time workers shall be compensated full pay at their regular rate of pay even if transferred to a lower-rated job. An employee's refusal to perform such work shall not warrant or justify any immediate or future disciplinary action.
- Employees shall not be required to work on any new or unfamiliar job until they have received adequate instruction in the performance of the job, and the hazards involved. In addition, management must judge whether the employee is capable of working safely.

Union Responsibility

- Employees and their representatives shall comply with all orders, rules, regulations, standards specified in the OSHA Act—particularly observing all safety rules, codes, regulations, and safe work practices as well as using protective and safety equipment as specified therein.

Discrimination

- No employees shall be discharged or discriminated against because such employee filed a complaint or otherwise became involved in any proceeding relating to the Occupational Safety and Health Act of 1970 or other actions related to safety and health.

Release Time for Union Representatives

Employee Protections

- The Union and individual employees may exercise all their legal rights to secure a safe and healthful workplace, without threats, loss of pay, or other reprisals of any kind. The exercise of these legal rights shall in no way supercede or nullify the rights guaranteed in the master contract.
- Union representatives of the joint-committee, upon request, will be allowed to leave their work for the purpose of performing their safety and health duties without a loss of time or pay.

Union Access to Information

- Management will provide the union with the results of all tests for toxicity levels and all medical test of employees with the employees approval.
- Management will provide the union with the results of all government inspections and all correspondence relating thereto.
- Management will provide the union with all accident records and all available information on the morbidity and mortality of all present and former employees.

Arbitration

- Should the joint-committee not be able to resolve a dispute pertaining to safety and health, then either side shall have the right to submit the question to immediate and binding arbitration provisions of the contract agreement.

Both labor and management are in position to play a useful role in upgrading safety and health throughout industry. Through a cooperative effort, a thorough hazard assessment of all workplaces can be initiated, safety and health hazards identified, and joint solutions arrived at. This activity, along with cooperation at the bargaining table will establish a relationship which will guarantee the highest level of job safety and health to workers throughout the nation.

Cooperation in Training and Education

Throughout this Chapter mention was made repeatedly that the strongest deterrent to hazards in the workplace is the joint effort made by both labor and management. The safety and health clauses in contracts, and the operation of joint safety and health committees both imply a need for experienced and knowledgeable people to meet the stated objectives. Thus, the proper training and education of workers and their representatives is of critical importance.

Since 1973, the Federal government, recognizing the need for the upgrading of workers knowledge and skills in assessing hazards in the workplace, along with the concomitant need to maintain a cooperative atmosphere between labor and management began to fund demonstration projects aimed at accomplishing both objectives. Among the earliest projects in this area was the Building and Construction Trades Department of the AFL-CIO project involving safety and health education and training of employee and employer representatives in the construction industry. This particular project demonstrated that two hundred people representing the National Constructor's Association and the seventeen affiliated unions of the Building and Construction Trades Department, could sit side-by-side and learn how to cooperatively identify and deal with hazards encountered in the construction workplace.

The model educational program methodology developed during this project demonstrated that a rational living and learning environment in which information is exchanged enables the participants to grow intellectually through close interaction. The concept of experience-sharing integrated throughout all program method, afforded the participants in this program the opportunity to better understand the basis for attitudes existing among their peers, even when such attitudes were in contrast to their own.

It stands to reason that if money is wisely spent to continue training and educating the people who can benefit from it the most—joint labor/ management groups—a much higher payoff will be realized in the future in lowering deaths, injuries, and illnesses while guaranteeing a safer and healthful workplace for all workers.

Cooperation in Standards Adoption, Deletion, and Modification

Collaboration between labor and management has still another monumental benefit. Through a joint analysis of jobs and the hazardous factors associated with these jobs, teams consisting of members of labor and management are in a position to bring a tremendous amount of experience and knowledge to bear on the reform of the existing safety and health standards.

In instances when members of the crafts sat side by side with their counterparts in management and reviewed the hazards associated with a particular job or job task, it became obvious, before long, that some of the safety and health standards are on target, with respect to their adequacy and usefulness. In other cases it was observed that the standards lack certain elements which, if modified adequately, would render them useful in preventing accidents. In still other cases, the requirements of the job coupled with the limitations set by the standard produce an incompatible situation where nobody is helped and often somebody is injured or perhaps killed. In instances like this, the team has an argument for having the standard deleted from the total standards package. Finally, when labor and management put their heads together to study the issue of workplace hazard control, they continually encounter problems to which no standard addresses. In cases like this, the team is able to recommend to OSHA the adoption, deletion or modification of standards in order to arrive at workable guidelines for the effective location, and control of hazards in the workplace.

During the years to come, a greater need will exist for those governed by safety and health standards to step up and make their demands for standards that make sense, have a purpose in accident reduction, and are compatible with specific industry demands. In so doing, safety and health standards will take on a more credible meaning, will be used with greater frequency, and perhaps accomplish what they were supposed to in the first place—reduce deaths, and injuries and illnesses to workers and damage to or loss of equipment, material, and workplace facilities, to say nothing of excessive costs involved with such losses.

Bibliography

"Consultative Document—Safety Representatives and Safety Committees," Health and Safety Commission, Baynards House, 1 Chepstow Place, Westbourne Grove, London W2 4TF.

"Contract Clauses for Occupational Health and Safety," Industrial Health and Safety Project Urban Planning Aid, 639 Mass. Ave., Cambridge, Mass., 02139.

Goldberg, J. P.; Ahern, E., Haber; W.; Oswald, R. A.; "Federal Policies and Worker Status Since the Thirties," Industrial Relations Research Association Series, 7226 Social Science Bldg., University of Wisconsin, Madison, Wisconsin, 1976.

Kochan, 7. A., Dyer, L., "The Effectiveness of Union-Management Safety and Health Committees," W. E. Upjohn Institute for Employment Research, Cornell University, 1977.

Notes

1. "Safety Program Practices in High Versus Low Accident Rate Companies" Interim Report U.S. Dept. H. E. W., National Institute for Occupational Safety & Health—June,1975.
2. BNA Basic Patterns in Union Contracts, 123–126 (8th ed. 1975).
3. BNA Basic Patterns in Union Contracts, 123–126 (8th ed. 1975).
4. Gerace v. Johns Manville, Corp., 95 LRRM 3282 (PA. Ct. CM. Pl. 1977).
5. "OSHA & the Unions—Bargaining on Job Safety & Health—A BNA Special Report-Bureau of National Affairs Inc., Washington, D.C. 1973.

Safety and Health Technical Section 12

Occupational Health and Industrial Hygiene

Unit 1

Occupational Diseases

For the purpose of this section, an *occupational disease is defined in this chapter as a disease caused by environmental factors, the exposure of which is peculiar to a particular process, trade, or occupation, and to which a worker is not ordinarily subjected or exposed outside of or away from such employment.* Occupational diseases include acute and chronic problem situations caused by inhalation, absorption, ingestion, or direct contact with a harmful substance or physical force. For the purpose of clarity, an *acute* situation is one caused by a single absorption or contact with a high initial dose experienced over a short period of time. A *chronic* situation, on the other hand, is characterized by multiple absorptions or contacts with lower doses over a longer period of time.

Industrial hygiene, as it will be referred to in this section, is *that speciality area devoted to the recognition, evaluation, and control of those environmental factors or stressors arising in or from the workplace which may cause sickness, impaired health and well being, or significant discomfort or inefficiency among worker or among the citizens of the community.* Figure 105 illustrates several environmental stressors which have the capacity to cause occupational diseases. The objectives of industrial hygiene are to prevent organic or systemic damage to workers as a result of: inhaling dusts, mists, fumes, gases, vapors and smokes; excessive heat and cold; noise; electromagnetic radiation; chemicals contacting the skin and eyes; poor body position; vibration; overexertion; and inadequate illumination. Perhaps another important objective is to stimulate the improvement of working conditions and equipment to promote the increased efficiency of personnel in performing the work assigned.

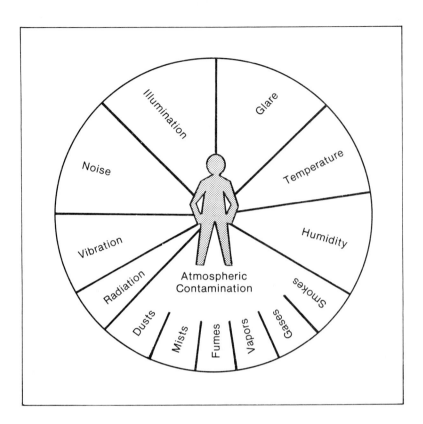

Figure 105. Environmen-
tal stressors.

How They Are Caused

Generally speaking occupational diseases are caused by: (1) Air polluted with dusts, gases, vapors, mists, etc., where these contaminants are routed to the bloodstream via the lungs; (2) contact with allergens, corrosives, carcinogens, bacteria, solvents, etc., which can produce skin diseases; (3) physical agents e.g., noise, (causing hearing loss), heat (causing heat stroke and exhaustion); lasers (causing eye and other organic damage); (4) microwaves; (5) ionizing radiation; (6) vibration; (7) Micro-organisms. (See Figure 105 and Figure 106.)

Problems Associated with Occupational Health Hazards

Problems associated with occupational health hazards may be grouped into the following five categories: (1) they cover the whole range of human disorders e.g., lungs, blood, kidney, liver, skin, eyes, ears, brain, and nervous system; (2) they frequently escape detection; (3) they don't come with a label thus they can be easily be misdiagnosed by a physician; (4) they come slowly as a rule, over months and years and every worker is not affected by them. When they do manifest themselves, they may be irreversible; (5) new potential hazards are continually introduced through the use of new substances, new uses for old materials, new combinations of chemicals, and process changes.

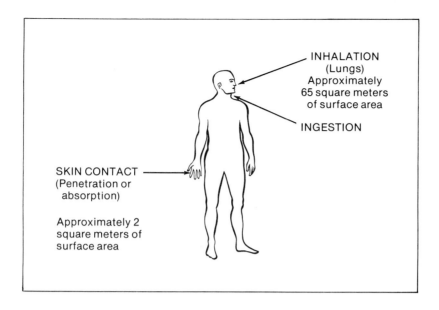

Figure 106. Portals of entry of toxic materials.

Examples of Occupational Diseases

Silicosis   A disease caused by breathing air containing free silica dust, and characterized fibrotic changes and the development of military nodulation in both lungs; shortness of breath; decreased chest expansion; and lessened capacity for work.

Hearing Loss   Chronic exposure to high noise and/or:
Vibration levels, causing physiological damage to the middle and inner ear. See Figure 107. Permissible noise levels and examples of common noise levels produced by several tools and machines are found in Tables 9 and 10. Figure 108 illustrates a worker's noise exposure being measured with a sound level meter.

Dermatitis   Skin exposure to acids, resins, oils, solvents, biological agents, physical agents, etc., resulting in reddening of the skin with mild itching to a rash or small eruptions with intense itching. Severe cases produce open or weeping sores.

Mercurial exzema   Prolonged exposure to mercury nitrate, resulting in corrosion and irritation of the skin.

Cancer   Induced by coal tar products, chromates, nickel refining and manufacture of some dyes.

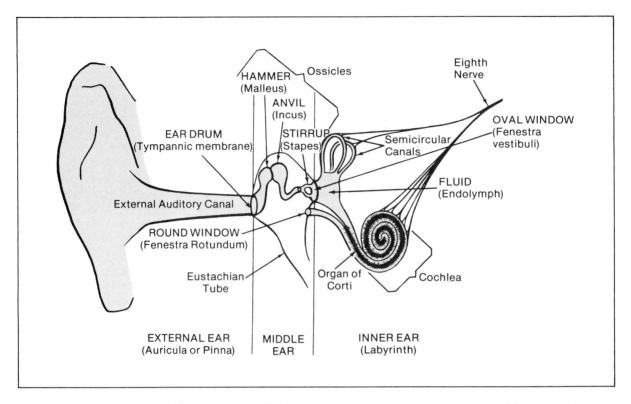

Figure 107. Illustrates the anatomy of the human ear. (Courtesy of American Foundrymen's Society)

Asbestosis "Evidence that asbestosis dust in the air will scar and destroy the lungs has been known for half a century. For the past thirty years, it has been a proven cause of cancer of the lungs, of the chest and abdominal cavities (mesothelioma), and of the stomach and intestines among workers. Usually exposure over a long period of time is necessary to produce an asbestos-related disease. But there is some evidence that even a single day of breathing large amounts of asbestos dust will harm the lungs."[1] Workers have been known to have their skin turn black—as a result of the chemical paranitroaniline being absorbed in dust form through their unbroken skin.

Paranitroaniline Converts the blood's oxygen-carrying hemoglobin, so it can no longer effectively carry oxygen to the blood tissues. Milder exposure—results in "blue lip" a blueing of lips and the flesh under fingernails.[2] Compounds of paranitroaniline are used in products such as corrosion inhibitors, gasoline, and red lipstick.

Tetrabrome Used as a fire retardant for fabric; has been known to make workers dizzy, lose their balance, become numb in their legs, and suffer weakening of their sexual functions.

TABLE 9
Permissible Noise Exposure

Duration per Day, Hours	Sound Level dB (A)* Slow Response
8	90
6	92
4	95
3	97
2	100
1½	102
1	105
½	110
¼ or less	115
Less than 1 second— impulsive or impact noise	140

TABLE 10
Intensity Level of Noises

Sound Level, dB	Common Noise
135	Jet engine
130	Riveting steel tank; sand blasting
120	Hydraulic press*
115	Punch press
110	Woodworking shop
105	Circular saw
102	Weaving room
100	Can manufacturing plant
97	Automatic screw machine
95	Inside subway
92	Diesel air compressor
90	20 ft. from subway train
80	Office tabulating machine
75	Busy street
70	Freight train (100 ft.)
60	Conversation (3 ft.)
50	Large office
40	Quiet office
30	Soft whisper (5 ft.)
0	Threshold of hearing

*At 120 dB and above, pain occurs.

Nitroglycerine   Chronic exposure to nitroglycerine causes an enlarging of the arteries to the heart. Withdrawal causes severe chest pains and eventual death.

Toxicity Vs. Hazard

Several times in this unit, the terms *toxicity* and *hazard* are used in our discussion of chemical, and biological agents.

The toxicity of a material is not synonymous with its health hazard. *Toxicity is the capacity of a material to produce injury or harm.* Toxicity is dependent on dose, rate, method and site of absorption, general state of health, in-

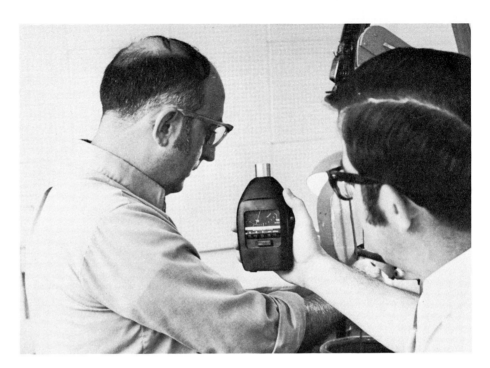

Figure 108. Worker's
noise exposure measured
with sound level meter.
(Courtesy General Radio
Company.)

dividual differences, diets, and temperatures. *Hazard* from the standpoint of occupational health and industrial hygiene is the possibility that a material will cause injury when a specific quantity is used under certain conditions without adequate controls. The key elements to be considered when evaluating a health hazard are: (1) how much of the material in contact with a body cell is required to produce injury? (2) the probability of the material being absorbed by the body to result in an injury, (3) rate of generation of airborne contaminant, (4) total time of contact, and, (5) control measures in use.

Threshold Limit Values (TLV)

According to the American Conference of Governmental Industrial Hygienists and NIOSH, these are exposure levels under which most people can work consistently for eight hours a day, five days a week, with no harmful effects.

Threshold Limit Values are quantitative estimates of the concentration in units such as parts per million (ppm) or milligrams per cubic meter (mg/m^3).

Problems with Threshold Limit Values

- T.L.V.'s are based on either judgement, opinion, or limited experimentation on laboratory animals. In few instances have these values been established as the result of human experience.
- Concentrations of chemicals rarely remain constant in the workplace throughout the work day.

Example: An adhesive maker working an eight hour shift spends eight fifteen-minute periods in a vat area where the concentration of Butanone is 350 ppm. He also spends five hours adjacent to the mixing vat where the Butanone concentration is 225 ppm. He spends the remainder of the work shift in another area of the plant, where the adhesive thinners are being poured into carboys and the average concentration of Acetone is 1,500 ppm. Is his exposure within the T.L.V. for Butanone and Acetone?

Answer:

$$(1) \quad \frac{(2)\ (350)\ +\ (5)\ (225)\ +\ (1)\ (0)}{8} = \frac{1825}{8} = 228 + \text{ppm}$$

The TLV for Butanone = 200 ppm. Therefore the worker is not within acceptable limits.

$$(2) \quad \frac{(7)\ (0)\ +\ (1)\ (1,500)}{8} = \frac{1500}{8} = 187.5\,\text{ppm}$$

The TLV for Acetone = 1,000 ppm. Therefore the worker is within acceptable limits of exposure.

- Most industrial environments contain mixtures of chemicals rather than single compounds.
- Individuals vary greatly in their sensitivity to toxic substances.
- We must keep the problem of individual variances in mind when we prescribe control measures, since most of the available controls are suited for the mythical average person. Those people whose sensitivity places them outside the mythical average must be cared for separately.

How Chemical, Physical and Biological Agents Enter the Body

Chemical and biological agents reach the body through inhalation, skin contact or ingestion. See Figure 106. Inhalation and skin contact are of considerable importance since the majority of occupational diseases result from breathing dusts, fumes, vapors, gases, mists, and from skin contact with chemical or biological materials.

Materials, when inhaled are frequently quickly absorbed in the blood or in the fluids of the lungs. When solvent vapors and gases are inhaled in sufficient quantities, they can produce injurious effects on a human organism in a relatively short period of time.

Occupational skin diseases (dermatoses) account for a high percentage of workmen's compensation claims. The most frequent cause of dermatitis occurs on individuals working with petroleum oils and grease, volatile solvents, explosives, alkalies, and materials encountered in metal plating.

The toxic action of solvents is illustrated in Figure 109. Chronic poisoning can occur if small amounts of toxic substances are swallowed daily. On the

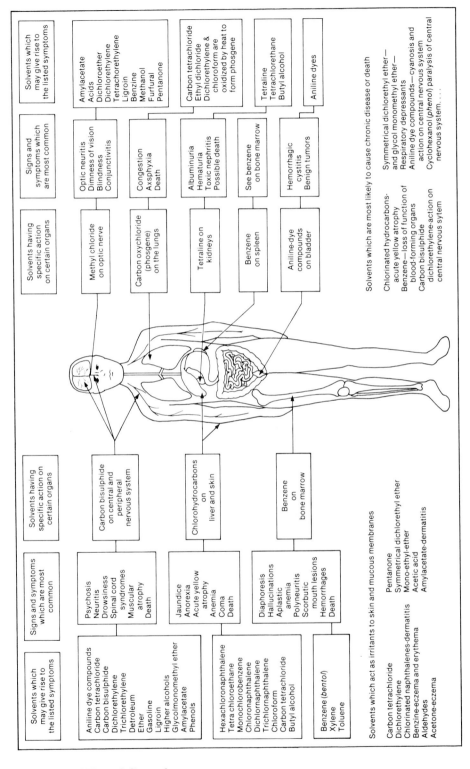

Figure 109. Toxic action of solvents. (From the Pennsylvania State Health Department, Division of Industrial Medicine.)

other hand, acute poisoning can occur if high concentrations of the agent is swallowed on initial dose.

Physical Agents, unlike the chemical and biological agents, do not have to enter the body to cause harm. Excessive environmental temperatures may affect the whole body by increasing the body heat load. High noise levels may be transmitted to the ear via the bony structure of the head and cause hearing loss.

Occupational health hazards which may adversely affect an employee are usually classified according to the following three categories: Category I—toxic chemical agents; Category II—biological agents; Category III—physical agents.

Category I—Toxic Chemical Agents

This category consists of gases and vapors, particulate matter, and miscellaneous substances. Gases are normally fluids which occupy the space of the exposure and can be liquified only by the combined effect of increased pressure and decreased temperature. Examples of common gases are oxygen, hydrogen, and nitrogen. Vapors, on the other hand, are distinguished from gases on the basis that vapors are the evaporation products of substances which are liquid at normal temperatures. Gases and vapors are classified as irritants, asphyxiants, and volatile drugs and druglike substances. In Figure 110 the worker is exposed to toxic vapors without adequate exhaust ventilation. In addition, the grounding system provided is ineffective.

Particulate matter is divided into solids and liquids. In the solid category, we find dusts, fumes, and smokes. In Figure 111 the welder is breathing high con-

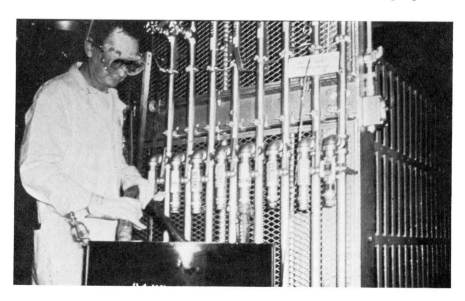

Figure 110.

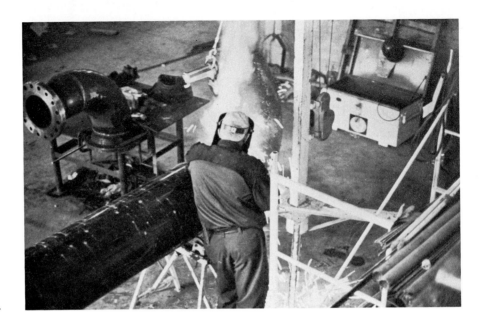

Figure 111.

centrations of welding fumes indicating a need for exhaust ventilation. These are all particulate matter, and the distinction between them is based on their particle size (measured in microns) and method of evolution. Dusts are formed from solid inorganic or organic materials reduced mechanically in size by processes such as grinding, crushing, blasting, drilling, and pulverizing. These particles may range in size from the visible to the submicroscopic. In air sampling work, our principle concern is with those particles below 50 microns (one micron = 1/25,000 inch), and particularly with those less than 10 microns, since these sizes are the ones that remain suspended in the atmosphere for a significant period of time. Figure 112 shows the larger particles of explosives dust attached to the ventilation hood. The worker is wearing a respirator to protect against the smaller particles.

Fumes are formed from solid materials, such as when lead is heated. A vapor is produced which condenses in the atmosphere, forming metallic particles. These particles, are very fine ranging in size from one micron to as small as 0.0001 micron, oxidize to lead oxide.

Smokes are usually considered to be the products of combustion of solid materials that are originally organic.

In addition to gases, vapors, and particulate matter, there are situations in which combinations of gases, dusts, fumes, and smokes may occur. In plants where several different processes are taking place at the same time in the same area, there is no way to prevent diffusion of the substances.

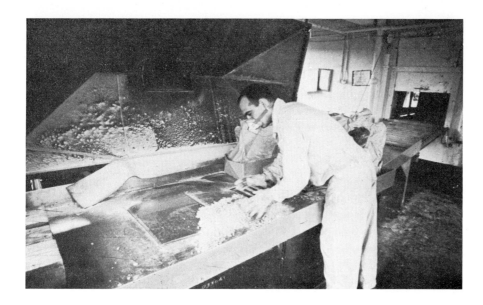

Figure 112.

Category II—Biological Agents   Certain bacteria, fungi, parasites, and microorganisms of occupational origin are known to cause illness, extreme discomfort, and even death in some circumstances. For example, bacterial infections may arise in workers in slaughter and meat packing plants who handle cattle infected with Bang's disease, and anthrax may develop in workers handling unsterilized wool and hair bristles imported from certain foreign countries.

Category III—Physical Agents   Exposure to environmental conditions or physical agents (encompass a field as large as the chemical agents) and are just as important from an occupational health viewpoint. Physical agents and conditions usually include radiation, noise, repeated motion, shock or vibration, temperature extremes and humidity, and illumination.

Industrial Noise

Perhaps the most perplexing of all the physical agents is noise. Noise has and still is a major source of compensable illnesses to workers.

Noise is produced when a vibrating source transmits its energy to molecules of air (gas) producing a variation in normal atmospheric pressure. As the energy is transmitted the pressure variations reach our ear drums and the vibrations are translated by our hearing system (Figure 107) into a sensation which we call sound. As the air is compressed and rarefied by the sound waves, a minute variation in barometric pressure that is sensed by the ear and by the pressure operated microphones used for the evaluation of the sound wave amplitude. The variation in normal atmospheric pressure characterizes a sound wave by the *rate* at which this variation occurs—the complete cyclic variation per second is the *frequency* of sound—referred to as *tone* or *pitch*. The frequency rate is designated as cycles per second or Hertz (cps or Hz).

A more common word used in noise measurement is the decibel (db)—a dimensionless unit. Decibels are measured on a logarithmic rather than a linear scale. Thus, an increase of 10 db represents an approximate 300 percent increase in sound pressure. A 100 db noise reading is three times as intense as a 90 db reading instead of about 10 percent more intense as might be expected.

The frequency range of speech ranges from 100–10,000 Hz, although the majority of speech sound ranges from 200–6,000 Hz.

The instrument which is most commonly used to measure the intensity of sound or noise is the sound level meter. See Figure 113. In the sound meter sound pressure levels are directly read as db, but are weighed by A, B, + D networks. These weighing networks respond to frequency ranges:

A scale: 400–12,000 Hz— discriminates quite severely against low frequencies.

B scale: 125–12,000 Hz— discriminates moderately against low frequencies.

C scale: 25–10,000 Hz— hardly discriminates at all against low frequencies.

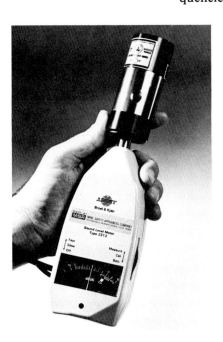

Figure 113. Sound level meter with calibrator. (Courtesy Mine Safety Appliances Co.)

The A scale weighing network is used for noise measurement because it responds most favorably with subjective response to loudness levels.

Hearing Damage

Hearing damage may be caused by one of three possibilities. First, high intensity sound pressure levels may penetrate the ear drum causing damage to the ear drum and the tiny bones in the middle ear. Secondly, lower sound pressure levels may cause damage to the bones in the middle ear due to excessive vibration. Thirdly, sound levels, above threshold (90 db by law although sound levels above 85 db is damaging to human hearing) slowly destroy the sound transmitting cells in the inner ear—preventing sound from reaching the auditory nerve to the brain. With continuous damage occurring in the inner ear (cochlea) permanent hearing disability will occur. Fourth, noise and vibration may be transmitted to the ear via bones in the skeletal system and cranium. Figure 114 illustrates a common mistake made by those attempting to provide worker protection from noise. Although the worker is equipped with an approved pair of ear muffs, the vibration coming from the impact tool is sufficient to cause noise to be transmitted to the worker's inner ear in spite of the ear protection. Shock mounting the impact tool along with the ear protectors would be a more effective alternative to the problem situation.

Controlling Noise Problems

The principles of controlling hazards discussed in Chapter 4 are applied again when attempts are made at noise abatement.

1. Substitute a quieter machine or machine components.
2. Reduce noise energy by decreasing the energy available for driving equipment.
3. Change the direction of the noise source,—e.g., changing the path of direction of sources of noise, e.g., mufflers, air silencers.
4. Use resilient (shock) mounts to cut down on vibration.
5. Increase the distance of the worker from the noise source. This is not always a practical alternative.
6. Use acoustical materials in an area to reduce revibrant noises—this technique is usually more effective for reducing noise levels for other workers in the area.

Control of noise requires a thorough study of the noise source, its environment, and so forth. In many instances, noise attenuation necessitates high dollar outlays. Although the most effective form of noise abatement lies with engineering the noise hazard out of the workplace, there are instances when this alternative cannot be chosen. Noise abatement on air fields would be a

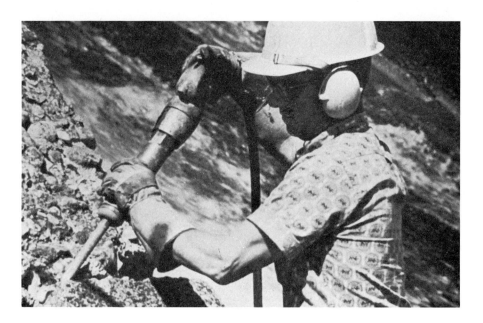

Figure 114.

good example. Nevertheless, when a noise problem cannot be engineered out, the employer has another (although less effective) alternative—personal protective equipment in the form of ear plugs, muffs, and helmets. A discussion of ear protective devices appears on page 461 of this chapter.

Appraising Health Hazards

The evaluation of health hazards is a prerequisite for making recommendations for control. The evaluation proceeds in two stages—a preliminary survey and a detailed study. The preliminary survey is made to determine which operations involve the use of or produce physical, chemical and biological agents which are hazardous to a worker's health. A detailed study is as its name implies, a more in-depth exploration into the health hazard problem by virtue of sampling, collection procedures, and analysis.

A preliminary survey is the first step in evaluating the occupational environment. During this survey, operating procedures should be observed in which potentially harmful materials are handled or equipment used in a manner that could result in excessive concentrations or dangerous levels which may cause harm to workers. This survey should include such considerations as: (1) general sanitation; (2) raw materials, products and by-products; (3) sources and types of air contaminants; (4) physical agents; (5) control measures in use. In preparation for the preliminary survey it is important to obtain a list of all chemicals which are used in the workplace. Once the list is obtained, it is necessary to determine which of the materials are toxic and to what extent. During the survey many potential health hazardous operations may be detected by visual observation. The most dusty operations can be spotted at this time. It must be remembered that the dust which cannot be seen by the unaided eye is the most hazardous, since it is of respirable size. Absence of a visible dust cloud does not mean that a dust-free atmosphere exists.

Sources of radiant heat, abnormal temperature and humidity, x-rays, and gamma rays should be noted. This information will be helpful during the conduct of the detailed study.

Detailed Study

Before a detailed study is conducted, to ascertain some or all of the hazards found during the preliminary survey, the analyst must realize that the degree of injury to an individual arising from occupational exposures depends on several factors: (1) nature of the substance or condition; (2) state of the material—solid, liquid, gas; (3) intensity of the exposure; (4) duration of the exposure; (5) individual susceptibility.

Analytical Procedures in Industrial Hygiene

Procedures employed in analyzing a collected sample may be chemical or physical. Chemical procedures include those in which a chemical reaction is employed to determine the amount of contaminant present. These methods in order of increasing sensitivity are as follows: (1) gravimetric; (2) volumetric; (3) volumetric with electrometric titration; (4) colormetric; (5) nephelometric. *Gravimetric methods* are those in which the collected contaminant is present in sufficient quantity to permit its weighing. *Volumetric procedures* are chemical procedures in which a known volume of standardized solution is permitted to react with the unknown amount of the contaminant. The amount of the unknown contaminant is always proportional to the amount of known solution used. *Volumetric determinations with electro- titration procedures* are similar in principle to the ordinary volumetric procedures with the exception that an electro-chemical change which takes place upon equilibrium in the titrating of the unknown solution is indicated electrically by a pair of electrodes and a potentiometer. *Colormetric procedures* are probably the most widely used methods in industrial hygiene chemical analysis because they provide micro-quantitative information relatively fast. The principle of colormetric methods is simple. It depends upon the formation of a colored compound or complex by the contaminant and a suitable reagent (usually organic). The reaction takes place in a solution which has known it to give the desired color and sensitivity. The compound or complex which results increases in its color intensity or changes its shade of color proportionally to increasing amounts of the contaminant. *Neptelometric Methods* are similar to colormetric but instead of a color reaction, a precipitate is formed. It is essential that this finely dispersed precipitate cause a turbidity which will remain stable for sufficient periods to enable an analysis to be made.

Physical methods employed in air analysis include optical methods (interferometer, photometric, spectrum absorption—ultraviolet, infrared), heat of combustion, thermal conductivity, vapor-pressure measurement, density measurement, refractive-index measurement, absorption, electrical conductivity.

During the conduct of the detailed study the following sampling review process may be of value.

Air Samples

1. Base the decision to sample an atmosphere for particular contaminants upon the results of a preliminary survey.
2. Evaluate the environment with reference to hygienic standards.
3. Determine contamination from a process, in order to study that process.
4. Appraise the performance of a given piece of equipment used to control the process.
5. Correlate environmental conditions with medical findings, in order to establish threshold limit values.
6. Make the sample collected representative of the working environment, and weighed it in direct proportion to the time the worker spends at various operations.
7. Divide the samples of air taken for industrial purposes into two major groups:
    a. Group 1—Grab Sample; "instantaneous." These samples are usually collected by means of evacuated flasks.
    b. Group 2—Continuous Sample. These samples are usually taken over the entire workday and/or weeks.

Measurement of Physical Agents

1. Nearly all physical agents are evaluated by means of direct reading instruments. Specific instruments are required for the particular physical agent to be evaluated.
    a. Noise—Intensity may be determined by means of a :
        (1) Sound level meter (Figure 113)
        (2) Sound survey meter
        (3) Octave band analyzer
        (4) Noise dosimeter
        (5) Sound level recorder
    b. Illumination—Instruments are available for measuring the quantity (illumination levels) and quality (brightness contrasts, glare and reflectance) of illumination.

    c.   Heat Stress—Four factors are needed to determine whether or not workers are exposed to heat stress:
- (1) ambient air temperature dry bulb thermometer
- (2) relative humidity wet bulb thermometer
- (3) radiant heat globe thermometer
- (4) air volocity indicator

    d.   When all of the above are calculated, they are compared with effective temperature charts listed in various heat standards.

    e.   The next step in evaluating the occupational environment is to compare results of air sample analysis or data with standards.
- (1) The American Conference of Governmental Industrial Hygienists, annually published, TLV's, covers, vapors, gases, mists, and dusts.
- (2) Standards and proposed standards for temperature, humidity and heat stress are found in various sources including NIOSH criteria documents.

    f.   All tests to determine duration will be based on an 8 hour work day.

Occupational Health Information Dissemination

So far in this unit, the discussion of worker's diseases has been limited to the workplace. Admittedly, the health of workers during their employment is our primary concern. However, there is another area—an extension of the workplace—where a great deal of assistance is needed. It is providing the worker's private physicians with information which will increase the physician's capacity to assess the symptoms of their patients more accurately.

The following case history demonstrates this point:

A carpenter working on the inside trim of a new house under construction began to lose weight and finally was hospitalized. After a few days in the hospital he gained his weight back and was released. The physicians at the hospital, having run numerous tests on the worker, were unable to determine the cause of the problem. When the carpenter returned to the job again, he started to lose weight again and felt generally bad. As it was learned later, the house was air conditioned and in order to conserve energy the air was recycled.

Upon receiving a complaint about this problem from the carpenter's local union, the State Industrial Hygienist came to examine the situation. When the hygienist entered the house he could smell what he thought was pentachlorophenol—a wood preservative which has a pharmological effect of causing people to lose weight. It also increases a persons metabolism causing the body to burn food faster, speed up the heart beat, and raise body temperature. The air samples which indicated that pentachlorophenol was at or slightly above its TLV, served to verify the hygienist's initial assumption. It was also determined that a paint containing pentachlorophenol was used on all the redwood interior finish in the house. The manufacturer intended that the paint would be used for exterior use but had not so indicated that on the label of the can. This is an example which shows that had not the hygienist known about the specific effects of chemical exposures and what could cause them, the carpenter might have suffered irreparable damage.

A case similar to this one involved a worker who used his hands to stir a 15 gallon can of pentachlorophenol. In this case, before anybody could do anything about it, the worker died.

Several labor unions have accepted this challenge of making the effects of toxic substances known to their membership. The United Association of Journeymen and Apprentices of the Plumbing and Pipe Fitting Industry and the International Association of Fire Fighters, for example, have embarked on projects to make known to the workers they represent the symptoms of substances and materials encountered during their work.

The following examples show how such health information is prepared for dissemination to workers and their physicians.

Ammonia: Irritating to the skin and eyes; can cause dermatitis; kidney damage; may induce vomiting; can cause cancer; shortness of breath, pulmonary edema; obstructive ventilatory dysfunction; lung congestion; irritation to trachea, bronchial tubes, nose and throat and lung tissue; fibrosis, bronchitis; mental confusion.

Asbestos: Stomach cancer; intestinal cancer; respiratory tract cancers; pneumoconiosis/pneumonitis; obstructive ventilatory dysfunction; lung congestion; lung cancer; irritation to trachea and bronchial tubes; irritation to nose and throat; irritation to lung tissue; emphysema.

Carbon Monoxide: Dizziness, headaches, nausea; drowsiness; unconsciousness; irritation to nose and throat; vomiting; myocardial alterations; tissue hypoxia.

With information like this available to workers and their physicians, everybody gains. The workers gains greater assurance and confidence in his physician's diagnoses and medical cures. The physician benefits by being able to diagnose symptoms (effects) with a far better insight into their causes (problems). The employer also benefits from such a system. Once the employer learns that one of his workers has become ill because of contact with or exposure to an agent in the workplace, action can be initiated. Using one or more of the sampling techniques mentioned in this unit, along with other assessment procedures, the employer can begin to determine if a problem exists, to what extent it exists, the number of people exposed, and what needs to be done to correct it.

Personal Protective Equipment   Unit 2

In Chapter 4 we discussed the methods of controlling hazards encountered in the workplace. It was pointed out that among all the control alternatives to choose from, personal protective equipment has to be listed as the last line of defense. However, there are two times when protective equipment is a likely candidate as a control alternative. First, as an interim measure, while the hazard is being engineered out of the workplace. Second, when there is no other means available to control the hazard's destructive effect by conventional control strategies. Using ear muffs on air fields to protect workers is a good example. The most serious weakness of protective equipment is that it does nothing to eliminate or reduce the hazard, but instead merely sets up a defense against it. Failure of the defense mechanism means immediate exposure of the worker to the full intensity of the hazard's destructive effect.

Given the fact that the hazard control specialist must employ the use of personal protective equipment, perhaps the following six factors will be helpful. First, a clear understanding of the hazard's potential to cause harm must be had. Second, the degree of protection should be proportionate to the seriousness of the hazard. It would be a poor decision to require workers to wear self-contained breathing apparatus when a particulate filter respirator would suffice. Third, protection must be considered, along with the equipment's capacity to interfere with worker performance. Here, trade-offs are often made between worker demands for freedom and the capacity of the work process to produce harm. Many times, situations will appear where the hazard control specialist, having exhausted all his alternatives, will have to recommend a protective device with which the workers will not be happy. In instances like this, the hazard control specialist will have to take extra care to be sure that the workers understand his dilemma and make the compromise necessary to assure their own protection; Fourth, the equipment must be acceptable and approved by a national testing agency, i.e., American National Standards Institute (ANSI), Mine Safety and Health Administration (MSHA), etc.; Fifth and Sixth, the subjects of equipment quality and cost enters the picture. In the selection of personal protective equipment, it should be the rule, except under rare circumstances, that the highest quality item be purhcased, given the cost constraints. Experience has shown that the better protective item will last longer, provide better fit, require less maintenance, and over the long run, be more cost/effective. Many people have, in the past, made the mistake of purchasing "bargain" equipment only to find that the "bargain" equipment ended up costing them more in the long run. On the subject of equipment quality, it should be noted that NIOSH, in its reports on tests of various items of protective equipment have determined that; even though equipment meets the criteria for approval, a wide margin may exist in quality between the equipment at the top of the list and those that barely got in under the wire.

Problems That Hamper the Effectiveness of Personal Protective Equipment

The six most common problems which hamper the effectiveness of personal protective equipment include: (1) Purchasing the incorrect type of equipment for the hazard at hand, e.g., choosing a dust respirator when a combination respirator is required. (2) Purchasing non-approved equipment. This should not be too much of a problem any longer, with the pressure of OSHA and NIOSH making it unwise for an employer to use anything else but approved equipment. However, there are records which show that where non-approved equipment is selected, equipment malfunctions and other problems may occur being responsible for avoidable personnel injuries and illnesses. (3) Failing to maintain equipment. A great many personal protective devices throughout industry are in various stages of disrepair. Poorly-maintained equipment is a likely candidate to fail when the time comes that a worker may depend upon it for his life. An example of equipment failure due to deterioration would be the surface breakdown of natural rubber (used for electrical insulated gloves) into a series of interlacing cracks, by the action of ozone in the air. When this happens, the insulative properties of the gloves are destroyed. (4) Ignoring equipment that has become ineffective. This problem is very closely associated with (3) above, since well-maintained equipment is less likely to become ineffective without the wearer knowing about it, than equipment that is not cared for properly and does not receive the proper preventive maintenance. However, even with good care and maintenance, protective equipment can still malfunction and fail. (5) Improper fitting protective equipment that doesn't fit properly cannot afford its designed protection. The ear plug that doesn't fill-up the space in the outer ear will permit sound to "leak" around the protective plug and damage the inner ear. The respirator facepiece that doesn't conform to the contours of the workers face, will allow toxic gases, vapors, etc., in the air to be inhaled by the worker—perhaps damaging the worker's lungs; (6) Failing to standardize equipment. Those who have brought more than one brand of a particular type of protective equipment into the workplace have witnessed problems concerning training workers in the equipment's usage, maintenance practices, and so forth. Control becomes extremely difficult. To eliminate these problems, the brands of protective devices, e.g., hard hats, respirators, etc., should be kept to a minimum. The ideal situation is to have only one brand of each.

The following is designed to introduce the reader to various kinds of protective devices.

Head Injuries

In 1971, the National Safety Council reported that there were 160,000 occupation head, face, and neck injuries—excluding the eyes which accounted for 7 percent of all injuries and 8 percent of the workmen's compensation paid.

In 1970, a review of New York State's Workmen's Compensation Records showed that out of 117,000 injury cases, 2,564 were head injuries which accounted for more than $6.9 million in compensation paid to claimants. Out of the total 2,564 cases of head injuries: 1107 cases were caused by the injured's head being struck by objects. Those 1107 cases averaged $2,755 per cases; 320 cases were caused when the injured fell to different levels. These 320 cases averages $4,226 per case, 306 cases were caused when the injured fell on the same level. These 306 cases averaged $2,406 per case.

The curious thing about these statistics is that the cases which appear (on the basis of amount of compensation paid) to be the most serious, were caused in situational modes where the hard hat was not able to do much good—side impact injuries.

Types of Head Injuries

Basically head injuries fall into two classifications: those occuring from slow compression—e.g., a head squeezed under a vehicle when a jack slowly collapsed, and those occurring from dynamic situations—e.g., a head struck by a falling object. According to Omaya[3] the dynamic situation is more complex. This is the way the head is commonly injured in falls and impacts. Two components that can injure are the inertial loading the impact itself, which produces the contact phenomena. In cases of indirect impact, such as a fall on the buttocks (which has been known to cause brain damage) or in certain instances of severe whiplash, the only cause of injury is inertial loading. In Omaya's experiments, it was found that the contact phenomena of the impact, shock waves, and the skull fracture scarcely contributed to the global or diffuse brain injury. Such components do contribute to local damage, and local damage, of course, can add to the more diffuse phenomena induced by inertial loads. In conclusion, it can be said that the major problem associated with head impact is the damage which occurs to the brain, despite the common idea that skull fracture is the most important. Omaya points out that brain damage can occur with no visible fracture to the cranial structure.

Head Protection

The worker's head must be protected against impact blows, flying particles, and falling objects. This protection is provided by specially-designed head gear that protects the wearer's head against forces of impact, thus preventing injury to the head, neck and back.

Head protective gear should be of durable construction to provide high impact-resistance and bump protection, have good abrasion qualities and, in some cases, have a dielectric strength to protect the wearer at certain types of operations. See Figure 115. More detailed information concerning head protection specifications can be found in American National Standard Institute's Z89 Standard.

There are two types of head protective devices on the market. One consists of an outer shell and the traditional suspension system. The other, a new development, consists of an outer shell lined with an energy-absorbing mate-

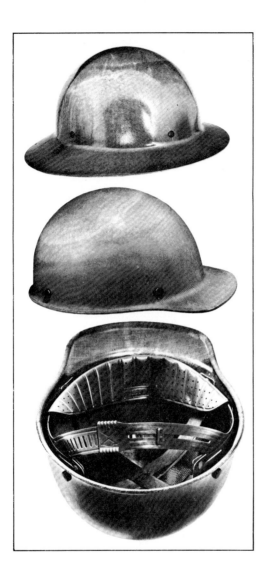

Figure 115. Industrial hard hats. (Courtesy Mine Safety Appliances Co.)

rial. Theoretically, this type can be worn without a suspension. However, this hard hat has not been very popular, as it is said to be uncomfortably warm, and in fact does not meet the existing standard for head protection. In both cases, the shells are designed to cushion the impact forces, deflect blows, and distribute the impact forces over a large area. Materials available for the new shell type have water, acid, and fire-resistant qualities and most are non-conductors of electricity. Plastics and fiber glass are among the materials commonly used.

Suspension systems perform a separate function. This web-type network, located inside the outer shell, supports the helmet on the wearer's head and prevents the shell from striking the worker's head when it is subjected to the forces of impact. The theory behind this system is that the longer the time duration it takes the forces of impact to reach the skull, the lesser the concussive effect. Suspension networks are made from various materials, although cloth and synthetic types are most common. The purchasing agent should examine suspension systems carefully before purchase, because, although a particular suspension may meet the ANSI standard, wide variances exist from one product to another.

Hard hats designed with a shell and a liner made of an energy-absorbing material conform to a different theory of head protection.

This theory indicates that the shorter the time duration of the forces of impact, the higher the pressure must be, in order to result in concussive effect. Therefore, this hard hat is capable of withstanding high impact with minimal concussive effect to the wearer's skull, by absorbing the energies transmitted and dissipating them over the surface of the liner. This theory deviates from that of hard hats using the web-types suspension networks, in that the suspension type depends upon a longer impact time duration, to absorb the shock before it reaches the skull.

This type of head gear consists of a hard shell, which will not be deformed excessively due to impact, and a liner, which will absorb the energies transmitted to it by the shell. Experiments indicate that greater impact can be sustained with the energy absorbing liner than with the suspension type.

In addition, it does not matter which part of the hard hat is subjected to impact, because adequate protection is provided on all part of the shell. Perhaps some day this type of head protection will be commonly used in the workplace.

Regardless of the type of head protective device selected, care will be required to keep the device in serviceable condition, because worn or damaged hats cannot provide the protection for which they were designed.

Care of Hard Hats

Following are guides for the proper care and maintenance of protective head gear:

- Suspension systems should be frequently inspected to detect deteriorated suspension system once found, deteriorated suspension systems must be replaced with brand new ones.
- Chemicals, oils, and petroleum products must be removed from shell materials as soon as possible, because these agents attack and soften certain shell materials and reduce their impact and dielectric protection. If it ever becomes necessary to repaint a hard hat, the manufacturer should be consulted regarding the choice of paints for a particular shell material.
- To assure the proper protection, the suspension network must leave 1 1/4 inches between the top of the wearer's head and the apex of the shell. The suspension lace, if present, should always be tied with a square knot.

- Hard hats that are damaged or do not fit properly should be replaced.
- For electrical work, hard hats should be tested periodically in acid, according to the ANSI Z 89.2, 1971, standard.
- Ventilation holes must never be drilled in the shell of a hard hat, as the holes will weaken its structural integrity.
- Proper care and maintenance of hard hats will assure their dependability in providing the protective function.
- Figure 116 illustrates a summary of the performance requirements for head gear as listed by the American National Standards Institute's Z89.1 and Z89.2 standards.

Eye Protection

Injury to eyes and loss of sight has plagued workers since their professions began. The National Safety Council estimates that approximately 100 industrial eye injuries occur each working day in the United States—of these, 10 result in partial or total loss of eyesight.

Workers are frequently exposed to physical and chemical agents that are capable of causing serious eye injury. The following are examples of injury—producing operations: cutting action of flying chips; air-borne dirt and debris; the impact of large and small flying particles generated by specialized cutting tools and splashing chemicals; bright light, injurious radiation. See Figure 117.

Figure 116. Protective requirements for head gear. (Courtesy of the American National Standards Institute.)

	CLASS			
	A	**B**	**C**	**D**
Description	General Use Limited Voltage	High Voltage Protection	General Use Metallic, No Voltage Protection	Firefighter Service
Material to be	Water Resistant Slow Burning	Water Resistant Slow Burning	Water Resistant Slow Burning	Fire Resistant
Insulation Resistance	2200 Volts 60 cps one minute 3 ma max. leakage	20,000 Volts 60 cps one minute 3 ma max. leakage	Not Applicable	2200 Volts 60 cps one minute 3 ma. max. leakage
Flammability	3 in./min.	3 in./min.	Not Applicable	Self Extinguishing
Water Absorption (by wt.)	5% max.	0.5% max.	5% max.	5% max.
Impact Energy	40 ft.-lb.	40 ft.lb.	40 ft.lb.	40 ft.-lb.
Impact Force **Avg.** **Attenuation** **Max.**	850 lbs. 1000 lbs.	850 lbs. 1000 lbs.	850 lbs. 1000 lbs.	850 lbs. 1000 lbs.
Weight, oz. max.	15	15.5	15	30
Penetration Resistance	3/8" max.	3/8" max.	7/16" max.	3/8" max.
Standard	Z89.1-1969	Z89.2-1971	Z89.1-1969	Z89.1-1969

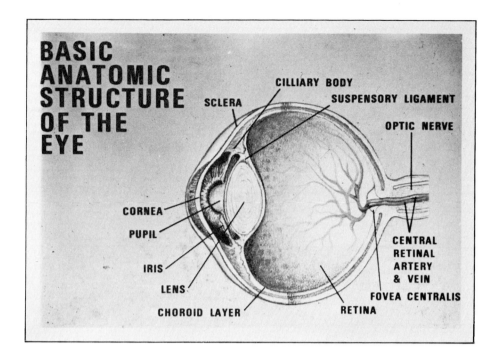

BASIC ANATOMIC STRUCTURE OF THE EYE

SCLERA

CILLIARY BODY

SUSPENSORY LIGAMENT

OPTIC NERVE

CORNEA

PUPIL

IRIS

LENS

CHOROID LAYER

CENTRAL RETINAL ARTERY & VEIN

FOVEA CENTRALIS

RETINA

Figure 117.

As with many other articles of personal protective equipment, some workers are reluctant to wear eye protection. Some of the reasons, which were valid in the past for rejecting eye protection—e.g., uncomfortable fit, distorted vision, fogging lenses, etc., are no longer justified, as modern eye protection has been significantly improved over their predecessors.

The selection of proper eyewear is not a simple task, because there are many products available, and each is specially designed to provide a particular type of protection (see Table 11.) The following points of information are offered to guide the evaluator toward proper eyewear selection.

Before a selection is made, consideration must be given to the extent of the hazard to be guarded against, the ability of the eye-protective material to afford this protection, and the types of eye-protective devices that fit the work objective. The types of eye-protective devices available include goggles, full face-shields and half face shields. Each performs a specific task. Figure 118 illustrates recommended eye and face protectors for use in industry, schools and colleges. Figure 119 illustrates a face shield/hard hat arrangement which nearly caused a worker to lose his eyes. When the employer decided that eye protection was necessary, he arbitrarily selected a face shield which seemed to meet his objectives for protection. However, he failed to consider that during a normal work day the worker frequently had to look above his head to align the materials he was working with. At the time of the accident, when a valve controlling a molten tar-like material failed, the molten tar spilled onto the

TABLE 11

Selected Properties of Eye-Wear Plastic Materials

	Acrylic	Polycarbonate	Polystyrene
Tensile strength (psi)	8,000-11,000	8,000- 9,500	3,500- 6,500
Flexural stranges (psi)	12,000-17,000	11,000-13,000	5,000-10,000
Impact strength (foot pounds)	0.4-0.5	12-16	.015-11.0
Hardness, Rockwell	M80-M100	M70-R118	M35-70 R50-100
Resistance to heat	140-200F.	250F.	140-175F.
Effect of sunlight	Very slight	Slight color change, slight embrittlement	Some strength loss
Effect of weak acids	Practically nil	None	None
Effect of strong acids	Attacked only by high concentrations of oxidizing acids	Attacked slightly	Attacked by oxidizing acids

worker's face shield. The space created at the point where the face shield came in contact with the bezel attached to the hard hat's brim, allowed the molten tar to enter the inside of the face shield causing burns to the worker's face. This situation illustrates that care must be taken before chosing any form of protective equipment and the employer must fully understand the capacity of the hazard to produce harm and the capabilities and limitations of the protective equipment to provide the desired protection.

Comfort Is Important

Regardless of which type of eye protection is selected, it is mandatory that the device fit the worker properly and comfortably. Uncomfortable or incorrect fitting eyewear will end up in a worker's pocket, thus negating its usefulness. A good rule to determine proper fit is to have the evaluator wear the protective device for a trial period. If it is uncomfortable to him, then it can well be expected to be the same for the worker. The edges of the device, which bear against the face, should be smooth and free from irregularities that might exert undue pressure or cause discomfort. Coupled with fit is vision. The device should be designed to afford an effective angle of vision of at least 105 degrees, and it should be made of materials that offer an acceptable degree of scratch-resistance.

Plastic is probably the most common material used for lens manufacture. This material combines mechanical strength and lightness of weight with impact-resistance. Of the many types of plastics on the market, the acrylics

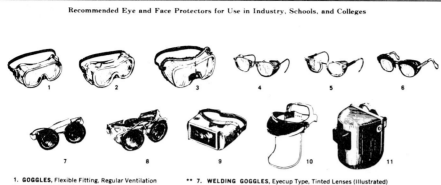

Recommended Eye and Face Protectors for Use in Industry, Schools, and Colleges

1. **GOGGLES**, Flexible Fitting, Regular Ventilation
2. **GOGGLES**, Flexible Fitting, Hooded Ventilation
3. **GOGGLES**, Cushioned Fitting, Rigid Body
*4. **SPECTACLES**, Metal Frame, with Sideshields
*5. **SPECTACLES**, Plastic Frame, with Sideshields
*6. **SPECTACLES**, Metal-Plastic Frame, with Sideshields

** 7. **WELDING GOGGLES**, Eyecup Type, Tinted Lenses (Illustrated)
7A. **CHIPPING GOGGLES**, Eyecup Type, Clear Safety Lenses (Not Illustrated)
** 8. **WELDING GOGGLES**, Coverspec Type Tinted Lenses (Illustrated)
8A. **CHIPPING GOGGLES**, Coverspec Type, Clear Safety Lenses (Not Illustrated)
** 9. **WELDING GOGGLES**, Coverspec Type, Tinted Plate Lens
10. **FACE SHIELD** (Available with Plastic or Mesh Window)
11. **WELDING HELMETS

*Non-sideshield spectacles are available for limited hazard use requiring only frontal protection.
**See appendix chart "Selection of Shade Numbers for Welding Filters."

APPLICATIONS		
OPERATION	**HAZARDS**	**RECOMMENDED PROTECTORS:** Bold Type Numbers Signify Preferred Protection
ACETYLENE—BURNING ACETYLENE—CUTTING ACETYLENE—WELDING	SPARKS, HARMFUL RAYS, MOLTEN METAL, FLYING PARTICLES	7, **8**, 9
CHEMICAL HANDLING	SPLASH, ACID BURNS, FUMES	**2**, 10 (For severe exposure add **10** over **2**)
CHIPPING	FLYING PARTICLES	**1**, **3**, 4, 5, 6, 7A, 8A
ELECTRIC (ARC) WELDING	SPARKS, INTENSE RAYS, MOLTEN METAL	9, **11** (**11** in combination with 4, 5, 6, in tinted lenses, advisable)
FURNACE OPERATIONS	GLARE, HEAT, MOLTEN METAL	7, **8**, 9 (For severe exposure add 10)
GRINDING—LIGHT	FLYING PARTICLES	**1**, **3**, 4, 5, 6, 10
GRINDING—HEAVY	FLYING PARTICLES	**1**, **3**, 7A, 8A (For severe exposure add 10)
LABORATORY	CHEMICAL SPLASH, GLASS BREAKAGE	**2** (10 when in combination with **4, 5, 6**)
MACHINING	FLYING PARTICLES	**1**, **3**, 4, 5, 6, 10
MOLTEN METALS	HEAT, GLARE, SPARKS, SPLASH	7, **8** (10 in combination with **4, 5, 6**, in tinted lenses)
SPOT WELDING	FLYING PARTICLES, SPARKS	**1**, **3**, 4, 5, 6, 10

This material is reproduced with permission from American National Standard "Occupational and Educational Eye and Face Protection, Practice for" Z87.1 copyright 1968 by the American National Standards Institute, copies of which may be purchased from the American National Standards Institute at 1430 Broadway, New York, New York 10018.

Figure 118. Selection chart.

and polycarbonates are probably the best for lens material. A common selection is the polycarbonates, because they combine tensile strength, impact-resistance, and resistance to heat and acids with lightness of weight and durability. This material offers excellent protection against impact and hot-metal and chemical splash hazards. However, there are certain chemicals that attack and weaken the polycarbonates. See Table 11.

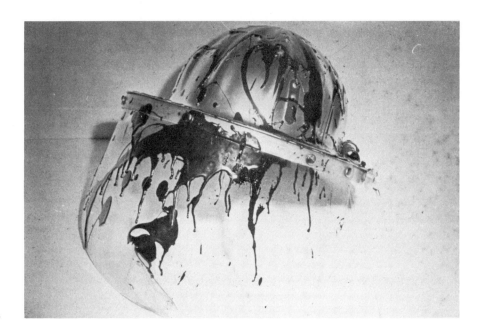

Figure 119.

Ventilation Is Necessary

Eye protective devices should be designed to permit the circulation of air behind the lens. Many operations involved contact with heat and water, and fogging becomes a problem. If a goggle type is selected, ventilation openings should be baffled or screened to prevent the direct passage of dust or liquids into the interior of the device. See Figure 120.

The lens should have the capacity to withstand at least 150 degrees F for one hour without noticeable distortion. All pertinent details concerning eye protection standards will be found in the American National Standard Institute's Z87.1 Standard.

Once selected, eye protective devices must be maintained to remain serviceable. Pitted or scratched lenses reduce vision and seriously reduce protection. When lenses are in this condition, they should be replaced immediately.

Workers Needing Corrective Lenses

Workers requiring corrective lenses must wear one of the following:(1) Spectacles with protective lenses which provide optical correction; (2) Goggles over corrected spectacles; (3) Goggles which incorporate corrective lenses mounted behind the protective lens.

Under no circumstances should a worker be allowed to wear contact lenses in places where eye hazards exist. Besides not having the capacity to provide the needed protection, there is additional rationale. Should the contact lense be shattered or a chemical substance get under the lens, serious eye damage may result.

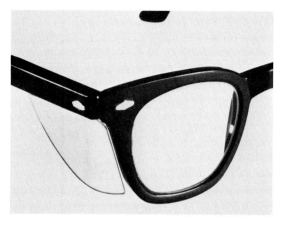

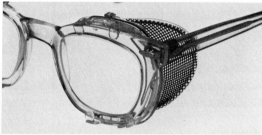

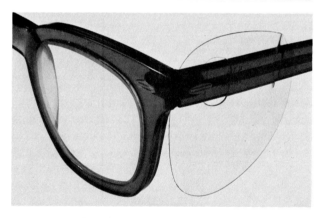

Figure 120. (Courtesy of Mine Safety Appliances Co.)

Respiratory Protection

The hazard control specialist who is establishing a respiratory protective program should take the time to assess his organization's particular needs. He should be certain that he understands why he is using respiratory protective equipment, what levels of contaminant he is guarding against, what the various types of respiratory equipment are that will provide this protection, how effective the protection will be, how much it will cost for the initial purchase, how much maintenance will be required, and what the cost of the maintenance will be. Answers to these questions, will require a study of the workplace and work processes, a careful reading of ANSI Z.88.2 *Practices for*

Respiratory Protection and a gathering of information from suppliers of respiratory equipment.

When selecting respiratory protective devices, consideration must be given to the specific types of hazards involved, because the effectiveness of such devices are limited to specific hazardous atmospheric conditions; i.e., oxygen deficiency, gaseous contaminants, particulate contaminants (dust, fumes, mists, fogs), or combinations of gaseous and particulate contaminants.

To do this the evaluator must consider: The *nature* of the hazard (oxygen deficiency or toxic air contaminant); *severity* (is the atmosphere immediately dangerous to life?); *type* of contaminant (gas, vapor, kind of particulate); *concentration* (is the contaminant concentration above safe levels? If so, how much above?); *period of protection* required (how long is the protection required?). Other factors determining the type of device procured are: *Location* of contaminated area (above ground, below ground, obstacles necessitating maneuvering, time duration between entering and leaving contaminated area), *activity of wearer* (the amount of freedom and flexibility needed by wearer to perform his tasks).

Respiratory protection, may be classified into three classes: Air purifying respirators; self-contained breathing devices; supplied air respirators.

Class I—Air Purifying Respirators

Class I air purifying respirators include two types: *gas masks and chemical cartridge respirators*. Gas masks consist of a facepiece, a canister containing an appropriate filtering material, a flexible tube leading from the facepiece to the canister and a harness system. The filtering material in each canister is designed to remove certain contaminants, such as chlorine, carbon monoxide, organic vapors, etc. Figure 121 illustrates the M.S.A. Type N Canister designed to provide protection against carbon monoxide. Gas Masks work on the principle of drawing contaminated air through the bottom of the canister, filtering it, and allowing air, free from the contaminant which the canister is capable of filtering, to reach the breathing zone of the user. See Figure 122. Gas masks are selected according to the level and specific type of contaminant present. Table 12 Color Code for Gas Masks will help in the selection of the proper canister to be used for a specific contaminant.

Gas Masks may be desirable because they are light weight, allow freedom of movement, and do a good job when used within their limitations. However, gas masks are limited to use in environments which contain at least 16 percent oxygen.

Chemical Cartridge Respirators

Chemical cartridge respirators are designed for use with dusts, fumes, or mists in combination with organic vapors. Included in this category of respirators is the particulate filter and

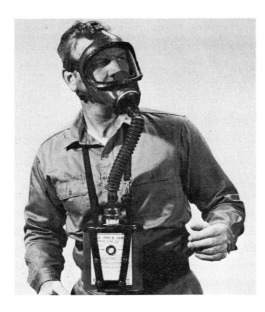

Figure 121. Type N Canister gas mask. (Courtesy Mine Safety Appliances Co.)

TABLE 12

Color Code for Gas Mask Canisters (ANSI K13.1—1967)

Atmospheric Contaminants To be Protected Against	Colors Assigned*
Acid Gases	White
Hydrocyanic acid gas	White with ½-inch green stripe completely around the canister near the bottom
Chlorine gas	White with ½-inch yellow stripe completely around the canister nead the bottom
Organic vapors	Black
Ammonia gas	Green
Carbon monoxide	Blue
Acid gases and organic vapors	Yellow
Hydrocyanic acid gas and chloropicrin vapor	Yellow with ½-inch blue stripe completely around the canister near the bottom
Acid gases and ammonia gas	Green with ½-inch white stripe completely around the canister near the bottom
Acid gases, organic vapors, and ammonia gas	Brown
Radioactive materials (excepting tritium and noble gases)	Purple (magenta)
Particulates (dusts, fumes, mists, fogs, or smokes) in combination with any of the above gases or vapors	Canister color for contaminants, as designated above with ½-inch gray stripe completely around the canister near the top
All of the above atmospheric contaminants	Red with ½-inch gray stripe completely around the canister near the top

*Gray shall not be assigned as the main color for a canister designed to remove gases or vapors.
Note: Orange shall be used as a complete body or stripe color to represent gases not included in this table. The used will need to refer to the canister label to determine the degree of protection the canister will afford.

This material is reproduced with permission from American National Standard Identification of Gas-Mask Canisters K 13.1-1967 copyright 1967 by the American National Standards Institute, copies of which may be purchased from the American National Standards Institute at 1430 Broadway, New York, New York 10018.

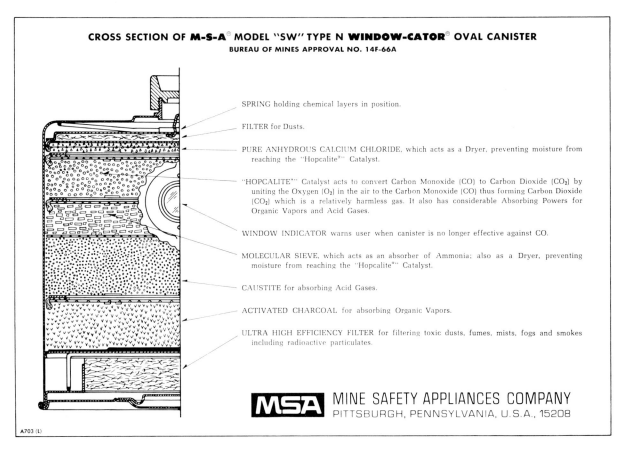

MSA MINE SAFETY APPLIANCES COMPANY
PITTSBURGH, PENNSYLVANIA, U.S.A., 15208

Figure 122. combination filter varieties. The *particulate (mechanical) filter respirator* can be designed to give satisfactory protection agianst any kind of particle. See Figure 123 and 123 A. However, the major items to be considered are the resistance to breathing offered by the filtering element, the adaption of the facepiece to faces of various sizes and shapes, and the fineness of the particles to be filtered out. Particulate filter respirators will remove particles of 0.3 microns (1/83,333 of an inch). A micron equals approximately 1/25,000 of an inch. *Combination Respirators.* The combination chemical and mechanical filter respirators Figure 124 utilize dust, mist, or fume filters with a chemical cartridge for duel or multiple exposure. Chemical cartridges do not last indefinitely. Once exhausted, they must be changed.

Class II—Supplied Air Respirators

This type of respirator supplies air to the user, through a facepiece via a tube from a source free of hazardous substances. One type of supplied air respirator is called a *Hose Mask*. Hose Masks fit over the face and have a

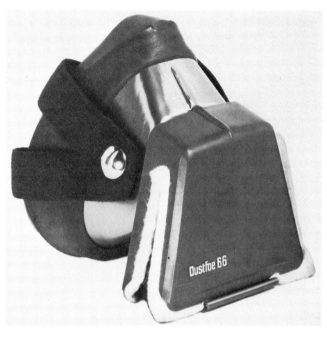

Figure 123. Mechanical filter respirator. (Courtesy **Mine** Safety Appliance Co.)

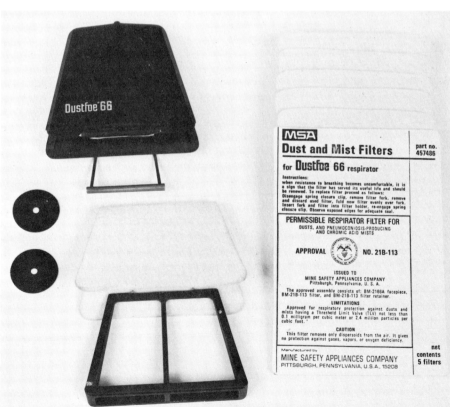

Figure 123a.

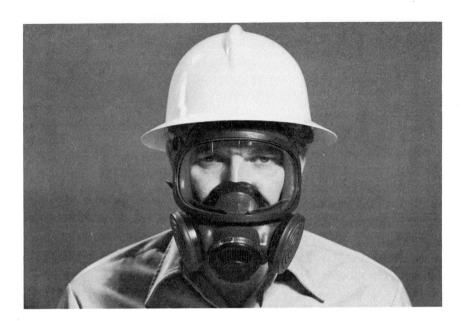

Figure 124. Combination respirator. (Courtesy Mine Safety Appliance Co.)

pressure hose for air supplied by a power-driven blower from an independent source which is known to be uncontaminated. The maximum length of hose approved by the U.S. Bureau of Mines and NIOSH is 300 feet. The OSHA Standards require that "in areas where the wearer, with failure of the respirator, could be overcome by a toxic or oxygen-deficient atmosphere, at least one additonal worker shall be present. Communication shall be maintained between both or all individuals present. Planning shall be such that one individual will be unaffected by any likely incident and have the proper rescue equipment to be able to assist the other(s) in case of an emergency." NIOSH recommends that hose-masks with blowers not be used in environments which are immediately harmful to life. The reason behind this recommendation is that if the blower fails, a significant negative pressure will develop in the facepiece permitting hazardous substances to leak in. Another type of supplied air respirator is called an *Air Line Respirator*. It is different from the hose mask in that it uses a compressed ailine from either a cylinder or a compressor for its oxygen supply, instead of a power-driven blower that is used for the hose masks. See Figure 125. A factor in favor of the supplied air respirator is that a positive pressure can be applied to the face mask, greatly reducing the chance of hazardous substances leaking into the apparatus. On the other hand, these respirators restrict movement about the workplace, and if the air line should be punctured, the user is immediately exposed to the damaging effects of the hazard. Thus, that is the reason why these respirators cannot be used in environments which are immediately dangerous to life and health. A point to remember about air line respirators is that the air received in the facepiece must be free from contaminants. Poorly designed or maintained compressors,

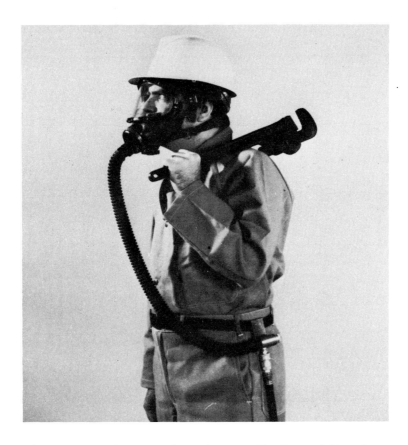

Figure 125. Constant flow
air-line respirator . . .

or compressors that are set-up in contaminated areas will substantially reduce
the air quality to be provided to the user.

Class III—Self-Contained Breathing Devices

Self-contained breathing devices are selected for work in a hazardous atmosphere, deficient in oxygen, where the worker will not be hampered by long
hoses, or threatened, should remote air supply either become contaminated or
fail.

There are two main classes of self-contained breathing devices: The Closed
Circuit Device and the Open Circuit Device. The most efficient type of closed
circuit (recirculating) device uses compressed air See Figure 126. The user
breathes oxygen from the air tank on his back. When the user exhales, his ex-
haled breath is directed to a reservoir breathing bag where the carbon is
separated from the oxygen, via a chemical cartridge. The remaining oxygen is
then available to be rebreathed. The Closed Circuit device provides for the
most efficient use of oxygen.

The Second Class of Self-contained breathing devices is called an Open Circuit Device, See Figures 127, 128 & 129. This device uses a cylinder of com-

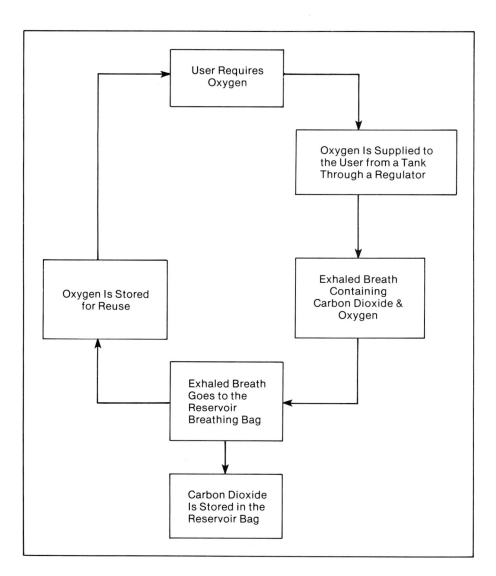

Figure 126. Closed circuit system.

pressed air that is carried on the users' back, and a mask and hose assembly with an exhalation valve. This type of breathing device is designed to provide up to thirty minutes of air to the user, depending on how hard he is working, and how much air he requires. A general "rule of thumb" to use in calculating the depletion time for an air cylinder is that a worker, working under moderate to heavy conditions, will require approximately 100 psi of air per minute. Thus, a 2,000 psi cylinder would last approximately twenty minutes, before it would have to be replaced. Figure 130 illustrates the components of one type of self-contained breathing appartus.

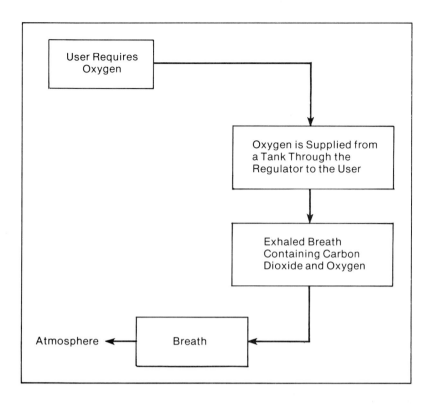

Figure 127. Open circuit system.

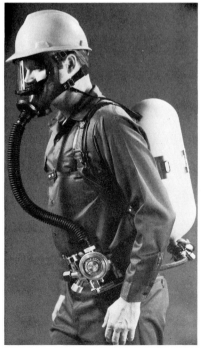

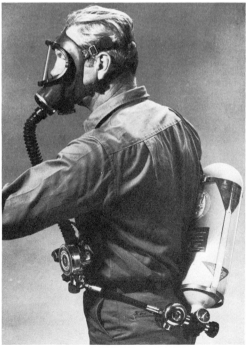

Figure 128. (left) Air mask TM 30-minute unit.

Figure 129. Air Cub TM 15-minute unit.

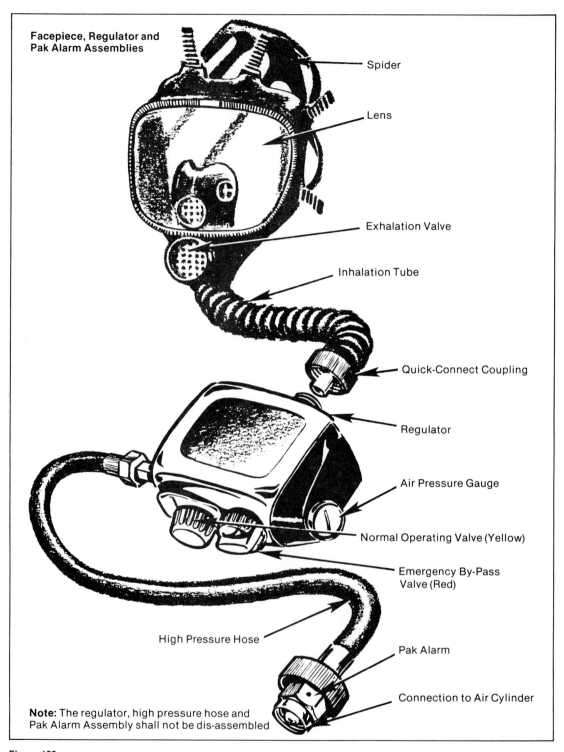

Facepiece, Regulator and Pak Alarm Assemblies

Spider

Lens

Exhalation Valve

Inhalation Tube

Quick-Connect Coupling

Regulator

Air Pressure Gauge

Normal Operating Valve (Yellow)

Emergency By-Pass Valve (Red)

High Pressure Hose

Pak Alarm

Connection to Air Cylinder

Note: The regulator, high pressure hose and Pak Alarm Assembly shall not be dis-assembled

Figure 130.

Figure 130. *Continued.*

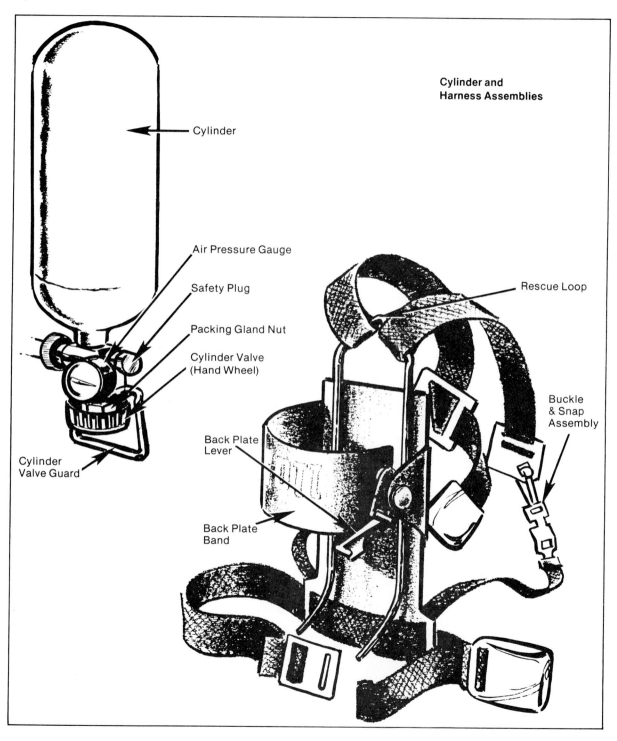

**Cylinder and
Harness Assemblies**

Cylinder

Air Pressure Gauge

Safety Plug

Packing Gland Nut

Cylinder Valve
(Hand Wheel)

Cylinder
Valve Guard

Rescue Loop

Buckle
& Snap
Assembly

Back Plate
Lever

Back Plate
Band

Positive Pressure—Open Circuit—Variety

A positive pressure, open circuit, self-contained breathing device is very similar to the standard Open Circuit variety except that constant air pressure is maintained in the wearer's facepiece. Pressure demand devices are preferred, since they reduce the possibility of hazardous substances leaking into the facepiece. See Figure 131.

Training

After selecting breathing apparatus, a training program must be instituted, to assure that the equipment will be used and maintained properly. It is essential that this training include explanations of the principles of operation, the capabilities and limitations of the equipment, the recognition of faulty functioning of equipment, instructions on what to do if the equipment malfunctions, and maintenance practices. Figure 132 illustrates a self-contained breathing device which was found with its harness assembly twisted and with its cylinder empty.

Another consideration is the proper fit of breathing apparatus face pieces. It is important for the worker to understand that if the face piece leaks, because it does not fit properly, protection is minimized.

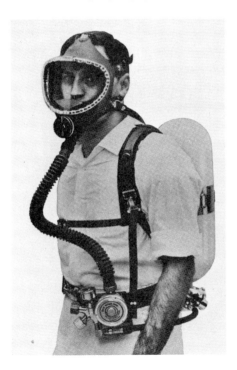

Figure 131. MSA pressure demand appartus. (Courtesy Mine Safety Appliance Co.)

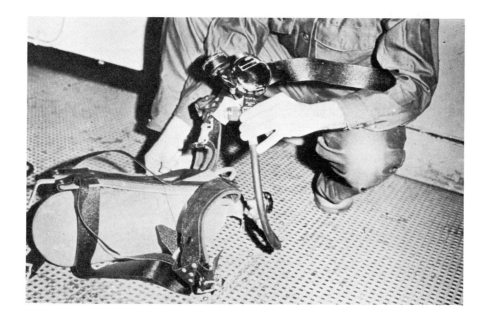

Figure 132. Self-contained
breathing apparatus
which was stored with
tangled harness assembly
and low air pressure in
cylinder.

Workers should also be instructed that it is their responsibility to guard against damage to the respiratory equipment and to report malfunctions to responsible persons as soon as possible.

Selecting the Proper Respirator

The information in Figure 133 will be of value in assisting the hazard control specialist in selecting the proper respirator for the problem at hand.

There are three main groups of ear protective devices: (1) plug or insert type; (2) cup of muff type; (3) enclosure which compeletely surrounds the head.

Ear Plugs or Inserts are classified as *aural*—those which are inserted into the ear canal and *superaural*—those which seal the external edges of the ear canal. Ear plugs, properly fitted, generally reduce noise reaching the ear by 25-30 decibels (DB) in the higher frequencies providing protection against sound levels of 115 to 120 db. See Figure 134. However, a slight leak will lower the ear plugs attenuator capacity as much as 15 db in some frequencies.

Ear Muffs are designed to cover the external ear and to provide an acoustic barrier. The amount of attenuation provided by ear muffs depends on the differences in ear muff design, head size and shape of the user, etc. The more effective ear muff may reduce noise approximately 10 to 15 decibels more than ear plugs, making them effective against sound levels of 130 to 135 db. See Figures 135 , 136, and 136a.

A combination of ear plugs and ear muffs give 3 to 5 more db of protection.

Ear Protection

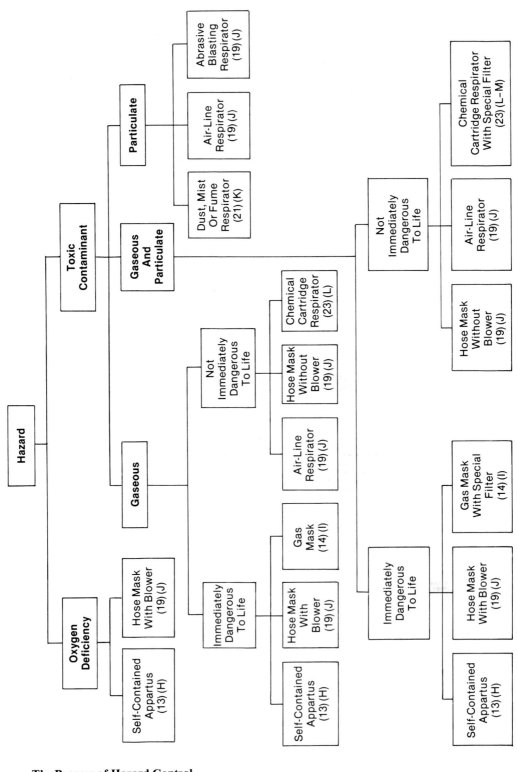

Figure 133. Outline for selecting respiratory protective devices. (Based on Bureau of Mines Information Circular 7792. Numbers in parentheses refer to Bureau of Mines Schedules; letter in parentheses refer to Subpart of NIOSH/MESA 30 CFR Part 11.)

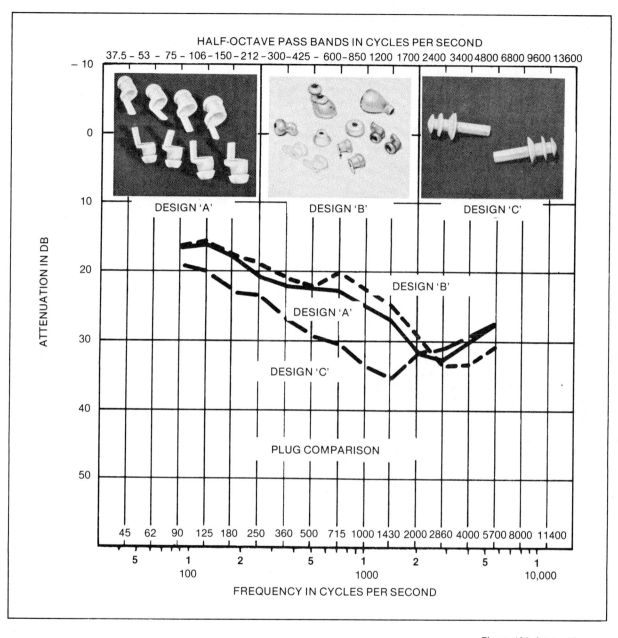

HALF-OCTAVE PASS BANDS IN CYCLES PER SECOND

DESIGN 'A' DESIGN 'B' DESIGN 'C'

PLUG COMPARISON

Figure 134. Attenuation (noise-reducing) characteristics of plug or insert type ear protection. Curves are for plugs of design shown in photographs above. (Courtesy of the National Safety Council.)

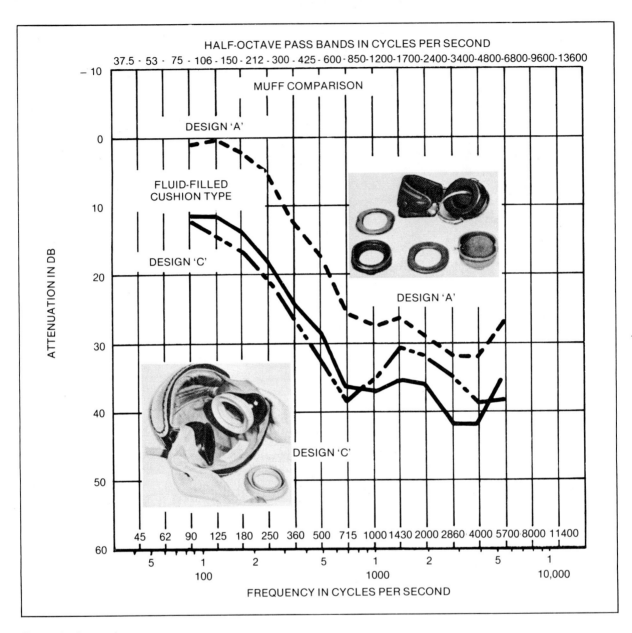

Figure 135. Attenuation characteristics of cup or muff type ear protectors. (Data from J. C. Webster and E. R. Rubin, U.S. Navy Electronics Laboratory. Courtesy of the National Safety Council.)

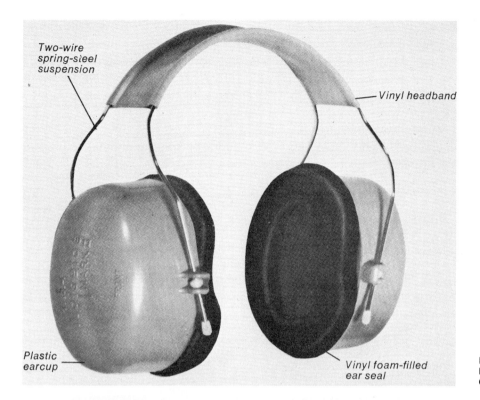

Two-wire spring-steel suspension

Vinyl headband

Plastic earcup

Vinyl foam-filled ear seal

Figure 136. (Courtesy Mine Safety Appliance Co.)

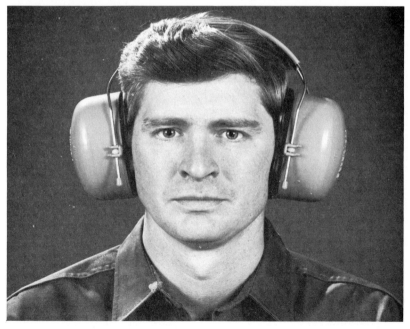

Figure 136a. (Courtesy Mine Safety Appliance Co.)

Protective Footwear, like any other article of protective equipment, must be selected after the full extent of the hazard is assessed.

Table 13 demonstrates that there are three classifications of safety toe footwear (classes 25, 50 and 75) which protect against various impact forces in foot pounds. Figures 137 and 138 illustrate the toe box system in safety toe footwear.

Should a worker have his safety toe box stressed under impact, the shoe should be brought to the appropriate authority for examination before its use is continued.

TABLE 13

Minimum Requirements for Men's Safety Toe Footwear

Classification	Compression Pounds	Impact, Foot Pounds	Clearance Inches
75	2,500	75	16/32
50	1,750	50	16/32
25	1,000	25	16/32

This material is reproduced with permission from American National Standard "Men's Safety-Toe Footwear" Z41.1 copyright 1967 by the American National Standards Institute, copies of which may be purchased from the American National Standards Institute at 1430 Broadway, New York, New York 10018.

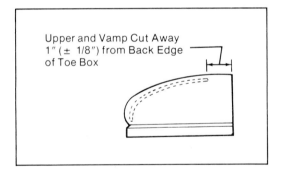

Figure 137. Toe box prepared for impact testing. (This material is reproduced with permission from American National Standard "Men's Safety-Toe Footwear" Z41.1 copyright 1967 by the American National Standards Institute, copies of which may be purchased from the American National Standards Institute at 1430 Broadway, New York, New York 10018.)

Upper and Vamp Cut Away 1″ (± 1/8″) from Back Edge of Toe Box

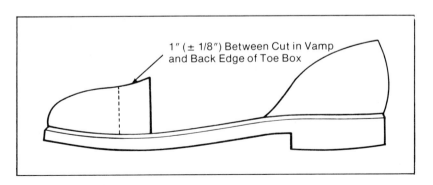

Figure 138. Footwear with vamp and upper cut away to facilitate compression testing. (This material is reproduced with permission from American National Standard "Men's Safety-Toe Footwear" Z41.1 copyright 1967 by the American National Standards Institute, copies of which may be purchased from the American National Standards Institute at 1430 Broadway, New York, New York 10018.)

1″ (± 1/8″) Between Cut in Vamp and Back Edge of Toe Box

The specific intent of this section is to: Arouse a conscious awareness of the dangers involved with using, transporting and storing hazardous materials and substances that can be injurious to the health of the industrial worker.

The Problem

The amazing progress of science and technology in our time has endowed mankind with virtually unlimited capability to produce materials and substances designed to make industry and the home easier to work and live in.

Progress does not always come without complications. In fact, man often pays quite severely for the effects of his inventions. Year after year, disasters of significant magnitude occur throughout the nation, many initiated by materials, which, from this point on, will be referred to as "hazardous."

The term, hazardous materials, has taken on so many varied definitions that it is extremely difficult to distinguish between those materials that have and do not have hazard potential. Certainly a truckload of 1, 3-butadiene cylinders can be readily recognized as being of high hazard potential because of butadiene's flammability, rapid vaporization, and easy-burning characteristics at normal temperatures and pressures, and because it is unstable and may form potentially explosive mixtures with water. In fact, this material is labeled as a flammable gas, indicating the hazard potential of its contents.

On the other hand, what about calcium carbide? Is calcium carbide dangerous? It is obvious to those who are familiar with basic chemistry that calcium carbide, under a proper set of circumstances, could be hazardous to health, especially if it comes into contact with water. Would safety or emergency personnel be aware of what they are up against? Experience indicates that they often wouldn't.

This is one example of the need for complete knowledge of the materials and substances used on the job, and transported throughout the country.

Several years ago a disaster occurred involving a train derailment that included eight tank cars loaded with vinyl chloride. When the vinyl chloride tanks were punctured and the material began to escape on the ground, decisions had to be—and were—made rapidly. On the advice of a chemist, an estimated 17,000 to 21,000 persons were evacuated from the area, primarily because it was feared that the vinyl chloride, if ignited, would generate phosgene gas. Later it was determined that the evacuation was not required, because the purported danger from phosgene gas did not justify the action in this particular circumstance. In fact, had emergency control personnel, trained hose streams on the vinyl chloride tanks (which had been impinged upon by flame for almost ten hours), the explosion and associated losses could have been averted. This is a clear case where information on a material labeled as "hazardous" was not sufficient.

When information was called for on vinyl chloride, this is what was received: "Vinyl Chloride—a colorless, sweet-smelling flammable gas at ordinary temperatures . . . forms explosive mixtures in air . . . gas is heavier than air and may travel a considerable distance to a source of ignition . . . will flash back . . . fires involving chloride result in the production of hydrogen chloride gas, phosgene gas, carbon dioxide, and water."

After the disaster, it was determined that, under conditions such as those detailed, the combustion of vinyl chloride could produce no detectable amount of phosgene. In this case, the reported danger from phosgene obscured the fact that the real danger associated with burning vinyl chloride is the hydrogen gas which is produced.

The conclusion drawn as a result of this case indicates that no accurate assessment of the burning vinyl chloride situation was made.

The situation described does not stand alone. Similar castrophies have happened at other places throughout the nation. A butane gas tank explosion in Illinois; an ammonium nitrate explosion in Texas City that resulted in $50 million damage and 561 deaths; the detonation in a building containing ammonium nitrate, pesticides, and other materials in Vernon, MO, and similar instances point out the necessity of complete knowledge of properties of hazardous materials to deal effectively and safely with potential catastrophic situations involving hazardous materials.

Materials with Known Potential

In addition to the problem of controlling hazardous materials where (in an emergency state) some hazard data are available, no matter how incomplete, there are situations where materials, that are normally thought of as being of one hazard classification for which control measures have been specified, present hazards of an entirely different class. For example, ethers are normally thought of as being flammable liquid fire hazards. However, their chemical instability may allow them to form organic peroxides, which are detonable.

Chlorine is another example of a material that presents unpredicted hazards. Chlorine is classified as a nonflammable compressed gas. However, chlorine is an oxidizing agent that can increase the ignition risk of other materials. Although chlorine would have a zero fire hazard, it could be the very trigger to a large-scale catastrophe. For example, if gasoline or LP gas should combine with chlorine during an emergency situation, a serious fire or explosion could occur resulting in the production of hydrogen chloride, phosgene, and similar toxic or irritant combustion gases. The last example can illustrate the magnitude of synergistic effects of chemical reactions, where the resultant problem has greater hazard potential than either of its constituents.

Hazardous Materials

Although some of the problems involved with hazardous materials have been suggested, the most paramount one remains to be discussed—the ability to identify a hazardous material.

Under certain circumstances, almost any material could be classified as hazardous. This premise can certainly cause confusion and it's use in hazard control is inadequate.

An example of this problem revealed itself recently during a discussion concerning compressed oxygen. The question was posed—"Is compressed oxygen to be classified as a hazardous material?" Answers were varied. Some felt that it was; others disagreed. The fact of the matter is that compressed oxygen may not be normally thought of as being a hazardous material. However, in a particular emergency state, under certain conditions, it does have high hazard potential and should be treated with respect.

Before Setting Controls

So far it seems obvious that as the first step before proper controls can be set, the term hazardous material must be precisely defined. Many definitions have been developed over the years. However, in almost every case, these definitions railed to cover all the materials that could have detrimental effects on people, property, or the environment.

The following definition is offered as an attempt to identify materials that are detrimental to workers, emergency personnel, the workplace, and the environment.

A hazardous material is any element, compound, or combination thereof, that is flammable, corrosive, poisonous, detonable, toxic, radioactive, an oxidizer, and etiological agent or is highly reactive, and that, because of handling, storing, processing, packaging, or transporting, may have detrimental effects upon operating and emergency personnel, equipment, the workplace, and/or the environment.

Hazardous Materials—Definition Breakdown

Flammable materials are readily ignitable in their designed operational state or when inadvertently released in the atmosphere.

Examples: Gasoline—all conditions; kerosene—when heated to flash point or under pressure.

Detonable materials, when subjected to heat, shock, friction, or electrical discharges, may violently decompose, creating shock waves.

Examples: TNT, dynamite, blasting caps.

Toxic materials, when released into the environment, have the capacity to be detrimental to man when sufficient quantities of the material are ingested, absorbed through the skin, or inhaled.

Examples: Phosgene, chlorine, sulphur dioxide.

Corrosive materials have the capacity to disintegrate or otherwise destroy living tissue or materially damage structures, vehicles, cargo, or containers or are likely to cause fire when in contact with organic matter or with certain chemicals.

Poisons

Oxidizers are agents that, when mixed with any element, compound, or combination thereof have the capacity to cause fire or explosion.

Examples: Perchlorates, nitrates.

Radioactive materials or combination of materials are those spontaneously emitting ionizing radiation.

Example: Radium.

Highly reactives are any element, compounds or combination thereof that, when mixed with certain other elements, compounds, or combinations thereof, have the capacity to spontaneously ignite, explode, polymerize, or generate toxic or flammable gases.

Examples: Calcium carbide, perchloric acid.

Etiological agents are agents that cause disease.

Examples: Anthrax-producing agents.

These definitions have been specifically designed to cover all types of materials that have detrimental effects on the industrial worker, energency personnel, and the community at large. If all materials that fit these definitions could be recognized and the necessary safety measures taken when dealing with them, deaths, injuries, and damage to the workplace would be considerably reduced.

Knowledge of the properties of each material or substance deemed hazardous must be available to all personnel. The worker must know what he is working with, or is exposed to, and understand exactly what precautions are necessary to protect his health and safety.

One way of providing this information is via special hazardous materials information sheets (see Table 14). These data sources should be provided for each hazardous material in the workplace. Each first line supervisor should have them in his or her possession, and the problems concerning each should be made available to his workers.

To construct these data sheets, information on hazards of industrial chemicals can be acquired from the manufacturer of the chemical, and from the following sources:

- Sax, I., "Dangerous Properties of Industrial Materials," Reinhold Publishing Co., New York 10000.

TABLE 14

Toluene (C$_6$H$_5$CH$_3$)

Other Names: Toluol, Methylbenzene, Phenylmethane.

Uses: Toluene is used extensively as the basic material in the manufacture of many important organic chemicals—such as explosives and dyes—and as a solvent for a wide variety of gums, resins, and fats.

Physical Properties:
Toluene is a colorless, flammable liquid with an odor similar to benzene

Molecular Weight—92.13	Specific Gravity—0.866 at 20.4C
Vapor Pressure—30 mm Hg @ 68F	Boiling Point—230.7F (110.4C)
Flash Point (closed cup)—40F	Auto-ignition Temperature—1,026F

Explosive Limits (by volume in air)—from 1.27 to 6.75 percent
Density (at 68F)—3.14 (air equaling 1)
The TLV for prolonged exposure to toluene vapors is 200 ppm in air.

Hazardous Properties:
Health Hazards (physiological effects)—Toluene vapors can cause irritation of the eyes, nose, and throat as well as headaches, dizziness, lack of coordination, sleepiness, or unconsciousness. Prolonged or repeated skin contact will produce dermatitis. Toluene is also harmful if swallowed.

First Aid
Vapor inhalation—Immediately remove the victim from the contaminated atmosphere, and contact the medical department.
Skin contact—Flush the affected areas immediately with soap and water for at least five minutes, removing clothing and shoes if they have become contaminated. Contact the medical department as quickly as possible.
Eye contact—Irrigate immediately with water for at least 15 minutes, holding eyelids apart to insure water contact with all eye and lid tissue surfaces. **Do not rub!** Call the medical department at once.
Ingestion—Call the medical department immediately.

Precautions
Personal Protection—Avoid contact with the skin. Wear protective clothing and equipment as required. Do not rely on protective creams to afford adequate protection. Do not use to clean hands, arms, or other portions of the skin. Avoid prolonged or repeated breathing of toluene vapor.
Protective Facilities—Provide ventilation for operations where toluene is being sprayed, heated, or agitated by air or mechanical means. Never work with any solvent in a confined area or space without mechanical ventilation and respiratory protection. Provide electrical equipment of the explosion-proof type where toluene is used or stored.
Fire Protection—Keep containers closed when not in use, and keep them away from heat, fire, or spark sources—such as exposed flame heaters or electrical heaters of any type, welding or cutting torches, lead or solder pots, flare pots, lighted smoking materials, etc. Notify the appropriate department when toluene is being used. Keep toluene in approved cans, and never store more than one day's supply on the job.

Labeling: All containers shall be clearly identified and have approved label warnings.

Storage: Toluene should be stored in a cool, well ventilated area away from possible sources of heat, fire, or sparks. Drums or tanks for storing toluene should be grounded to prevent the accumulation of static electricity. When toluene is being dispensed, the receiving container should also be grounded. The grounding must be of an approved type.

One way of providing details on an especially hazardous material is with an information sheet on the material. Each first line supervisor should have copies of these information sheets. The sheet can be printed on standard size paper and kept (alphabetically by material name) in a notebook for referral.

- Manufacturing Chemists Association, Chem Card Manual, 1825 Connecticut Ave., N.W., Washington, D.C. 20009.
- Association American Railroads, Bureau of Explosives, Dangerous Articles Emergency Guide, 2 Penn Plaza, New York 10000.
- National Safety Council, Alphabetical Index Industrial Safety Data Sheets, 425 N. Michigan Ave., Chicago 60626
- U.S. Army Chemical Center, Hazardous Commerical Chemical Data, For McClellan, Alabama—November, 1970.
- National Fire Protection Association, Fire Protection Guide on Hazardous Materials, 60 Batterymarch St., Boston, 02110.

Data sheets should be brief and easy to read, but still provide essential information.

Available Systems

Many agencies and industrial firms have taken available information on hazardous materials and catalogued it for ready reference. Others have developed systems for identifying certain kinds of hazardous materials. Each of these is available for the asking. Representatives of these systems are:

The Department of Transportation—System for the Transportation of Hazardous Materials.[4]

DOT has devised a system to promote uniform enforcement of law and to minimize the dangers to life and property incident to the transportation of explosives and other dangerous articles by common carriers engaged in interstate or foreign commerce.

The system is one of single hazard identification. The classes are divided into the following:

Class 1—Explosives
Class 2—Flammable and nonflammable compressed gas
Class 3—Flammable liquid
Class 4—Flammable solid
Class 5—Oxidizing material
Class 6—Poisons
Class 7—Corrosive liquids

A drawback with this system is that dangerous articles having more than one hazardous characteristic, as defined by the DOT regulations, must be classified according to the greatest hazard present, except those articles that are also poisons, Class B[1] or D[2], which must be classified according to both dangerous characteristics.

Often a material will have several equally serious hazards. Which one should receive recognition? A good example of this would be acrylonitrile, which according to DOT is classified as a flammable liquid. However, NFPA rates this same material as a Class 2 Reactive material (because it polymerizes). Hydrogen sulfide is another. DOT classifies it as a flammable gas; NFPA as a serious Health and Flammability hazard. Sometimes these same problems of classification face the industrial worker. There have been times when a plant manager has ordered solvents to be used for some industrial process and later found out that the solvent presented hazards not previously considered. What happened? Suppose the chemical used in the solvent was carbon tetrachloride (CCL_4), as to flammability, it won't burn and can be considered safe from that standpoint. Most people know CCL_4 is an extinguishing agent. However, from a health standpoint, CCL_4 is hazardous—in that it has the ability to cause damage to the liver, skin, respiratory tract, etc. In addition it produces phosgene gas when it comes in contact with heated metals. This situation could be averted if the manufacturer is asked to supply any hazardous material data concerning the solvent prior to plant personnel using it in the workplace.

NFPA System

National Fire Protection Association—Hazard Identification System— NFPA 704 M. (2)

The NFPA system consists of a diamond-shaped figure divided into four quadrants, in three of which are designated numerals that indicate the severity of the hazard (see Figure 139 and Table 15). The bottom space is reserved for special information. In this space there may be a (W) with a line drawn through its center. This symbol indicates that water should not be used on the material because of its reactive characteristics (see Figure 139).

This same space may also be used to indicate that the chemical is subject to polymerization under some emergency conditions (P) or to identify a radiation hazard.

The diamond-shaped diagram allows workers to identify the "flammability," "reactivity," and "health" hazards of a chemical by indicating the degree of hazard or extreme danger from zero (meaning no particular concern) to four (indicating severe hazard or extreme danger). See Figure 140.

University of Minnesota

The University of Minnesota has developed a system for labeling hazardous materials that is based on the NFPA 704M System. However, they have added additional information (see Figure 141). If a system such as this were to be used throughout the workplace to identify hazardous materials, and all workers were educated in its use, a step forward would be taken to reduce the number of injuries and deaths resulting from hazardous materials.

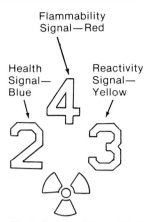

Flammability
Signal—Red

Health
Signal—
Blue

Reactivity
Signal—
Yellow

Fig. 1. For Use Where White Background is Not Necessary.

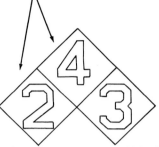

White Adhesive-Backed Plastic Background Pieces—One Needed for Each Numeral, Three Needed for Each Complete Signal.

Fig. 2. For Use Where White Background is Used With Numerals Made From Adhesive-Backed Plastic.

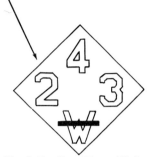

White Painted Background, or, White Paper or Card Stock

Fig. 3. For Use Where White Background is Used With Painted Numerals or, For Use When Signal is in the Form of Sign or Placard.

ARRANGEMENT AND ORDER OF SIGNALS —OPTICAL FORM OF APPLICATION

Distance at Which Signals Must be Legible	Size of Signals Required
50 feet	1″
75 feet	2″
100 feet	3″
200 feet	4″
300 feet	6″

NOTE:
This shows the correct spatial arrangement and order of signals used for identification of materials by hazard.

IDENTIFICATION OF MATERIALS BY HAZARD SIGNAL ARRANGEMENT

Figure 139. Illustrates the NFPA Hazard Identification System, which consists of a diamond-shaped figure divided into four quandrants. Three of the numerals indicate the severity of the hazard, and the bottom quadrant is reserved for special information. Reproduced by permission from "Identification System of Fire Hazards of Materials" (NFPA No. 704M), 1969 edition, copyright National Fire Protection Association, 60 Batterymarch Street, Boston, Mass.)

MCA's CHEMTREC

The Manufacturing Chemists' Association (MCA) has developed a system called Chemical Transportation Emergency Center (CHEMTREC).

This facility, which went into effect on September 5, 1971, is designed to provide immediate action response information to the scene of a chemical transportation accident, on receipt of a phone call identifying the product involved. The service is available twenty-four hours a day, seven days a week.

Once the call is placed, CHEMTREC will provide the caller with response/action information for the product or products, and tell what to do in case of spills, leaks, fire, and exposure. This informs the caller of the hazards, if any, and provides sufficient information to take immediate first steps in controlling the emergency. CHEMTREC's toll free telephone number is (800) 424–9300. This system, as well as other information from the MCA is valuable in controlling hazardous materials used in the workplace.

TABLE 15

Hazard Identification System

Identification of Health Hazard Color Code: BLUE		Identification of Flammability Color Code: RED		Identification of Reactivity (Stability) Color Code: YELLOW	
	Type of Possible Injury		Susceptibility of Materials to Burning		Susceptibility to Release of Energy
Signal		Signal		Signal	
4	Materials which on very short exposure could cause death or major residual injury even though prompt medical treatment were given.	4	Materials which will rapidly or completely vaporize at atmospheric pressure and normal ambient temperature, or which are readily dispersed in air and which will burn readily.	4	Materials which in themselves are readily capable of detonation or of explosive decomposition or reaction at normal temperatures and pressures.
3	Materials which on short exposure could cause serious temporary or residual injury even though prompt medical treatment were given.	3	Liquids and solids that can be ignited under almost all ambient temperature conditions.	3	Materials which in themselves are capable of detonation or explosive reaction but require a strong initiating source or which must be heated under confinement, before initiation or which react explosively with water.
2	Materials which on intense or continued exposure could cause temporary incapacitation or possible residual injury unless prompt medical treatment is given.	2	Materials that must be moderately heated or exposed to relatively high ambient temperatures before ignition can occur.	2	Materials which in themselves are normally unstable and readily undergo violent chemical change but do not detonate. Also materials which may react violently with water or which may form potentially explosive mixtures with water.
1	Materials which on exposure would cause irritation but only minor residual injury even if no treatment is given.	1	Materials that must be pre-heated before ignition can occur.	1	Materials which in themselves are normally stable, but which can become unstable at elevated temperatures and pressures or whch may react with water with some release of energy but not violently.
0		0	Materials that will not burn.	0	Materials which in themselves are normally stable, even under fire exposure conditions, and which are not reactive with water.

Table 15 lists the NFPA numerical designations of specific types of hazards. The numbers, themselves, are color-coded as follows: blue indicates a health hazard; red indicates a flammable hazard; yellow denotes the reactivity of a particular substance.

Reproduced by permission from "Identification System of Fire Hazards of Materials" ((NFPA No. 704M), 1969 edition, copyright National Fire Protection Association, 60 Batterymarch Street, Boston, Mass.

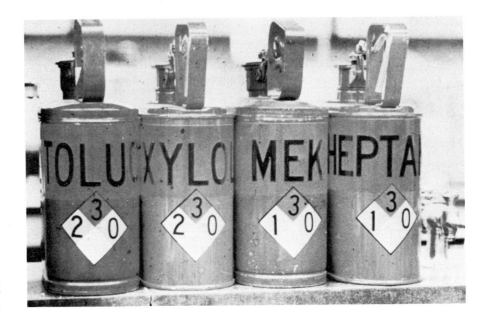

Figure 140. Hazardous chemical marked for worker recognition.

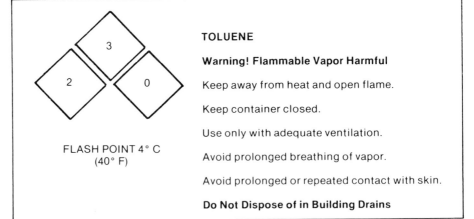

Figure 141. Is an example of a hazardous material labeling system that was developed by the University of Minnesota. It was based on the NFPA system, but it adds information about the substance. (Courtesy University of Minnesota.)

FLASH POINT 4° C
(40° F)

TOLUENE

Warning! Flammable Vapor Harmful

Keep away from heat and open flame.

Keep container closed.

Use only with adequate ventilation.

Avoid prolonged breathing of vapor.

Avoid prolonged or repeated contact with skin.

Do Not Dispose of in Building Drains

Other Organizations

Information concerning hazardous materials may also be acquired from such organizations as the Nuclear Safety Information Center, National Pollution Response Center, U.S. Coast Guard, National Safety Council (Chemical Data Sheets), and Railway Systems and Management Association.

If hazardous materials must be used in the workplaces, they must be properly controlled. The hazard control specialist, the supervisors, and the worker himself must be interested enough to learn about the hazard potential of the materials they are working with and the necessary safeguards to control their use.

References

For materials outline or mentioned here, write to the source:

1. The Department of Transportation
    400 Seventh St., S.W.
    Washington, D.C. 20590
2. National Fire Protection Association
    60 Batterymatch St.
    Boston 02110
3. Nuclear Safety Information Center
    Oak Ridge National Library Box Y
    Oak Ridge, Tenn. 37830
4. National Pollution Response Center, U.S. Coast Guard
    400 Seventh St., S.W.
    Washington, D.C. 20591
5. U.S. Coast Guard
    400 Seventh St., S.W.
    Washington, D.C. 20591
6. The National Safety Council, (Chemical Data Sheets)
    425 N. Michigan Ave.
    Chicago, Illinois 60611
7. Railway Systems and Management Association
    163 E. Walton St.
    Chicago, Illinois 60611
8. Manufacturing Chemists' Association
    1825 Connecticut Ave., N.W.
    Washington, D.C. 20009

Unit 4 Fire Protection

Introduction

Fire Loss to Industry

The National Fire Prevention and Control Administration estimates that fire killed approximately 7,800 people in the United States during 1976. Property destroyed by fire during 1971 totaled approximately $3.35 billion. Table 16 presents estimates of numbers of fires and corresponding losses by type of fire for 1976. Table 17 presents estimates of numbers of fires and corresponding dollar losses for elected property uses for 1976. In both tables, the dollar amounts include only direct property damage resulting from fire, and no adjustments were made for monetary inflation.

Ignition Sources

A study made by the Factory Mutual Engineering Corporation of almost 25,000 industrial fires, reported over a ten-year period indicates that the majority of fires have their origins traced to the following general causes:

1. 23% electrical
2. 18% smoking
3. 10% friction
4. 8% overheated materials
5. 7% hot surfaces
6. 7% burner flames
7. 5% combustion sparks
8. 4% spontaneous ignition
9. 4% cutting and welding
10. 3% exposure
11. 3% incendiarism
12. 2% mechanical sparks
13. 2% molten substances
14. 1% chemical action
15. 1% static sparks
16. 1% lightening
17. 1% miscellaneous

Electrical (23%)   Electrical fires are the leading cause of industrial fires. They are caused by electrical arcing, short circuits, overheated electrical equipment, etc.

TABLE 16

Estimated United States Fires and Property Loss by Type of Fire, 1976

Type of Fire	Number of Fires	Property Loss
Building	964,200	$2,656,400,000
Vehicle	492,900	215,200,000
Brush and rubbish, outside buildings	1,127,600	19,900,000
Other	354,400	468,500,000
TOTALS:	2,939,100	$3,360,000,000

These estimates are based on data reported to the NFPA by the public fire service. No adjustments were made for unreported fires and losses. Dollar figures represent direct property loss only and were not adjusted for monetary inflation. With the exception of brief excerpts for news or editorial purposes, no reproduction of this table or any part thereof is permitted without the express written consent of the National Fire Protection Association.

TABLE 17

Estimated United States Fires and Property Losses for Selected Property Uses, 1976*

Property Use	Number of Fires		Property Loss	
Public Assembly		37,700		$ 188,900,000
Educational		23,500		159,700,000
Institutional		24,100		25,300,000
Residential		665,400		1,433,000,000
One-and two-family dwellings	451,200		940,400,000	
Apartments	159,600		319,800,000	
Hotels and motels	16,000		62,500,000	
Mobile homes	16,800		59,200,000	
Other residential	21,800		51,100,000	
Stores and offices		76,300		508,000,000
Industry, utility, defense**		50,000		289,400,000
Storage**		42,300		235,400,000

*Since this table does not present results for all property users, the statistics presented should not be totaled to obtain estimates of overall U.S. fire experience.

**Since some incidents for these property uses are handled only by private fire brigades or fixed suppression systems and are not reported to the NFPA, the results represent only a portion of U.S. fire experience.

These estimates are based on data reported to the NFPA by the public fire service. No adjustments were made for unreported fires and losses. Dollar figures represent direct property loss only and where not adjusted for monetary inflation. With the exception of brief excerpts for news or editorial purposes, no reproduction of this table or any part thereof is permitted without the express written consent of the National Fire Protection Association.

Taken from "A Study of United States Fire Experience," 1976, Fire Journal, National Fire Prevention and Control Administration, 1977.

Smoking (18%)　　Fires started by careless or neglectful workers who do not abide by the rules which prohibit them from smoking in dangerous areas of which contain flammable liquids, gases, vapors, dusts, fibers, etc.

Friction (10%)　　Fires caused by heat produced by inadequate lubrication, cutting or grinding operations, maladjustment of power drives and conveyors, etc. Friction can be created by two moving parts, or one moving and one stationary such as a conveyor system.

Overheated Materials (8%)　　Caused by processes or operations which require heating of flammable materials, liquids, and ordinary combustibles.

Hot Surfaces (7%)　　Conduction, convention, and radiation of heat from boilers, furnaces, forges, which ignite flammable liquids and combustibles.

Burner Flames (7%)　　Improper use or poor maintenance of portable torches, boilers, driers, and portable heating equipment.

Combustible Sparks (5%)　　Sparks released from foundry cupolas, furnaces, incinerators, etc.

Spontaneous Ignition (4%)　　When combustibles and oxygen in the air are heated sufficiently, reaction begins and continues until the combustible reaches a temperature at which the reaction becomes self-sustaining. This temperature level is known as the "ignition point" or "ignition temperature." For convenience substances subject to spontaneous ignition have been divided into four groups:

1. Group 1—Substances not themselves combustible, but which may cause ignition. (Wetting calcium oxide, and unslaked lime, in the presence of combustibles).
2. Group 2—Substances having ignition points below ordinary temperatures. (Reaction of sodium and potassium with water).
3. Group 3—Combustible substances which may undergo sufficient oxidation at ordinary temperatures to reach their ignition point. (Easily oxidized vegetable oils which generate heat sufficient to cause ignition).
4. Group 4—Organic combustible substances subject to microbial thermogenesis, including agricultural products such as hay or grain.

Cutting & Welding (4%)   Most commonly caused by sparks and hot metal from cutting and welding operations or by defective gauges or deteriorated gas lines on welding apparatus.

Exposure (3%)   Fires occurring from converted or radiated heat from adjoining or nearby properties.

Incendiarism (3%)   Fires started maliciously by employees, intruders and arsonists.

Mechanical Sparks (2%)   Sparks generated by metal in machines, grinding, and crushing operations.

Molten Substances (2%)   Fires caused by molten metal released from a ruptured furnace or by molten metal spilled during handling.

Chemical Action (1%)   Chemicals reacting with other chemicals or materials; decomposition of unstable chemicals.

Static Sparks (1%)   Sparks resulting from the contact and separation of materials which ignite flammable vapors, dusts, and fibers, etc. These static charges are generated on agitation and mixing equipment, belts, splash filling of tanks, etc.

Chemistry of Fire

Fire is the combining of oxygen and fuel in proper proportions and at the proper temperature to sustain combustion.

Combustion is the process of the chemical union of fuel and oxygen at a rapid rate as the result of applied heat, producing light and heat.

To produce combustion there must be: (a) Fuel, (b) Oxygen (air), (c) Heat, and (d) Uninhibited chain reaction (see Figure 142).

Fuel   Wood, paper, coal, gas, are just a few of the products we think of as fuels. However, from the chemical standpoint, we consider only the common fuel elements: carbon (C), the most common of the fuels, is found in almost a pure state in coal, coke, lignite, and peat. It is also found with other fuels, such

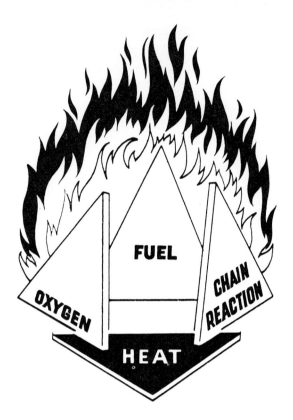

as fat, petroleum, natural gas, and wood; hydrogen (H) is commonly found in compound with carbon and other elements. Liquified fuel material and gases contain significant portions of hydrogen; finally, sulphur (S) is a good burning fuel and is found with other fuels—carbon and hydrogen.

Oxygen   This factor in combustion is furnished in the air (which consists of about 21% oxygen). A fire started in a place where fresh air is scarce will smolder and not adequately blaze because oxygen is not available in sufficient quantities for complete combustion.

Heat   Fuel will not burn, or the union of oxygen and fuel will not take place, until it reaches a certain temperature. This temperature depends on the type of fuel. For example, hydrogen will ignite as there are other factors which determine the point at which fuel will burn, such as: (a) the surface exposed; (b) the vapor present; (c) presence or absence of other fuels; and (d) nature of nearby fuels.

Heat may be produced by friction, by an electric spark, by chemical action, by the rays of the sun or by heat from other burning materials.

Uninhibited Chain Reaction · This factor is used by proponents of the Tetrahedron Theory of Fire, which emphasizes the need for the chemical reactions between the fuel and oxidizer to progress without interference.

Classes of Fires

The National Fire Protection Association has categorized fire into four general classifications.

Class A Fires This class of fires occurs in materials such as wood, cellulose, paper, excelsior, etc. Class A fires are extinguished by bringing the burning materials below their ignition temperature with the quenching and cooling effects of water. Under certain circumstances, these fires may be extinguished by the blanketing or smothering effects of dry chemical and carbon dioxide fire extinguishers.

Class B Fires Class B Fires are those that occur in the vapor-air mixture over the surface of flammable liquids such as oil, greases, alcohol, kerosene, gasoline, etc. Class B fires are most successfully extinguished by limiting of the air which supports combustion. Fire extinguishers of the dry chemical, carbon dioxide, foam, halogenated hydrocarbon agents, and fog streams of water are recommended for this type of fire.

Class C Fires Those which involve electrical equipment are Class C Fires. The extinguishing agents recommended are dry chemical, carbon dioxide, compressed gas and vaporizing liquid.

Class D Fires This class is reserved for fires occurring in combustible metals such as magnesium, lithium, sodium, and aluminum. Special extinguishing methods and agents are used, such as graphite base type.

Transmission of Fires

Conduction Heat is conveyed by matter without any visible motion of the matter itself. It is the passing on of heat from the hotter to the colder particles of the material.

Convection Heat is transferred by the motion of heated matter, for example, in a current of hot air or the flow of hot water through pipes.

Radiation   Heat is propagated like light, by a wave motion, traveling in all directions in straight lines until they are absorbed or reflected by another object. The heat of the fire may be sufficient to start fires across wide streets.

Static Electricity

Theory

1. Static electricity is generated by the contact and separation of dissimilar material. See Figure 143.
2. One such body takes a positive charge and the other a negative charge. The charges remain on the outer surface of the bodies unless they come in contact with or near a less charged body, uncharged or oppositely charged body. At such time the charge may pass from one body to another in order to be neutralized. When sufficient charge has accumulated to break down the resistance of the atmosphere, a spark or electrical charge may be formed.
3. Static electricity means electricity at rest on the surface of a body, as distinguished from the commonly recognized type of electricity known as electricity in motion.

Processes Where Static Electricity is a Hazard

1. Processes that involve the storage and handling of flaable gases and liquids, combustible fibers and dusts and similar easily ignitable materials can be subject to the fire hazard of static electricity. See Figures 144 and 145.
2. Static electricity is also generated on moving parts of equipment such as power transmission belts. See Figure 146.

Fire Detection Systems

1. Heat Detectors.
   a. Fixed temperature.
   b. Rate of rise.
2. Smoke Detectors.
3. Ionization Detectors.

Fire Extinguishing Systems

1. Water Systems.
   a. Automatic sprinklers.
      (1) Wet pipe (See Figure 147, and Table 18).
         (a) Upfeed system, Figure 148.
         (b) Downfeed system, Figure 149.

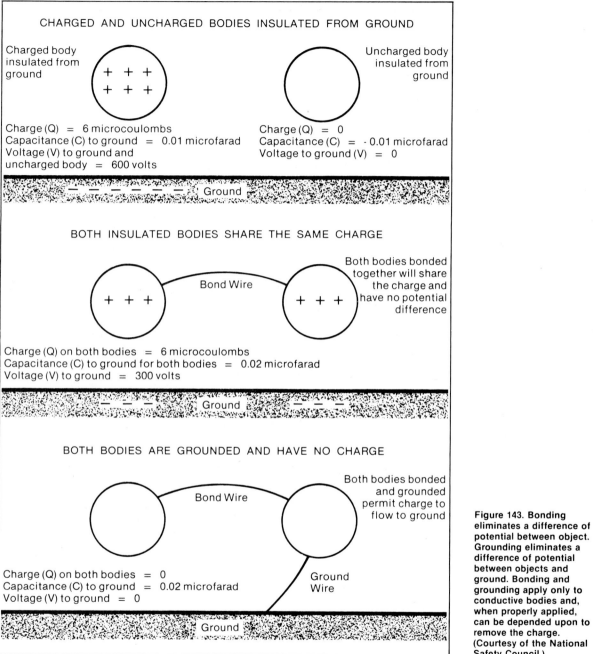

CHARGED AND UNCHARGED BODIES INSULATED FROM GROUND

Charged body insulated from ground

Uncharged body insulated from ground

Charge (Q) = 6 microcoulombs
Capacitance (C) to ground = 0.01 microfarad
Voltage (V) to ground and uncharged body = 600 volts

Charge (Q) = 0
Capacitance (C) = - 0.01 microfarad
Voltage to ground (V) = 0

Ground

BOTH INSULATED BODIES SHARE THE SAME CHARGE

Bond Wire

Both bodies bonded together will share the charge and have no potential difference

Charge (Q) on both bodies = 6 microcoulombs
Capacitance (C) to ground for both bodies = 0.02 microfarad
Voltage (V) to ground = 300 volts

Ground

BOTH BODIES ARE GROUNDED AND HAVE NO CHARGE

Bond Wire

Both bodies bonded and grounded permit charge to flow to ground

Charge (Q) on both bodies = 0
Capacitance (C) to ground = 0.02 microfarad
Voltage (V) to ground = 0

Ground Wire

Ground

Figure 143. Bonding eliminates a difference of potential between object. Grounding eliminates a difference of potential between objects and ground. Bonding and grounding apply only to conductive bodies and, when properly applied, can be depended upon to remove the charge. (Courtesy of the National Safety Council.)

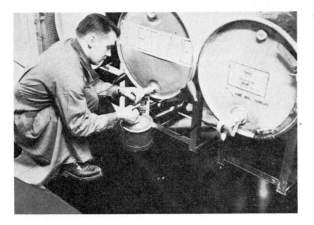

Figure 144. Typical arrangement for maximum safety. (Courtesy of the National Safety Council.)

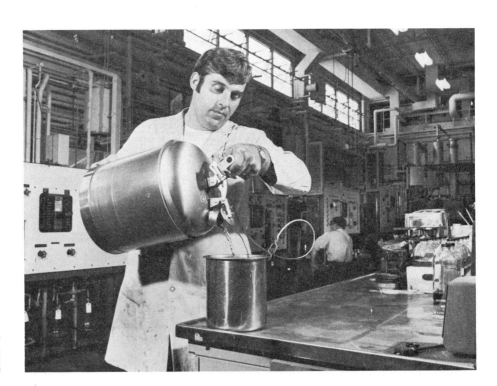

Figure 145. Pour can bonded to container. (Courtesy of the National Safety Council.)

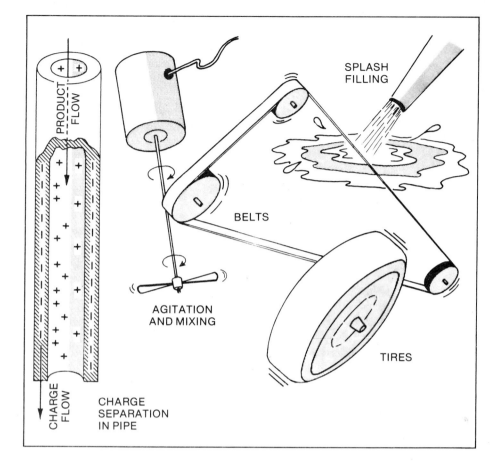

PRODUCT
FLOW

CHARGE
FLOW

CHARGE
SEPARATION
IN PIPE

AGITATION
AND MIXING

BELTS

SPLASH
FILLING

TIRES

Figure 146. Typical static-producing situations, including charge separation in pipe. (Courtesy of the National Safety Council.)

(2) Dry pipe.

(3) Deluge.

2. Foam Systems.

a. Chemical foam.

Formed by the chemical reaction in which bubbles of CO_2 gas and a foaming agent combine to produce and expand froth. Used on Class B fires.

b. Mechanical foam.

This consists of bubbles of air which are produced when air and water are mechanically agitated with a foam-making agent. Mechanical foam is used on Class B fires.

c. High expansion foam.

This consists of tiny foam bubbles filled with air which are created by a fan blowing air through a mesh over which a detergent base solution is flowing. High expansion foam is used where water damage is a problem, or where access to an area is infeasible.

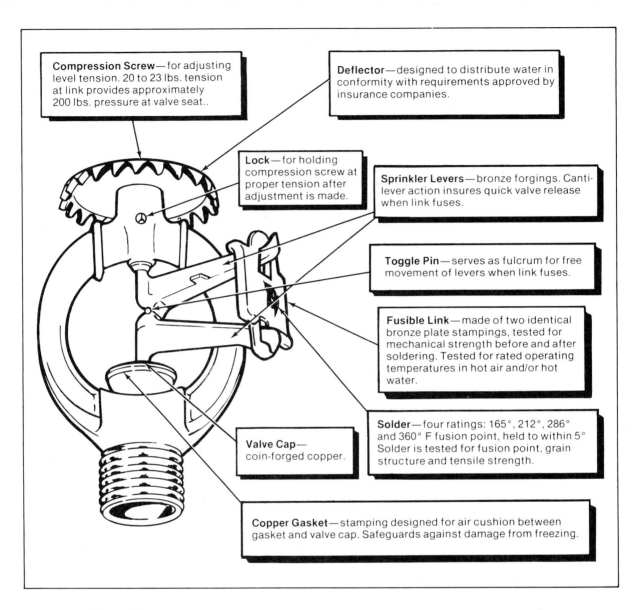

Compression Screw—for adjusting level tension. 20 to 23 lbs. tension at link provides approximately 200 lbs. pressure at valve seat..

Deflector—designed to distribute water in conformity with requirements approved by insurance companies.

Lock—for holding compression screw at proper tension after adjustment is made.

Sprinkler Levers—bronze forgings. Cantilever action insures quick valve release when link fuses.

Toggle Pin—serves as fulcrum for free movement of levers when link fuses.

Fusible Link—made of two identical bronze plate stampings, tested for mechanical strength before and after soldering. Tested for rated operating temperatures in hot air and/or hot water.

Solder—four ratings: 165°, 212°, 286° and 360° F fusion point, held to within 5° Solder is tested for fusion point, grain structure and tensile strength.

Valve Cap— coin-forged copper.

Copper Gasket—stamping designed for air cushion between gasket and valve cap. Safeguards against damage from freezing.

Figure 147.

488   **The Process of Hazard Control**

TABLE 18

Rating	Operating Temperature (F)	Color	Maximum Ceiling Temperature (F)
Ordinary	135-170	uncolored*	100
Intermediate	175-225	white*	150
High	250-300	blue	225
Extra high	325-375	red	300
Very extra high	400-475	green	375
Ultra high	500-575	orange	475

*The 135°F sprinklers of some manufacturers are half black and half uncolored. The 175°F sprinklers of the same manufacturers are yellow.

Reproduced by permission from "Sprinkler Systems," (NFPA Standard No. 13, Table 3651), 1972 edition, copyright National Fire Protection Association, 60 Batterymarch Street, Boston, Mass.

3. Carbon Dioxide Systems.

Found in either a storage tank of CO_2 or a group of CO_2 compressed gas cylinders with appropriate piping, this is used on Class B and C fires.

4. Dry Chemical Systems.

This consists of an agent which is neither toxic nor a conductor of electricity, nor does it freeze. An example of this is sodium bicarbonate.

5. Water Spray Systems (Fog).

Consisting of spray nozzles, a water supply and appropriate piping, the water spray systems are used for exposure protection of buildings, tanks and control of Class B flammable liquid fires.

6. Steam Systems.

Steam jet systems may be utilized to smother some fires which are in closed containers or in confined spaces. It is practicable only when a large supply of steam is continuously available.

Portable Fire Extinguishers

1. Classes of Fire Extinguishers.
   a. Class A extinguishers.

   For ordinary combustibles (wood, paper, etc.) where extinguishment is accomplished by quenching—cooling the material below its ignition temperature.
   b. Class B extinguishers.

   For flammable liquids (gasoline, paint, oil, grease, etc.) which demand a smothering action for quick extinguishment.

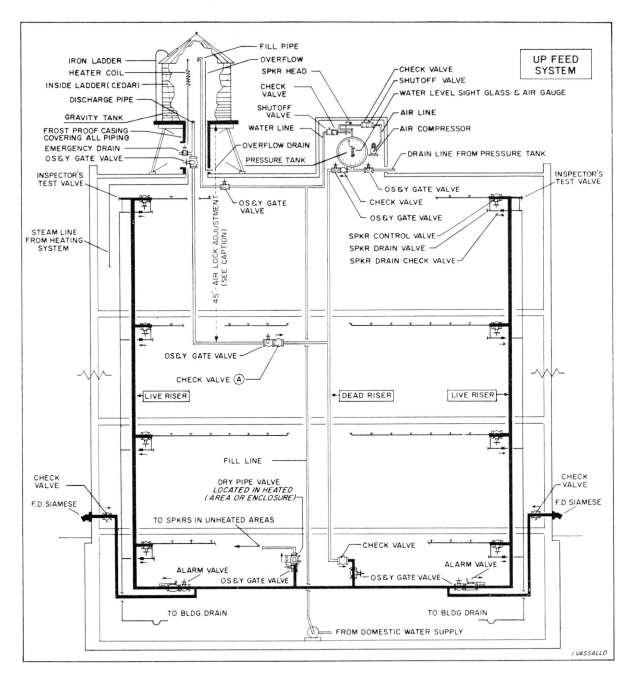

Figure 148. Typical Upfeed System showing arrangement of pressure and gravity tank feeds into sprinkler piping. Sprinkler piping shown in solid black indicates flow of water when supplied by fire department through F. D. siamese connection. Water cannot enter tanks due to check valve indicated at base of dead riser. Where sprinklers are operating after the pressure tank is empty, there will be 15 p.s.i. residual pressure on the tank side of check valve. (A). The excess pressure on the gravity tank side (45) $\times$ .434 = 19.5 p.s.i.) opens the check valve and allows the water from the gravity tank to enter the sprinkler system pipes. (Courtesy Milton Brodey, New York City Fire Department.)

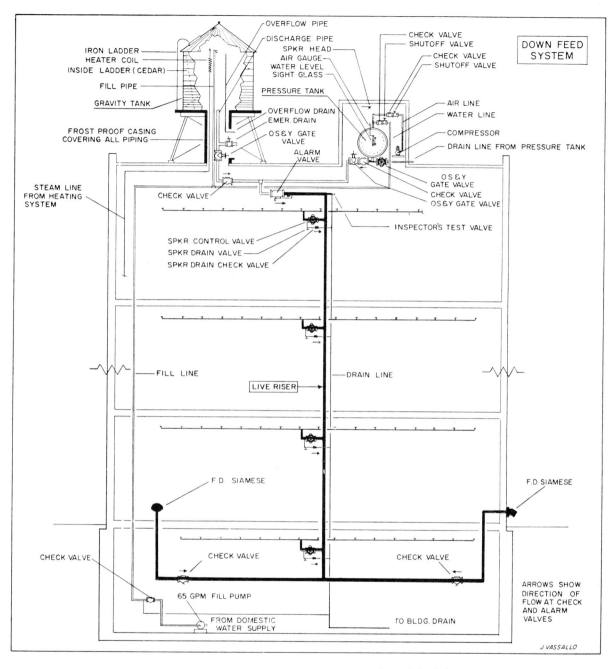

Figure 149. Typical Downfeed System showing arrangement of pressure and gravity tank feeds in sprinkler piping. Sprinkler piping shown in solid black indicates flow of water when supplied by Fire Dept. through F. D. siamese connection. Water cannot enter tanks due to alarm valve check, but must enter sprinkler system for use on fire. Floor control valves in both types of systems are generally located in center, or side center, portion of protected building. In both Downfeed and Upfeed systems, about 50% of installations will be as shown in diagram. In the remainder, the gravity tank will be mounted directly over the pressure tank house. In systems using only a gravity or a pressure tank, the piping is essentially the same. (Courtesy Milton Brodey, New York City Fire Department.)

c. Class C extinguishers.
For live electrical fires (motors, switches, appliances, etc.) The extinguishing agent used in this class of extinguisher is nonconductive.

d. Class D extinguishers.
For fires in combustible metals, such as magnesium, potassium, powdered aluminum, sodium, etc.

Hydrostatic Testing for Extinguishers

See Table 19.

TABLE 19

Hydrostatic Test Interval for Extinguishers

Hydrostatic Test Pressure Requirements—Non-ICC Shells, Shells Not Specified in U.S. Department of Transportation Regulations. (Formerly Interstate Commerce Commission)

Extinguisher type	Test interval year	Original factory test pressure	Requires hydrostatic test pressure
All dry chemical and dry powder		400 p.s.i. or greater	75% of factory test pressure
		350-399 p.s.i. below 350 p.s.i.	300 p.s.i. 75% of fracture test pressure
Foam—500 p.s.i. factory test		500	375
Foam—350 p.s.i. factory test		350	300
Soda-acid—500 p.s.i. factory test		500	375
Soda-acid—350 p.s.i. factory test		350	300
Stored-pressure or cartridge-operated water-type (including antifreeze and loaded-stream)		400 p.s.i. or greater 350-399 p.s.i below 350	75% of factory test pressure 300 p.s.i. 75% of factory test pressure
Soda-acid	5		
Cartridge-operated water and/or antifreeze	5		
Storage-pressure water and/or antifreeze	5		
Wetting agent	5		
Foam	5		
Loaded stream	5		
Dry chemical extinguishers with stainless steel shells, aluminum shells, or soldered-brass shells	5		
Carbon dioxide extinguishers	5		
Dry chemical extinguishers with brazed-brass shells, or mild-steel shell. .	12		
Bromotrifluoromethane	12		
Dry powder extinguishers for metal fires	12		

Reprinted from *Federal Register,* Vol. 36, No. 75, April 17, 1971.

Business organizations throughout the country are finding increasing uses for the laser to perform tasks which were at one time thought to be impossible. Although the laser has proven its usefulness and versatility, it is capable of inflicting serious injury to personnel and hence requires special precautions. While hazards associated with lasers are the particular concern of designers, technicians and others involved with its use, they are also the concern of the fire fighter personnel, particularly when they are called to control fire and/or explosions at laser installations. The intent of this section is to acquaint the reader with the uses and hazards associated with lasers and to set guides for effective and safe emergency operations.

Laser Characteristics

The laser, short for *light amplification by stimulated emission of radiation,* is a device which takes energy and organizes it into an intense beam of coherent, visible, infrared and/or ultraviolet light. When this beam is focused on a spot, it can create temperatures over 200 billion times hotter than an equivalent spot on the surface of the sun. The principle behind the laser operation is that light, when absorbed, is converted to heat. Laser light beams are unique from all other types of light in that, in addition to being coherent, they are monochromatic (one color) and are highly collimated (that is, the light is concentrated in a narrow beam for a long distance in the same plans of polarizations).[5]

Until now, the laser has been successfully used for various types of drilling, cutting, and welding operations, but its potential applications are unlimited. It has had particular success as a tool for drilling holes in diamonds, a task which formerly was time-consuming and expensive with conventional tools (see Figure 150). Lasers are also being used as surgical instruments, for lens-less three-dimensional photography (holography), as tools for aligning equipment used for digging tunnels and also for experimental types of communication equipment. A laser system or combination of systems may eventually replace telephone wires.

Hazards

The hazards associated with laser operations fall into two categories: hazards from the laser itself and hazards from associated equipment.

1. The beam: The primary hazard associated with the laser is the beam that it emits. Exposure to laser beams can result in burns and other physiological damage, the most serious occurring to the eyes. Beams in the ultraviolet and infrared ranges are not detectable by the human eye, thus compounding the hazard.

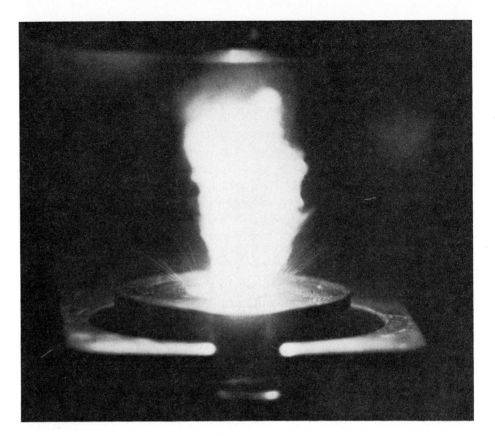

Figure 150. Laser vs Diamond. Plume of smoke rises from diamond in center of circular die as tremendous light energy of a laser beam strikes it. The beam is piercing a hole in the diamond die, used for drawing fine telephone wire at Western Electric's Buffalo, New York plant. (Courtesy of Western Electric News Features, January 1966.)

2. Electrical hazards: High voltages are associated with many types of lasers. These high voltages, coupled with improper safety procedures, have the potential to produce serious electrical shock and burns. Some high-voltage equipment, especially that exceeding 15,000 volts, may generate X-rays capable of inflicting injury to personnel.

3. Associated equipment: Cryogenic gases such as liquid nitrogen and liquid helium may be used as coolants for a solid-state laser crystal. These gases present many potential hazards, such as producing skin burns and displacing oxygen in the atmosphere. Installations using liquid nitrogen as a coolant should be adequately ventilated.

Many laser operations may be conducted in areas where flammable solvents and materials are located. These can be ignited by a laser beam if proper precautions are not taken.

4. Combustion by-products: Hazardous respirable materials, such as fumes, oxides, biological materials, carbon monoxide, carbon dioxide, ozone, lead and other metallic substances, may be generated when firing a laser. The contaminants produced depend to a large extent on the laser application.

5. Radiation: Ultraviolet and infrared radiation may be emitted from certain types of lasers. The fact that infrared radiation may not be visible to the naked eye contributes to the potential hazard. Although very high intensities from lasers may produce ionization in air and other materials, laser radiation should not be confused with ionizing radiation.

6. Fire and explosion: Laser capacitor banks and optical pump systems have been known to fail, resulting in explosions. The potential of a fire in the laser target area may be increased, as stated earlier, by the presence of combustible materials.

Exposure Hazard

The field of laser technology is relatively new. Thus, data concerning biological effects on man are far from complete. To add to the uncertainty, the hazard potential of low-powered lasers is not calculated to be the same as for the higher-powered ones. Research indicates that the type and extent of injury to those exposed to the laser beam depends on: (a) the area of the body hit by a direct or reflected laser beam; (b) the power of the laser; (c) wavelength, and (d) several other factors. To date, permissible exposures limits have been tentatively established by the American Conference of Governmental Industrial Hygienists.

With this in mind, we should consider all laser operations to be hazardous until we receive information to the contrary, and should design our operational methods accordingly.

Laser equipment presents two problems from a fire control standpoint. The first is the necessity of working at a fire or emergency in the laser area itself, and the second, having to operate in areas surrounding or adjacent to a laser area. In each case, many of the hazards associated with the laser and its equipment are the same.

Operations Guidelines

The following are guidelines for planning effective emergency operations at laser installations:

1. Inspection activities should be utilized to locate establishments using lasers. In particular, the location of laser areas, voltages used and power shutoff stations should be recorded and made available for emergency use.

2. Beam enclosures should be installed on laser equipment and a sign should be placed on every laser area door. These signs should include the type of laser, voltages and associated material, including cryogenic gases. Unlike radioactive materials, lasers do not have a universal warning symbol to indicate their hazard. In addition, no personnel monitoring devices, such as film badges of the type used to measure ionizing radiation, are available to measure laser radiation exposure.

Audible signals may be present at each laser room to indicate when the laser is operating, and there should be a power shutoff switch outside the room.

3. Many laser areas are in remote areas of establishment, away from employee travel routes. Exact location of lasers should be available for use by emergency personnel.

4. All power shall be deenergized and the residual charge in the capacitors bled off, before emergency personnel enter any area where lasers are present. If the situation is such that this is impossible extreme caution must be taken, and only those who are well-acquainted with the hazards involved and who are properly protected should be allowed to enter.

5. Under no circumstances should metal tools, and similar devices be brought inside laser equipment rooms unless power is deenergized.

6. In combating fires in laser installations, water in any form must not be directed against any electrical equipment without the advice of an expert. While the use of fog may be safe around electrical equipment, the water which drains away from the location may cause short circuits in other equipment.

7. As previously mentioned, cryogenic gases, such as liquid nitrogen and liquid helium used as coolants in some laser systems, are capable of producing skin burns upon contact. Personnel entering rooms where such gases are known to exist must wear proper equipment, such as head, eye, body, and hand protection. Self-contained breathing apparatus is mandatory in these areas since these cryogenics have the capability of displacing oxygen from the atmosphere.

8. Laser rooms should be well-lighted before workers enter. A well-lighted room prevents dilation of the pupils in a person's eyes. A dilated pupil makes a larger target for the laser beam to strike, creating the possibility of irreversible eye damage. Personnel exposed to any laser beam, particularly if they report consistent after-images of light, should be the immediate concern of medical authorities.

9. Personnel should never look directly at the head of a laser. An unsuspected pulsed beam could destroy the eye. If they must enter a laser room where electrical power cannot be deenergized, they must wear properly designed laser goggles capable of attenuating the emitted wavelength.

10. Personnel should never expose any part of their body to a laser beam. Protective gloves, clothing, and shields impervious to light must be used to prevent skin exposure.

11. Electrical-insulated gloves should be worn around laser electrical sources.

12. Emergency personnel may encounter safety interlocks at the entrance of laser areas. These interlocks are provided to prevent unauthorized or transient personnel from entering the area while the laser power supply is charged and capable of firing.

In conclusion, a knowledge of the hazards peculiar to laser operations and the necessary control measures to be taken will enable maintenance and emergency personnel to more effectively and safely accomplish their missions without injury.

Ground-Fault Circuit Interrupter (GFCI)   Unit 6

The ground-fault circuit interrupter (GFCI) is a fast-acting circuit breaker which senses small imbalances in the circuit caused by current leakage to ground and, in a fraction of a second, shuts off the electricity. The GFCI continually matches the amount of current going to an electrical device against the amount of current returning from the device along the electrical path. Whenever the amount "going" differs from the amount "returning" by approximately 5 milliamps (5/1000 ampere), the GFCI interrupts the electric power within as little as 1/40 of a second. See Figure 151. It is important to understand that a GFCI will not protect the user from line-to- line contact hazards nor is it intended as a substitute for good electrical safety procedures. The GFCI merely provides protection against the most common form of human electrical shock hazard—the line-to-ground fault. GFCI's are available in portable models for special protection of portable equipment. They are also available in permanently installed models in capacities to 70 amperes.

Machine Guarding   Unit 7

Types of Guards

Whenever the actions or motions of a machine present a hazard, it is essential that the operator and fellow workers be protected, by well-constructed, foolproof guards. See Figures 152, 153, 154. There are four kinds of guards:

1. Enclosure.
2. Interlocking.
3. Automatic.
4. Remote Control, Placement, Feeding, and Ejecting.

Enclosure Guards   The fixed enclosure guard is preferable to all other types because it prevents access to dangerous moving parts by enclosing them completely. The guard admits the stock but will not admit hands because the size of the feed opening is limited. The guard also restrains broken and flying

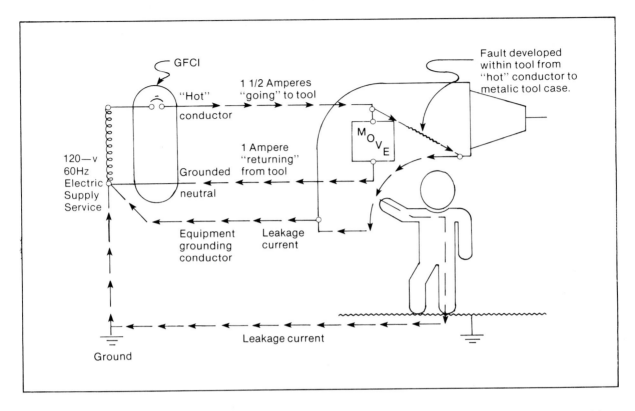

machine parts. See Figures 155, 156, 157 and 158. In Figure 159 a guard has been provided to protect a worker from the explosive forces of the material he is testing. The improper mounting of the guard along with the fact that his hand must be exposed to the hazard makes this attempt at control a poor one.

The adjustable enclosure guard forms a barrier which can be fitted around different sizes or shapes of the die. It requires frequent adjustment and careful maintenance.

Machine guards must be carefully designed to eliminate hazards, but must not create hazards of their own. They must be in accordance with recognized standards of construction and performance and should not interfere with production.

Interlocking Guards   When a fixed guard or enclosure is not practicable, an interlocking barrier should be considered as the first alternative. One type of interlocking guard consists of a barrier that shuts off or disengages power, preventing the machine from starting when the guard is open. It also prevents the opening of the guard while the machine is under power of coasting.

Another type of interlocking guard utilizes an electric contact or mechanical stop that activates a mechanical or electric brake. When any part of the

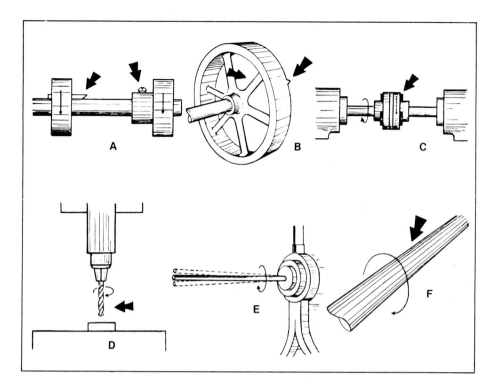

Figure 152. Rotating mechanisms, that can seize and wind up loose clothing, belts, hair, and the like, should be provided with guards: A—projecting key and setscrew; B—spokes and burrs; C— coupling bolts; D—bit and chuck; E—turning bar stock; and F—rotating shaft. (Courtesy of the National Safety Council.)

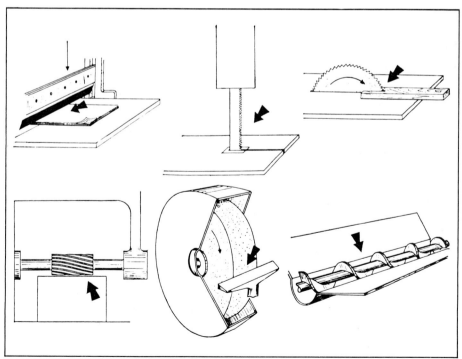

Figure 153. Protection against all variations of these common cutting and shearing mechanisms should be provided. (Courtesy of the National Safety Council.)

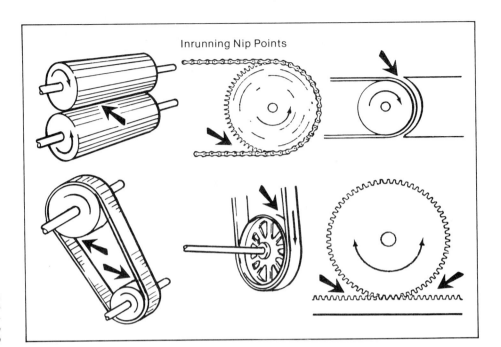

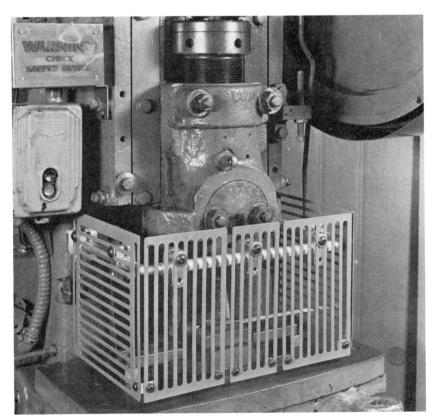

500   The Process of Hazard Control

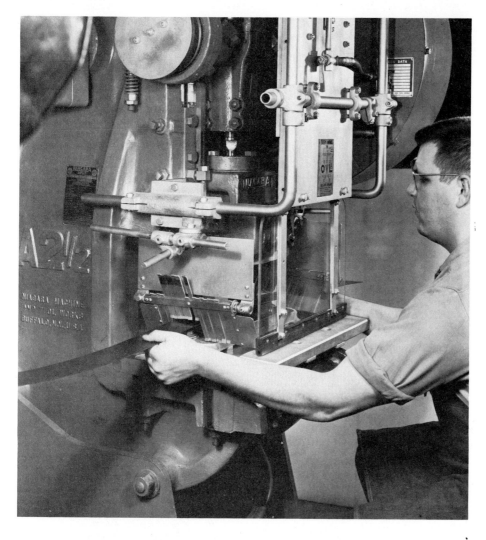

Figure 156.

operator's body enters the danger zone, the machine stops immediately. Both of these guards require careful adjustment and maintenance.

A third type of interlocking guard protects the operator with an electric eye beam that stops the machine or prevents it from being started if the operator's hands are in the danger zone.

Automatic Guards   When enclosure or interlocking guards are not practicable, an automatic guard may be used. Repeating its cycle as long as the machine is in motion, this guard actually pulls the operator's hands, arms, or body from the danger zone as the ram, plunger, or other tools close on the work being done.

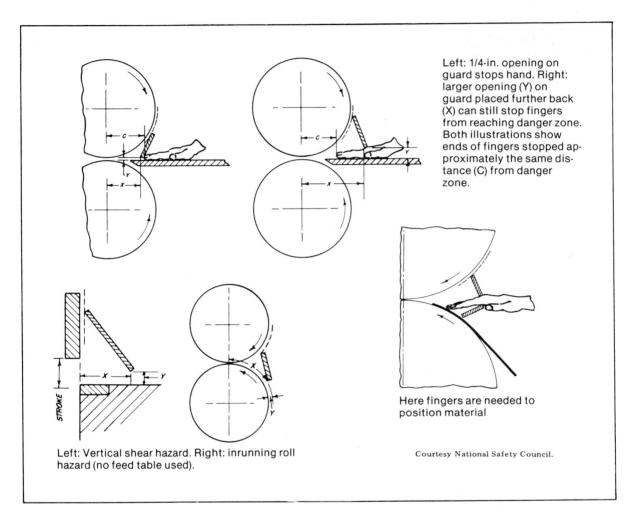

Left: 1/4-in. opening on guard stops hand. Right: larger opening (Y) on guard placed further back (X) can still stop fingers from reaching danger zone. Both illustrations show ends of fingers stopped approximately the same distance (C) from danger zone.

Here fingers are needed to position material

Left: Vertical shear hazard. Right: inrunning roll hazard (no feed table used).

Courtesy National Safety Council.

Figure 157. (Courtesy of the National Safety Council.)

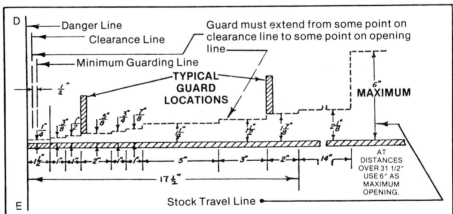

Figure 158. Sample guard locations are shown by vertical crosshatched blocks. Barriers placed to touch dashed line will wedge hand or forearm.

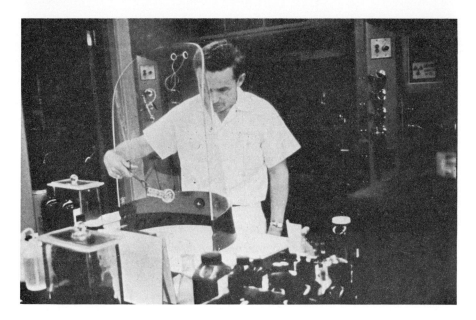

One common type of automatic guard consists of a moving barrier that is connected to the operating mechanism of the machine and pushes or lifts hands out of the danger zone.

A third type of automatic guarding consists of limiting the stroke of a machine. Plunger travel, for instance, may be limited to 3/8 of an inch or less so that fingers cannot enter between the pressure points. See Figure 158.

Remote Control, Placement, Feeding, Ejecting

Other methods may be used to protect the operator from dangerous points-of-operation. They may be used to complement another type of guard or as a substitute.

A two-handed trip system may be used to start a machine. These devices require the simultaneous action of both the operator's hands on electrical switches, air control valves, or mechanical levers. If two-handed trip systems are used on machines requiring more than one operator, each operator should have a separate set of controls.

Two-handed operating devices on presses with a noninterrupting stroke should require manual operation until the danger point in the cycle of the machine has ceased. The controls should be located so that it is impossible for the operator to move his hands from the controls to the hazard zone before the cycle is completed.

Stock may be fed automatically or semiautomatically by chutes, hoppers, conveyors, revolving dies, or dial feeds in conjunction with ram enclosures. This guard will not admit any part of the body to the danger zone.

Special jigs or feeding devices made of metal or wood may be used to handle stock and keep hands safe at the point-of-operation. Operators may also use long-handled tongs, vacuum lifters. Table 20 outlines point of operation protection from the standpoint of various guarding alternatives and the advantages and limitations of each alternative.

Application of Machine Guarding

The Occupational Safety and Health Administration (OSHA) republished in the Federal Register of June 27, 1974, a comprehensive set of machinery and machine guarding standards. The rules and regulations of the standards in Subpart O spell out clearly, in more detail than is possible here, the ways of providing the operator with protection from moving machine parts.

All employers of shops where machinery is used should be familiar with the standards that apply to the machines they use. Employees and students will find them of great personal benefit in the trades they have chosen. Figure 160 illustrates a gross violation of machine guarding. The worker is exposed to the cutting action of the saw without any protection. The exposed drive belts compound the problem.

Remembering that all mechanical action or motion, in varying degrees, is hazardous, and by understanding the basic techniques for guarding simple machinery, you will be better prepared to deal with the problems of more complex machinery. Following are some of the guarding techniques frequently found in industry.

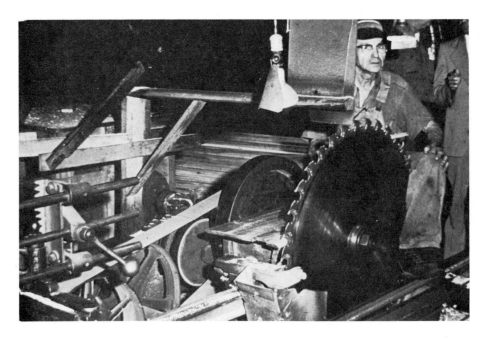

Figure 160.

TABLE 20

Point-of-Operation Protection

Type of Guarding Method	Action of Guard	Advantages	Limitatons	Typical Machines on Which Used
Enclosures or Barriers				
Complete, simple fixed enclosure	Barrier or enclosure which admits the stock but which will not admit hands into danger zone because of feed opening size, remote location, or unusual shape	Provides complete enclosure if kept in place Both hands free Generally permits increased production Easy to install Ideal for blanking on power presses Can be combined with automatic or semiautomatic feeds	Limited to specific operations May require special tools to remove jammed stock May interfere with visibility	Bread slicers Embossing presses Meat grinders Metal square shears Nip points of inrunning rubber, paper, textile rolls Paper corner cutters Power presses
Warning enclosures (usually adjustable to stock being fed)	Barrier or enclosure admits the operator's hand but warns him before danger zone is reached	Makes "hard to guard" machines safer Generally does not interfere with production Easy to install Admits varying sizes of stock	Hands may enter danger zone—enclosure not complete at all times Danger of operator not using guard Often requires frequent adjustment and careful maintenance	Band saws Circular saws Cloth cutters Dough brakes Ice Crushers Jointers Leather strippers Rock crushers Wood shapers
Barrier with electric contact or mechanical stop activating mechanicol or electric brake	Barrier quickly stops machine or prevents application of injurious pressure when any part of operator's body contacts it or approaches danger zone	Makes "hard to guard" machines safer Does not interfere with production	Requires careful adjustment and maintenance Possibility of minor injury before guard operates Operator can make guard inoperative.	Calenders Dough brakes Flat roll ironers Paper box corner stayers Paper box enders Power presses Rubber mills
Enclosure with electrical or mechanical interlock	Enclosure or barrier shuts off or disengages power and prevents starting of machine when guard is open; prevents opening of the guard while machine is under power or coasting. (Interlocks should not prevent manual operation or "inching" by remote control)	Does not interfere with production Hands are free; operation of guard is automatic Provides complete and positive enclosure	Requires careful adjustment and maintenance Operator may be able to make guard inoperative Does not protect in event of mechanical repeat	Dough brakes and mixers Foundry tumblers Laundry extractors, driers and tumblers Power presses Tanning drums Textile pickers, cards

Courtesy of the National Safety Council

TABLE 20. *Continued.*

Automatic or Semiautomatic Feed			
Nonmanual or partly manual loading of feed mechanism, with point of operation enclosed	Stock fed by chutes, hoppers, conveyors, movable dies, dial feed, rolls, etc. Enclosure will not admit any part of body	Generally increases production Operator cannot place hands in danger zone	Excessive installation cost for short run Requires skilled maintenance Not adaptable to variations in stock	Baking and candy machines Circular saws Power presses Textile pickers Wood planers Wood shapers

Hand Removal Devices			
Hand restraints	A fixed bar and cord or strap with hand attachments which, when worn and adjusted, do not permit an operator to reach into the point of operation.	Operator cannot place hands in danger zone Permits maximum hand feeding; can be used on higher-speed machines No obstruction to feeding a variety of stock Easy to install	Requires frequent inspection, maintenance, and adjustment to each operator Limits movement of operator May obstruct space around operator Does not permit blanking from hand-fed strip.	Embossing presses Power presses
Hand pullaway device	A cable-operated attachment on slide, connected to the operator's hands or arms to pull the hands back only if they remain in the danger zone; otherwise it does not interfere with normal operation.	Acts even in event of repeat Permits maximum hand feeding; can be used on higher-speed machines No obstruction to feeding a variety of stock Easy to install	Requires unusually good maintenance and adjustment to each operator Frequent inspection necessary Limits movement of operator May obstruct work space around operator Does not permit blanking from hand-fed strip stock	Embossing presses Power presses

Two-hand Trip			
Electric	Simultaneous pressure of two hands on switch buttons in series actuates machine	Can be adapted to multiple operation Operator's hands away from danger zone	Operator may try to reach into danger zone after tripping machine	Dough mixers Embossing presses Paper cutters Pressing machines Power presses Washing tumblers
Mechanical	Simultaneous pressure of two hands on air control valves, mechanical levers, controls interlocked with foot control, or the removal of solid blocks or stops permits normal operation of machine.	No obstruction to hand feeding Does not require adjustment Can be equipped with continuous pressure remote controls to permit "inching." Generally easy to install	Does not protect against mechanical repeat unless blocks or stops are used Some trips can be rendered unsafe by holding with the arm, blocking or tying down one control, thereby permitting one-hand operation Not used for some blanking operations.	

This unit is not intended to explore the details of all hazards associated with crane operations. Instead, several important areas have been chosen for discussion because of their demonstrated potential to cause catastrophic accident situations.

Wire Rope/Sheaves

Many accidents involving cranes is due to a failure or wire rope. Investigation of each of these cases reveal that the cause of wire rope failure is due to one of several reasons.

First, that the wire rope was used with broken wires. The OSHA Construction Safety Standards addresses this issue by stating that "wire rope shall be

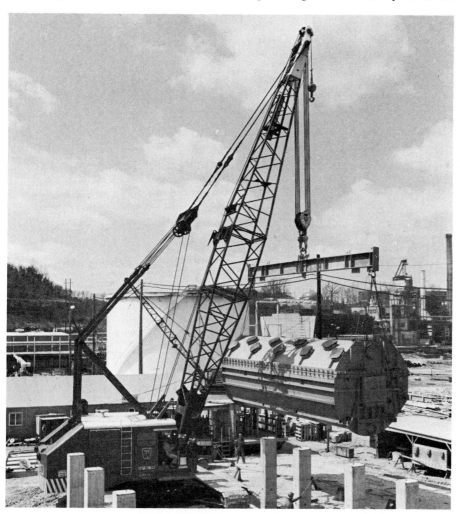

Figure 161. Lines of workers and the destruction of expensive material and equipment are dependent upon the structural intensity of the crane and its components as well as the skill of the operator.

taken out of service when six randomly distributed broken wires in one lay or three broken wires in one strand in one lay.'' See Figure 162.

Second, improper methods of clip installation. Figure 163 demonstrates the approved method of clip installation. Failures have occurred when operations have place the U-bolt over the live end of the rope, have staggered the placement of U-bolts, and when an insufficient number were used.

Third, when the wire rope has become flattened out due to crushing or pinching. The improper weld on the hoist drum in Figure 164 caused the flattening out and eventual breakage of the wire rope illustrated in Figure 165. Figure 166 illustrates another situation where, sharp cutting edges, can seriously damage wire rope to a point where it will fail under a load.

Fourth, when wire ropes are improperly matched to their sheaves. Rope which is too small will flatten out as it passes over the sheave causing it to weaken and fail. See Figure 167. A wire rope which is too large will pinch the sides of the sheave causing it to weaken and eventually fail. See Figure 167. In Figure 168, a sheave is illustrated which has been once subjected to the cutting action of a small diameter rope. During operation the rope cut an undersized groove in the sheave. Many accidents have occurred when, a sheave cut like this was later used with correct size rope. The sharp edges of the undersized groove severely damaged the wire rope to a point where it eventually failed.

Figure 169 illustrates a hazardous situation. The broken parts of the sheave housing illustrated belongs to the crane in Figure 170. The hazardous condition resulted from the combined conditions of vibration and cold soaking—(when ferrous metals are subjected to extreme cold a crystaline growth occurs in the steel causing it to weaken and eventually fail).

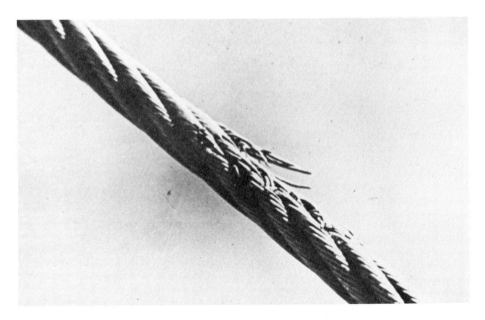

Figure 162.

STEP 1.

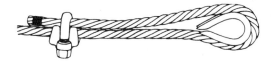

APPLY FIRST CLIP—one base width from dead end of wire rope—U-Bolt over dead end—live end rests in clip saddle. Tighten nuts evenly to recommended torque.

STEP 2.

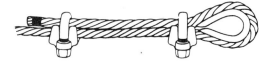

APPLY SECOND CLIP—nearest loop as possible—U-Bolt over dead end—turn on nuts firm but DO NOT TIGHTEN.

STEP 3.

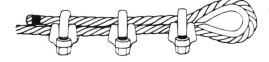

ALL OTHER CLIPS—Space equally between first two—this should be no more than one clip base apart—turn on nuts—take up rope slack—TIGHTEN ALL NUTS EVENLY ON ALL CLIPS to recommended torque.

Figure 163. Method of clip installation. (Courtesy of the National Safety Council.)

Hooks

Hooks used on cranes for lifting must be equipped with safety latches. Figure 171. OSHA standards state that "hooks require a daily visual inspection and a monthly signed inspection report." The standards go on to state that hooks with cracks or having more than 15 percent in excess of normal throat opening or more than 10 degrees twist from the plane of the unbent hook should be replaced. Figure 172 illustrates a 150 lb crane hook that failed during operations.

The situation in Figure 173 illustrates how workers are subjected to a high hazard situation because of improper use of equipment for the hoisting and lowering of materials.

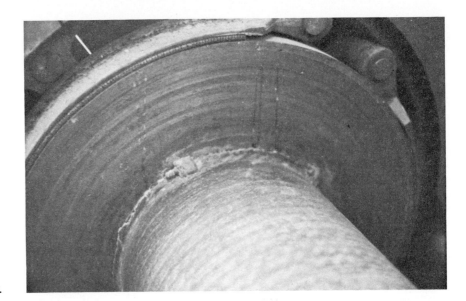

Figure 164.

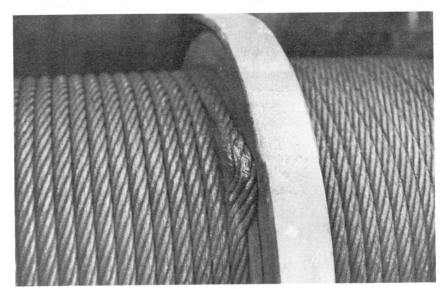

Figure 165.

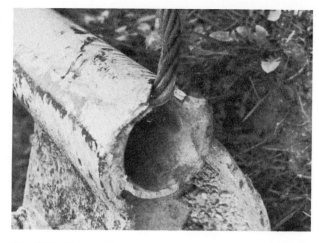

Figure 166.

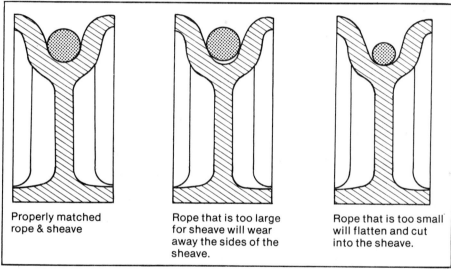

Properly matched rope & sheave

Rope that is too large for sheave will wear away the sides of the sheave.

Rope that is too small will flatten and cut into the sheave.

Figure 167.

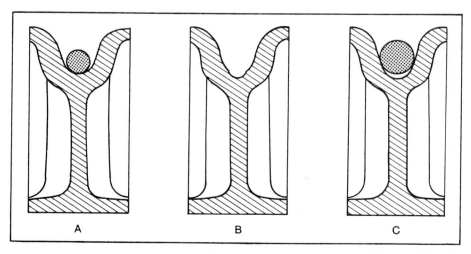

A

B

C

Figure 168.

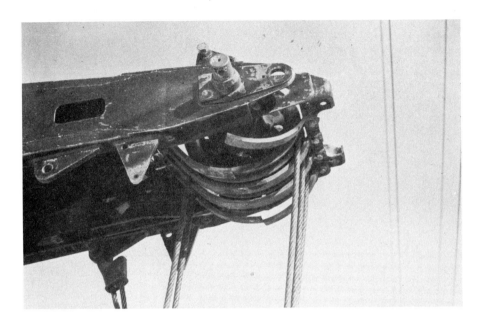

Figure 169. The effect of cold soaking on steel.

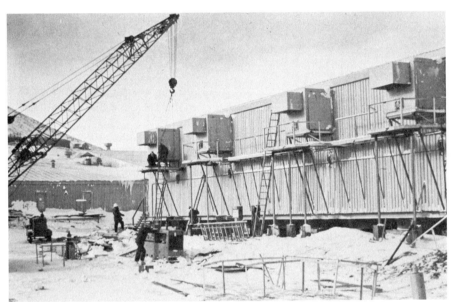

Figure 170. The lack of a safety latch on hook adds another dimension to the problem.

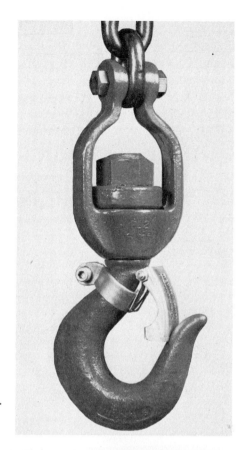

Figure 171. (Courtesy of The Warrington Company.)

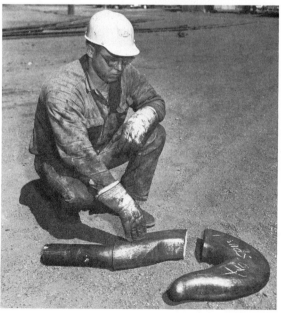

Figure 172. (Courtesy of the Colorado Fuel and Iron Company.)

Swing Radius of
Crane

Figure 174 illustrates a crane being operated without barricades which would prevent workers from being struck and crushed by the crane as it makes its swing. This situation has been responsible for many deaths to workers as the crane operator cannot see what is going on in the "blind spot" behind him. The OSHA regulations state that accessible areas within the swing radius of the rear of the rotating superstructure of the crane, either permanently or temporarily mounted, shall be barricaded in such a manner as to prevent a worker from being struck or crushed by the crane.

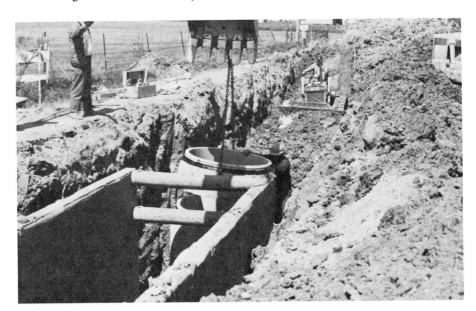

Figure 173. The absence of adequate shoring compounds the hazardous situation.

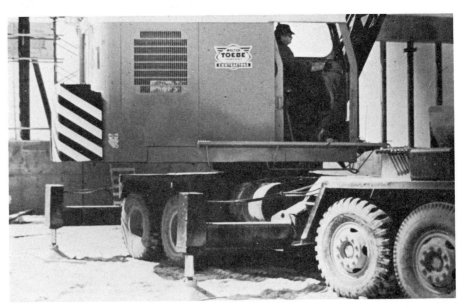

Figure 174.

514   The Process of Hazard Control

American National Standards Institute, Safety Standards, 1430 Broadway, New York, New York 10018.

Arnold, P. G., and Gross, E. E., "Handbook of Noise Measurement," 6th edition, General Radio Company, West Concord, Massachusetts.

Davidson, Ray, "Peril on the Job," Public Affairs Press, Washington, D.C.

Harris, Cyril M., "Handbook of Noise Control," New York, McGraw-Hill Book Company, 1962.

Longely, M. Y., Harris, R. L., and Lee, D. H. K. "Calculation of Complex Radiant Heat Load from Surrounding Radiator Surface Temperatures, Journal of the American Industrial Hygiene Association, 24:103–112, March-April, 1963.

Manufacturing Chemists Association, "Chemical Safety Data Sheets," 1825 Connecticut Ave., N.W., Washington, D.C. 20009.

Meidl, James H., "Flammable Hazardous Materials," Glencoe Press, Collier-Macmillan Limited, London.

National Fire Protection Association, "Fire Protection Guide on Hazardous Materials," 60 Batterymarch Street, Boston, Massachusetts 02110.

National Fire Protection Association, "Fire Protection Handbook," 60 Batterymarch Street, Boston, Massachusetts, 02110, 1969, 13th edition.

National Safety Council, "Accident Prevention Manual for Industrial Operations," 7th edition, 1974, N.S.C. Chicago, Illinois 60611.

"Occupational Diseases—A Guide to Their Recognition," Revised edition, June, 1977, U.S. Department of Health, Education, and Welfare, NIOSH, Publication No. 77–181.

Patty, F. A., "Industrial Hygiene and Toxicology," Vol. I, II, and III, Interscience Publishers, Inc., New York.

Sax, I., "Dangerous Properties of Industrial Materials," 1969, Reinhold Publishing Corp., New York.

U.S. Department of Labor, Bureau of Labor Standards, "Occupational Safety and Health Standards," Federal Register, Saturday, May 29, 1971, Vol. 36, No. 105, Washington, D.C., Revised October 18, 1972, Vol. 37, No. 202.

U.S. Department of Labor, Bureau of Labor Standards, "Safety and Health Regulations for Construction," Federal Register, Saturday, April 17, 1971, Vol. 36, No. 75, Washington, D.C., Revised December 16, 1972.

Bibliography

Notes

1. Industrial Union Department, AFL/CIO, "Facts and Analysis" Occupational Health and Safety, Asbestos (Part 1), March 28, 1971.
2. Ray Davidson, "Peril on the Job," Public Affairs Press, Washington, D.C.
3. A. K. Omaya, "Critique of Neural Trauma Research: Status and Possible Solutions" NIOSH Symposium on Personal Protection, pub. NIOSH 75–143 January, 1974.
4. Gases or liquids that are of such nature that a very small amount of it mixed with air is dangerous to life.
5. F. X. Worden; and W. C. Roberts; and J. P. Dunn; "Guidelines for Safe Use of Lasers," Western Electric Company.

Index